VETERINARY RADIOLOGICAL INTERPRETATION

Veterinary Radiological Interpretation

S. W. DOUGLAS, M.A., M.R.C.V.S., D.V.R.

and

H. D. WILLIAMSON, M.S.R.

School of Veterinary Medicine,
University of Cambridge

Photography by Josephine Patten

HEINEMANN VETERINARY BOOKS

First Published 1970
Reprinted 1975
Reprinted 1978

published by William Heinemann Medical Books Ltd, London

SBN 433 07800 6

Printed in Great Britain by
Redwood Burn Limited, Trowbridge & Esher

CONTENTS

This work is dedicated to G. C. Knight, F.R.C.V.S., D.V.R., whose early interest and enthusiasm for veterinary radiology laid the foundations upon which this book is based.

PREFACE

Although radiography has been employed as an aid to diagnosis for a comparatively short period in the history of medicine, it has now become such an integral part of medical science that every hospital has its own department of radiology. Such departments are staffed by radiographers whose training and equipment permit the consistent production of high quality radiographs, and by radiologists who have trained and specialised in the interpretation of the films.

In the field of veterinary medicine such specialisation can only be attempted at the teaching and research institutions, and the practitioner must himself have a knowledge of both radiography and radiology. For a number of reasons these subjects have formed a very minor part of the instruction given at the teaching schools in the past, and, while there are indications that this omission is now being remedied, there is still considerable need for guidance in these subjects. The reception given to the book "Principles of Veterinary Radiography" has encouraged the authors to publish this volume, which is intended as a complementary work, dealing with the general principles of radiology, for students and practitioners.

It is important that the radiologist should approach each film without any preconceived ideas and that he should systematically examine the radiograph recognising all normal and abnormal variations. Therefore, while the radiological findings in the common pathological conditions of animals are described, the emphasis of this book is on the general recognition of evidence of abnormality and pathology, rather than attempting to provide specific "blue prints" for the identification of every condition that might be recognised radiologically.

It must be accepted that up to the present, veterinary clinical radiology has been concerned almost solely with dogs and cats and, to a limited extent, the horse. The lack of the application of this technique to farm animals may well be remedied in the future, as various practical problems are overcome. However, in the first edition of this book, all references are to the dog, except where otherwise indicated.

It should also be stressed that, while radiography is a valuable aid in the investigation of the etiology of disease, it should never be employed as a "short cut" to diagnosis. Any attempt to draw final conclusions from radiographic examination alone, will lead, sooner or later, to errors. Radiography should only be employed where there is evidence that it may provide more significant information, and this information should be considered and interpreted finally in relation to all the other data concerning the case (history, clinical examination, laboratory findings, other specialised examinations, etc.).

The publication of radiographs always poses problems, since they inevitably lose some detail during reproduction. These difficulties are greater when dealing with clinical examples which, in the majority of instances, were not obtained with a view to publication. When films were not suitable, diagrams have been used to illustrate particular radiological features.

The illustrations and diagrams have all been obtained from cases seen and treated at the University of Cambridge School of Veterinary Medicine. The authors wish to express their gratitude to Professor Phillipson, M.A., M.R.C.V.S., PH.D., F.R.S.E. for permission and encouragement to use the radiographs and facilities of the School, and to thank their colleagues on the staff for advice and help in many ways.

A special word of appreciation must be expressed to Miss J. Clarke who has typed and retyped the manuscript and undertaken many of the routine tasks associated with the production of this volume.

Our thanks are also due to the publishers of the Journal of the American Veterinary Medical Association for permission to use the illustration on page 295.

S. W. DOUGLAS
H. D. WILLIAMSON

PART ONE

INTRODUCTION

CHAPTER 1

RADIOGRAPHIC FACTORS WHICH INFLUENCE RADIOLOGICAL INTERPRETATION

In the medical field the radiologist demands films of the highest radiographic standard before he will attempt to interpret them. Films that are not up to such standards are rejected and must be repeated until they are suitable.

While there are many inherent difficulties in the way of producing veterinary radiographs of optimum quality, one of the main stumbling blocks would appear to be the lack of a sufficiently critical approach by the veterinary surgeon who normally must be both radiographer and radiologist.

As a radiographer, he should be aware of the factors in radiographic technique which will influence the subsequent interpretation of the radiograph and then endeavour to produce films of the highest quality. As a radiologist, he should then critically examine the standard of the films produced, so that any shortcomings may be allowed for in the interpretation of the film, and so that such errors may be avoided in future radiography.

Provided that such a critical appraisal of the subject is made, the fact that the radiographer and radiologist are identical can contribute to establishing a high standard of both radiography and radiology. In those matters which are a question of personal preference (e.g., "light" or "dark" films), the radiographer should at least have no difficulty in knowing the wishes of the radiologist!

It is advisable therefore to commence by considering those qualities which the radiologist should expect to find in the X-ray films submitted to him by the radiographer, if he is to obtain the maximum information from them, and then to consider how radiographic technique affects the production of these qualities.

Ideally, these qualities are:

1. A minimum of magnification and distortion of the structure under examination.
2. Sharp delineation of detail.
3. Adequate contrast.
4. Correct exposure.

5. A sufficient number of projections to demonstrate the complete extent of the structure or lesion under investigation.
6. An absence of artifacts due to radiographic and processing faults.

Before considering the factors which influence each of these qualities in greater detail it should be remembered that they all depend upon the size, build and temperament of the animal patient, the characteristics of the equipment used, and the skill and experience of the radiographer.

1. MAGNIFICATION AND DISTORTION

Magnification and distortion are present in every clinical radiograph to a greater or lesser degree because the image is a two-dimensional representation of a three-dimensional structure which has been projected onto the film by the beam of radiation.

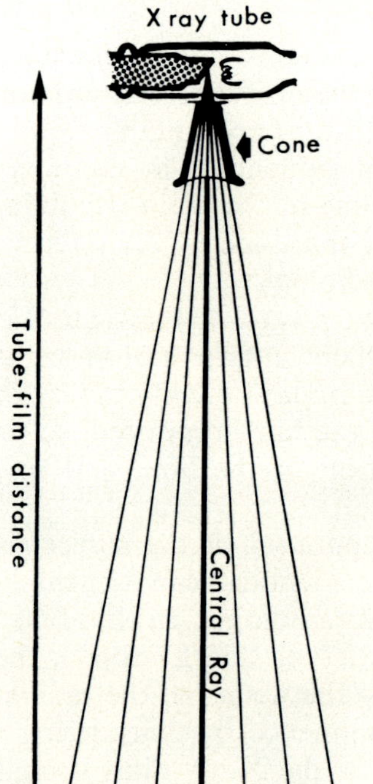

FIG. 1.1.

One of the most important concepts in radiography is that of the central ray. This is the path of radiation which forms the long axis of the X-ray beam and is the path of minimum distortion. All other rays diverge outwards at an ever increasing angle up to the periphery. Alignment of the patient to the central ray is the basis of radiographic positioning. Except in special cases, the X-ray film cassette is placed at right-angles to it and when a stationary grid is employed, the central ray must be aligned along its long axis.

The consequences of the divergence of the rays of the beam are two-fold:

(a) The intensity of the beam is reduced as the distance from the focal-spot is increased. This is an important consideration when assessing exposure factors.

(b) The image of an object placed in the beam will be magnified and may be distorted.

Magnification of the Image

An object placed directly in the path of the central ray will cast an evenly distributed shadow but the diverging rays passing around the periphery of the object will magnify it. The degree of magnification is dependent upon the distance of the

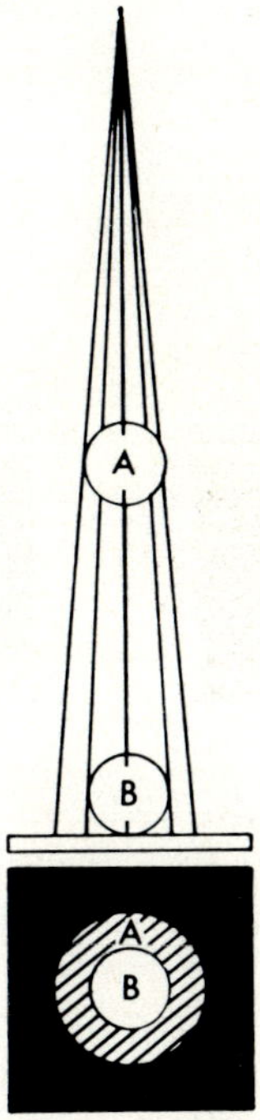

FIG. 1.2.

object from the film. This is greatest when the object is close to the tube (A), and least when the object is close to the film (B). It follows, therefore, that the limb or side of an animal under examination should be placed as near to the film cassette as possible.

The distance between the tube focal-spot and the film also greatly influences the magnification of the image. In Fig. 1.3.a, the tube-film distance is short (12″) and to cover the field, a large aperture cone must be used, with the consequence that the rays diverge at a wide angle and the image of an object of significant size placed in the beam will be enlarged.

If the tube-film distance is now increased to 30″ (Fig. 1.3.b) the area covered by the beam will be proportionately increased. The divergent peripheral rays can now be cut out by using a smaller cone or diaphragm so that only the almost parallel rays around the central ray are used to form the image.

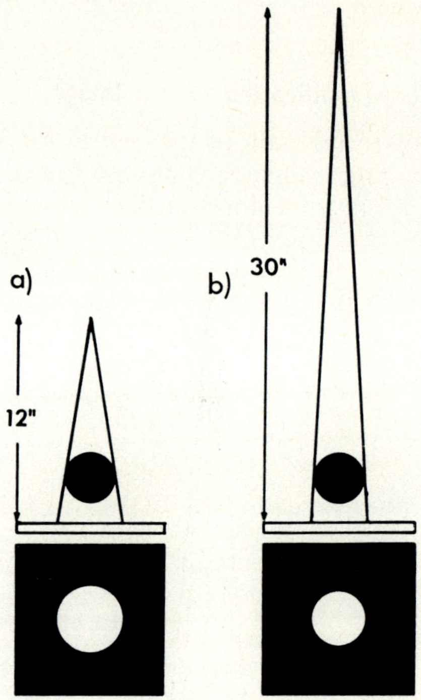

FIG. 1.3.

Thus, the magnification effect is also reduced by increasing the tube-film distance. In human chest radiography, a tube-film distance of 72″ is commonly used in conjunction with powerful X-ray apparatus. The tube-film distance commonly employed in veterinary practice is 30″, which represents a compromise between the magnification effect and the increased exposure required for longer tube-film distances. This distance is satisfactory for most purposes but the radiologist must remember that structures which are not close to the film will be enlarged (e.g., the uppermost kidney in a lateral view of the abdomen of a large dog).

Distortion of the Image

Geometrical distortion of the image occurs when:

(a) The central ray is not in line with the object.
(b) The central ray is not at a right-angle to the object and the film.
(c) The film is not at right-angles to the central ray.
(d) The object is not positioned parallel to the film.

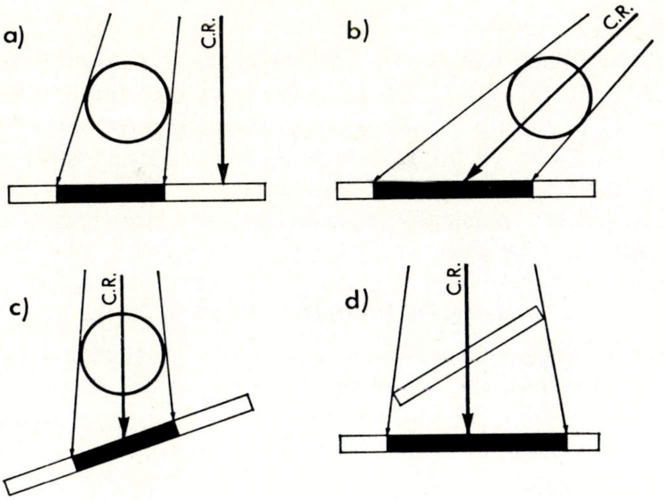

FIG. 1.4.

(a) Correct Alignment of the Central Ray

The object of radiographic positioning is to accurately display the part under examination. This includes orientating the part properly in relation to the beam so that the central ray passes through the area of major interest. For example, when radiographing the stifle joint it is important to check that the central ray will pass cleanly through the joint space. This is insured by first carefully orientating the stifle in relation to the film and then directing the central ray to the centring-point, which lies in the middle of the joint space. If the central ray is inaccurately directed to the centring-point, the oblique rays will pass through the joint space and distort its outline, making accurate diagnosis difficult.

A further example of the distorting properties of the diverging rays occurs when investigating the intervertebral discs. Even when the animal is properly positioned, only the disc spaces in the region of the central ray will be clearly and accurately visualised. The spaces on either side will be progressively distorted by the peripheral rays.

(b) Angulation of the Central Ray

Minimum distortion occurs when the central ray is at 90° to the film. For certain examinations the central ray is angled deliberately to project an overlying structure out of the way. This naturally causes some distortion of the image.

(c) Angulation of the Film

This cause of distortion is similar to (b). Error occurs mainly when the beam is directed horizontally and the film held vertically (e.g., in equine limb radiography).

(d) Orientation of the Object

Distortion of the image will occur if the object is not parallel to the film and at right angles to the central ray. This is especially true of the long bones which may require very careful positioning if an accurate image is required.

The fragments of fractured bones can lie at any angle, so more than one view is desirable if an accurate assessment is to be made. Similarly, superimposition of the fragments can completely mask the fracture line, and thus it is always desirable to obtain more than one projection.

2. RADIOGRAPHIC DEFINITION

The structures visualised on a radiograph should be clearly and sharply defined. If the outlines are blurred, i.e., there does not appear to be a clear dividing line between two adjacent tones, the film will be of poor diagnostic quality.

The causes of poor detail are listed below in decreasing order of importance:

(a) Movement blur.
(b) Scattered radiation.
(c) Focal spot size.
(d) The intensifying screens.
(e) The film emulsion.

(a) **Movement blur** is the most common reason for loss of detail. This is usually due to the patient moving during the exposure, although if the apparatus is unsteady and shaking it will produce the same effect. Movement blur can only be minimised by: using the shortest possible exposure time in conjunction with the use of fast films and screens, reassuring the conscious patient and making it comfortable, watching for the natural respiratory pause, or the use of sedation or general anaesthesia.

(b) **Scattered Radiation** When the primary beam interacts with the atomic structure of the patient and other materials it gives rise to secondary or scattered radiation which travels in all directions. This becomes a significant factor when the tube potential is over 65 kV. and the tissue thickness is over 12 cms., e.g., the average canine abdomen.

The main effect of scatter is to fog the film, thereby reducing contrast and definition. Where there is danger of serious degradation of the image (e.g., the radiography of the thicker parts of animals) a stationary grid must be employed to filter out the scatter although this necessitates a significant increase in exposure. Other aids to reduce the amount of scatter include the use of small cones to confine the beam to the essential area and a compression band to reduce the depth of tissue thickness.

(c) **Focal Spot Size** In most diagnostic self-rectified units the effective tube target size is between 1—1·5 sq.mm. This is adequate for the usual veterinary procedures. However, in certain circumstances, a penumbra can be projected, the exaggerated geometry of which is shown in Fig. 1.5.a.

The penumbral effect is most troublesome when it is necessary to visualise small details, not close to the film, which are of the same dimensions or smaller than the focal spot (Fig. 1.5.b and 1.5.c). In these circumstances a double image will be formed which tends to merge with the ground tone of the surrounding tissues and become invisible. This is one reason why small neoplastic foci in the lung fields may not be demonstrated radiographically.

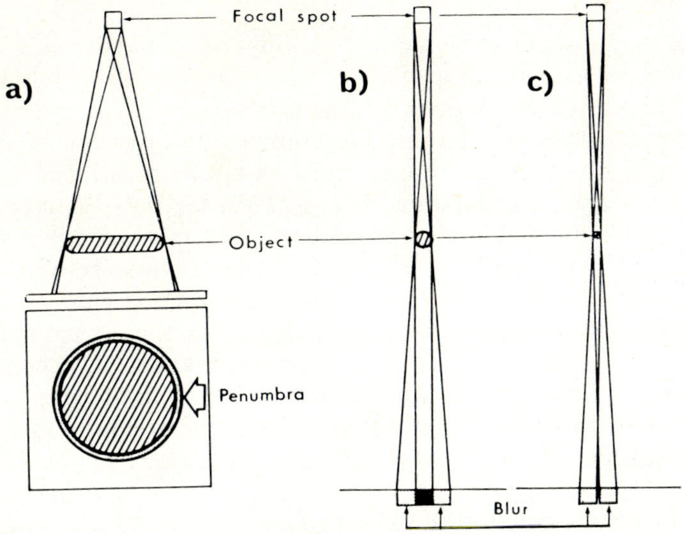

FIG. 1.5.

Similarly if the focal spot is pitted, due to overloading, the definition of the radiographs produced will be inferior.

Some modern portable units (e.g., Philips "Practix") are fitted with dual foci, enabling the operator to select either a fine focal spot for a thin subject, or a broad focal spot for a heavier subject.

(d) The Intensifying Screens Some loss of definition must be expected when intensifying screens are used because of the crystalline nature of the fluorescing surfaces. The degree to which definition is affected depends upon the size of the crystals used and the thickness of the coating. Very fine fluorescing crystals in intimate contact with the film emulsion produce the sharpest image. The emission from a thick coating of larger crystals (used in the faster screens) will result in a more diffuse image, but the light output will be greater, enabling a much shorter exposure time to be used and thus reducing the risk of blurring from movement.

(e) Film Emulsion Although grain is an important factor which affects normal photographic definition, it has little significance in general radiography. In general, the slower films have a finer grain.

3. CONTRAST

The word "contrast" means difference. In radiology the word is applied both to the actual differences in the radiant image caused by the differential absorption of the beam in its passage through the subject (subject contrast), and to the difference in adjacent densities, or tones, seen on the X-ray plate (visible or radiographic contrast). The degree of visual contrast is not the same as subject contrast on a radiograph but is deliberately exaggerated in the manufacture of the film emulsion.

(a) Subject Contrast

Radiological diagnosis depends upon the differences in radiopacity of the various structures of the body and radiopacity, in turn, depends upon the atomic number, density and thickness of the structure. The interaction of the photons of radiation with the atomic structure of the subject is complex and will not be dealt with here, but certain aspects which affect contrast must be briefly mentioned.

Bone is more opaque to radiation than soft tissues but this contrast effect also depends upon the applied kilovoltage and is most marked when the kV. is low (about 40—50). When the kV. is high (75+) the contrast between bone and soft tissue is much less. From this is derived the radiographic rule—to increase image contrast, lower the kilovoltage, and to decrease contrast, raise the kilovoltage.

The use of high kilovoltage also results in the production of high-energy, scattered radiation which degrades the visual image by causing scatter-fog on the film. A stationary grid must be used to filter out this unwanted radiation as well as the other aids to reduce scatter, i.e., cones or diaphragms and where applicable, compression bands.

Gas, fat and calcium are all of different radiopacity from soft tissues. Because of their presence in the body, the outline of organs of normal tissue density can usually be visualised. In certain cases artificial contrast can be created by introducing contrast agents.

(b) Visual Contrast

The translation of the subject contrasts into visual contrasts depend upon the recording medium, the use of intensifying screens, careful and optimum processing technique and the viewing facilities.

Film manufacturers deliberately prepare X-ray emulsions to double the contrast of the radiant image. Screen film emulsions are balanced to be used with intensifying screens which also enhance contrast. Non-screen film is also designed to give high contrast but is not suitable for recording thick areas of soft tissues.

It must be emphasised however that this increased contrast will not be achieved unless the film is processed under optimum conditions, following strictly the manufacturers' instructions concerning time and temperature of development, in properly prepared and maintained solutions.

The film should be viewed under suitable illumination (see Chapter 2).

The function of visible contrast is to enable detail to be clearly seen. The overall density of the X-ray image should neither be too dark nor too light, but the local densities should range from jet black, through a long range of clearly differentiated grey tones to clear film. Possibly the best characteristic of a good film is that it has "sparkle". A low contrast film on the other hand is dark, or dull and grey and individual structures do not stand out clearly.

The main causes of poor visual contrast are:

(a) Under or over-exposure.
(b) Under or over-development.
(c) Fog,
or a mixture of two or three of the above.

Fog has been defined as a density on a film which is not connected with the image. It can be caused by stray light, defective safe-lighting, poor or overlong storage of the films, over-development, stale developer, scattered radiation, or the film box being stored near a source of radiation.

Contrast is of prime concern to the radiographer who must be able to manipulate the various radiographic factors to produce a good diagnostic film.

4. CORRECT EXPOSURE

Correct exposure is the use of X-radiation of a certain penetrating power (kV), in sufficient quantity (milliampere-seconds or mAS), to produce a radiograph which, when correctly processed, shows an image of optimum quality of the part being examined.

The technique of selecting and varying the kV and mAS is considered in greater detail in "Principles of Veterinary Radiography".* It must be remembered, however, that while modern X-ray film allows of considerable latitude in the choice of exposure factors, errors in their selection can greatly reduce the diagnostic value of radiographs.

The authors have had the opportunity of examining a large number of radiographs produced in veterinary practice. Probably the commonest fault noted was that, although produced with the smaller types of apparatus, many showed evidence of over-exposure or of over-penetration, or of both of these faults. Thus films have been too dark to permit perception of significant detail, or over-penetration has obliterated fine bone structure or soft tissue detail.

In a correctly exposed film all the relevant detail of the structures penetrated should be present and easily perceptible, and the radiologist should check the radiographic technique by examining both the densest and the least radiopaque areas of the film for evidence of this. However, if the part being examined contains tissues which vary considerably in radiopacity it may not be possible to demonstrate them all adequately in one film. In these circumstances the radiographer must select his exposure factors according to the particular tissue he intends to visualise and, if necessary, expose a further film using other factors for the demonstration of other parts. Thus for lateral radiographs of the dog the factors selected for demonstration of the abdominal organs are likely to be of lower penetrating power than those chosen to show the lumbar vertebrae.

Finally it must be admitted that the exact degree of blackening and of penetration which is desirable in a radiograph is a matter of personal preference. Some radiologists prefer light films with fine detail and with subtle gradations in tone, while others, feeling that such films may occasionally fail to show sufficient detail in particularly

* Bailliere, Tindall and Cassell, London.

thin areas, prefer darker radiographs and, if necessary, use illumination of greater intensity to examine the densest portion of the film.

It is easy to assert that all films presented for diagnosis should be correctly exposed but in practice this is not easy to achieve. Exposure must be selected on the basis of experience and measurement of the part under examination. Factors are selected because they have produced reasonable results under similar conditions in the past and are adapted for variations in the size of other patients. It must be emphasised that while published data can act as a rough guide, only data derived from a particular unit used in conjunction with its own accessories are of any real value and a chart upon which a full record is kept of all exposures is therefore essential.

5. THE NEED TO TAKE SUFFICIENT PROJECTIONS

Since radiography involves the reproduction of a three-dimensional structure on a flat film, it is seldom that a single radiograph will enable the full extent of a lesion to be visualised. Normally two projections are sufficient but these must not be taken haphazardly but at a known angle to each other (usually at right angles) and to the patient. Knowing the projections the radiologist is then in a position to compare the two films and to build up a reasonably accurate three-dimensional concept of the part being examined.

In some circumstances additional projections may be necessary—e.g., small lesions at the edge of large structures (the canine skull or equine limb bones) may only be visualised by oblique projections.

6. ARTEFACTS DUE TO RADIOGRAPHIC AND PROCESSING FAULTS

The effect of radiographic faults on the subsequent interpretation of the film has been considered above. In addition, faulty or careless processing can blur the whole film or result in local marks which may be mistaken for a foreign body or other lesion.

As pointed out at the beginning of this chapter, it is important that, before attempting interpretation, the radiologist should critically examine the technical quality of each radiograph. Radiographic and processing errors can then be allowed for, and an attempt made to eliminate these in subsequent films. The following table lists the faults of this nature which may be recognised in a radiograph and suggests the most likely causes.

RADIOGRAPHIC AND PROCESSING FAULTS

Appearance of Image	Cause
(1) *Faults in Contrast and Detail*	
Image too dark. Poor contrast.	(a) Over-exposure. (b) Over-development. (c) Fog.

Appearance of Image	Cause
Image too light. Poor detail Background grey and translucent.	(a) Under-exposure. (b) Under-development.
Grey over-all image. Detail present, but contrast poor.	(a) Over-exposure and under-development. (b) Excess scattered radiation.
Fog (a density not connected with the actual image). Low contrast.	(a) Storage fog. Due to films being kept for too long, or in a damp place. (b) Chemical fog. Due to over-development, exhausted developer, or aerated or very fresh developer. (c) Light fog. Due to leakage of light into the darkroom or to defective safe-lights. Local fogging of the edge of film is likely to be due to leaving the lid off the film box or developing tank, or to faulty cassettes. (d) Scatter fog. Due to density of tissues and an absence of precautions to minimise scatter (coning down, grids, etc.). (e) Backscatter fog. Due to absence of lead shielding beneath non-screen film. (f) Streaky fog. Due to prolonged examination of film under safe-light during development.

(2) *Radiographic Technique Faults*

Blurring of image. Loss of detail.	Movement of patient or tube stand.
Localised blurring of detail.	Faulty screen contact.
Vignette effect (fall-off of density at the edge of the film).	Seen in association with the use of a grid. Due to the central ray not being aligned to the centre of the grid.

Appearance of Image	Cause
Distortion of grid lines at edge of film.	Damaged grid (usually due to it having been dropped).
Magnified image.	Object-film distance too long, or film-focal distance too short.
Distorted image.	Incorrect positioning of the part or of the central ray.

(3) *Radiographic Artifacts*

Stains (deposits or discolourations which obscure the image).	
(a) Colourless scum removable by washing.	Deposit of hypo after inadequate washing.
(b) Colourless scum *not* removable by washing.	Sludge formed in fixer as a result of contamination with developer.
(c) Yellowing and fading of image after storage.	Formation of silver sulphide—due to inadequate fixing and washing.
(d) Yellow-green scum with metallic lustre.	Insoluble oxidation products floating on top of exhausted developer.
(e) Dichroic stain (pink in transmitted light, yellow-green in reflected light).	Deposit of colloidal silver due to mixing of developer and hypo as a result of insufficient rinsing, or to exhausted fixer.
Localised light marks	
(a) Small and circular.	Bubbles on the film surface during development.
(b) Irregular.	Dust or other foreign material on the intensifying screens.
(c) Splashes.	Hypo splashed on to the film before development.
(d) Half-moon marks.	Buckling of film due to careless handling before exposure of film.

Appearance of Image	Cause
(e) Fine, light lines.	Cracks in the intensifying screens, or abrasion of the film after processing.
(f) White fingerprints.	Film handled with greasy or fixer contaminated fingers before processing.
(g) Blotchy marks (noted on all films used in one cassette).	Fungal growths on screen.
(h) Uneven lines (seen on non-screen film used in envelopes).	Pressure marks—usually due to the animal pawing the film.
Localised dark marks	
(a) Small and circular.	Pinholes in wrapping material.
(b) Splashes.	Splashes of developer or water on the film before development.
(c) Small, with comet tails.	Due to undissolved particles of developer obtained in powder form.
(d) Fine, dark lines.	Mechanical abrasion before development.
(e) Dotted or arborescent marks.	Static electricity discharged by friction in dry weather.
(f) Dark half-moons.	Handling marks occurring after exposure but before development.
Streaking	
(a) Steamers running from dark areas to light, or from light areas to dark.	Downward diffusion of exhausted developer from areas of high density, in a stagnant solution. Corrected by agitation of the film.
(b) Streamers running from one edge.	Dried chemicals on the bars of channel hangers becoming reactivated during processing.

CHAPTER 2

GENERAL PRINCIPLES OF RADIOLOGY

In the previous chapter the importance of producing radiographs of a high technical standard before attempting to read them was stressed. Similarly, unless the veterinary surgeon takes time and trouble to train himself in the art of viewing and interpreting a radiograph, a carefully produced film may be very largely wasted. If a radiologist is to obtain the maximum information from a radiograph the following conditions must be fulfilled:

(1) The film must be of a good radiographic standard.
(2) The film must be viewed under satisfactory conditions.
(3) The radiologist must be aware of the radiological anatomy of the part being examined, and of its normal variation with age, species and breed.
(4) The radiologist must be able to recognise and dismiss from his consideration artefacts arising in the patient (in addition to those due to the radiographic errors mentioned in the previous chapter).
(5) The radiologist must make a detailed and systematic examination of the *whole* film, identifying any significant variations from the normal and correlating these with pathological lesions or disease processes.

The first requirement has been discussed fully in the previous chapter, and the remaining points will now be considered:

(2) THE VIEWING OF RADIOGRAPHS

For obvious practical reasons films are usually examined while still wet. However, the wet film is swollen and as it dries it will contract and improve the definition. Therefore, when evaluating lesions of fine detail, final examination should be postponed until the dried radiograph is available.

Radiographs can only be satisfactorily viewed against a diffuse uniform source of illumination, such as that provided by the X-ray viewing box. Any attempt to "make do" with uneven sources of light (e.g., a window or room light) for detailed examination of a film can result in errors in interpretation. The standard radiographic viewing box has a screen measuring 17 by 14 inches, which is adequate for all normal radiographs. There is considerable advantage in having two such viewing boxes, or one with double this area, available, so that at least two films can be examined at the same time. This will enable the radiologist to compare a film showing suspected pathology with a "normal" of the same area, or to build up a three-dimensional concept of a lesion from films taken in two different planes. In certain viewing boxes the intensity of illumination can be varied and, while not essential, this refinement does facilitate the examination of films which vary in density. Inevitably some films will contain areas of such density that they cannot be visualised by the usual levels of illumination and some form of "spot light" may be necessary to show the details of such local areas. (An ordinary "Anglepoise" lamp containing a 60 watt pearl bulb is very suitable for this purpose.)

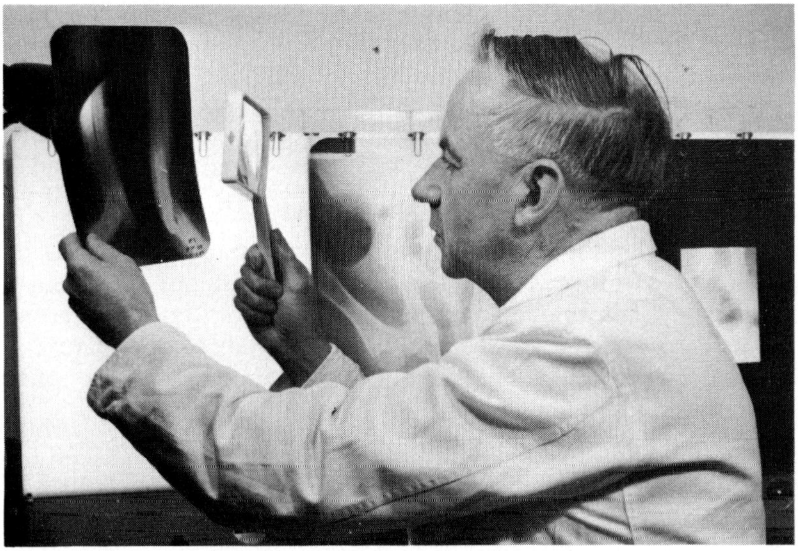

FIG. 2.1. The use of a spotlight to show detail in a dense radiograph.

If the illumination provided by the viewing box is to be utilised to the best advantage the position in which the box is placed must be chosen with care. A bright light falling on the front of a viewing box can render it useless for its purpose, and strong illumination around a viewing box (as will occur if it is placed in a window) can make accommodation of the radiologist's eyes to the radiograph difficult. A similar distracting glare can be troublesome when viewing a small radiograph on a standard illuminator, and it is surprising how much more radiological detail becomes apparent once such glare is eliminated. A series of cardboard masks which can be used to restrict the viewing area are useful for this purpose.

It can also be helpful to have a magnifying glass available when making a close inspection of films showing particularly fine detail (e.g., those produced with a small focus X-ray tube).

A small but important point that is often overlooked is that it is worth giving thought to the way in which the film is placed for viewing, and adopting a consistent method of doing this. While it might be expected that a lesion would appear just as obvious if the radiograph were placed upside down instead of the correct way up, such positioning can lead to errors in the estimated location of an abnormality, particularly if the film is examined hurriedly. Similarly, two views of the same or similar limbs cannot be satisfactorily compared if one of the radiographs is reversed. The most important reason, however, for adopting a consistent method of placing films on a viewing box, is that it aids familiarity with the normal radiographic anatomy of the part and enables one to carry an image of this in one's mind. Thus variations from the normal can be more readily appreciated when examining other films of the same area. While, as long as the same placing is adopted each time, the exact position used is of less importance, it can be helpful to always place the radiograph in such a way that it corresponds with the normal erect standing position of the patient. Where this is not possible (in respect of dorso-ventral and ventro-dorsal projections of the chest and abdomen), the authors have adopted medical usage and normally place the left of the film to the right of the viewing box (thus the medical radiologist always sees the film as though his patient was facing him). It will be found that such placing has been adopted throughout this book.

(3) NORMAL RADIOLOGICAL ANATOMY

While a knowledge of the normal anatomy of the common species of domestic animals is essential to the veterinary radiologist, it must not be assumed that this knowledge will render him immediately familiar with radiological anatomy. It has already been pointed out that a radiograph is a two-dimensional reproduction of three-dimensional structures. Therefore the anatomical features which can be appreciated in a radiograph are:

(a) The contour of the organ or structure—this is likely to alter significantly according to the plane in which the part has been radiographed (even slight oblique changes in any plane can result in marked differences).

(b) The internal structure of the part—both gross (e.g., the outline of the medullary cavity) and fine detail (e.g., the trabeculae of bone).

(c) Variations in the radio-density of the part being examined—this may be due to the nature of the tissue (e.g., increased when calcification occurs, decreased when gas is present) or to its thickness (thus a pulmonary blood vessel seen "end on" will be visible as a small dense mass, while in a lateral view it may be almost imperceptible).

Familiarity with these features of radiological anatomy can only be acquired as a result of experience of examining a large number of radiographic plates. While some useful studies of veterinary radiological anatomy have been published and will be referred to in the appropriate chapters, the radiographs with which they are illustrated inevitably lose detail during reproduction and are not so informative as original radiographs, and the radiologist would be well advised to build up his own library of normal anatomical films. Furthermore it must be remembered that radiological anatomy will vary not only with species, but with breed (cf. the limb bones of a Pekinese and a Greyhound) and age, and the library should include examples of these variations. The variations with age are particularly important with regard to the skeletal system of the young growing animal. The changing radiological picture of young bone which is associated with extending calcification, and the considerable radiological significance of the epiphyseal line will be discussed in the next chapter. Other "normal" anatomical variations will be considered, where appropriate, in subsequent chapters.

It can also be of considerable help to the radiologist to be able to refer to anatomical specimens (usually bones) of the part when examining a film. These will enable him to appreciate the differences in contour caused by rotation of the part, or to locate the position of a particular part of a larger structure (e.g., it is difficult at first to judge the position of the eye in a radiograph of a dog's head unless comparison is made with a skull).

(4) ANOMALOUS SHADOWS

When examining a film the radiologist has to be able to recognise apparent variations in contour and density which are due to artefacts and not of clinical significance. Changes of this nature which are associated with the radiographic technique have been considered in the previous chapter; but other confusing shadows are in fact normal structures within the patient's body but are not necessarily recognised as such by the inexperienced radiologist. Examples are:

(a) The particularly large dense shadows cast by the testicles and penis of the male dog.

(b) The small, but very dense, opacities due to minor bones, such as the transverse hyoid bone, or the clavicle in the cat, seen "end on" and which can easily be mistaken for foreign bodies.

(c) The mammary glands of the bitch which, because of their calcium content, can, when superimposed on the kidney area, be mistaken for kidney calculi.

(d) Lines, usually assumed to be due to skin folds, which are seen in radiographs of the chest. These, when superimposed on the lung fields, can simulate collapse of the lungs.

The common pitfalls of this nature which are associated with particular areas of the body will be listed in the appropriate subsequent chapters.

(5) THE EXAMINATION AND INTERPRETATION OF CLINICAL RADIOGRAPHS

Radiographic diagnosis does not depend on memorising certain gross radiological appearances and subsequently remembering and recognising these as being diagnostic of a particular condition. If the art of examining and interpreting radiographs is to be employed to the greatest advantage, it requires a careful painstaking approach to each film. The radiologist should endeavour to examine each film without any preconceived ideas as to the diagnosis, and without allowing his attention to be distracted by obvious major abnormalities. He should proceed to make a detailed routine examination of the whole film, noting every structure or tissue that can be identified and checking for evidence of normality or abnormality. Significant variation from the normal will be indicated by one or more of the following features:

(a) Displacement of the structure. This may show pathology of an adjacent organ (e.g., upward displacement of the trachea can be indicative of enlargement of a mediastinal lymphatic gland), or of the structure itself (e.g., a dislocated hip).

(b) Variation in the density of the tissue. The density may be increased (e.g., the lung parenchyma in pneumonia) or decreased (e.g., osteolysis in association with bone necrosis).
(c) A break or variation in the contour of the part (e.g., a fracture or a neoplastic enlargement of an organ).
(d) Variation in the detailed structure of the part or tissue (e.g., the marked narrowing of the bony cortex which occurs in association with juvenile osteoporosis).

A similar examination should be made of any other relevant films, and from radiographs taken in two or more planes it should be possible to build up a three-dimensional conceptio f the extent and nature of any lesion and to correlate this with the pathological changes which are known to occur with the lesion or disease suspected.

In some instances it will be necessary to study a series of radiographs taken over a period of time, before commenting as to whether the pathological processes observed are progressing or regressing.

Finally, the information gained from radiological examination must be compared with that obtained from clinical and laboratory examinations and the significance of the X-ray findings reassessed in the light of this further information.

Such detailed examination of radiographs will be time-consuming, particularly at first; but unless the veterinary surgeon is prepared to do just this, he will make mistakes and will not make the best use of the valuable aid to diagnosis provided by his X-ray apparatus.

PART TWO

THE SKELETAL SYSTEM

CHAPTER 3

GENERAL CONSIDERATIONS

In this chapter general features of the radiological investigation of the skeletal system are considered, in order to avoid unnecessary repetition when particular bones and joints are examined in greater detail in the next four chapters.

While bones and joints are closely interrelated it is more convenient at this stage to discuss them separately.

BONES

Radiography

Since bony structures are comparatively dense and distinct when compared with soft tissues and because the lesions encountered in bone are usually more easily recognised, appraisal of the radiological quality of films of the skeletal system is not always so critical as is desirable. The importance of the two following points must be born in mind both by the radiographer and the radiologist.

(1) Exposure Factors The kilovoltage selected must be sufficiently high to ensure penetration of the thickest parts of the bone and demonstration not only of the outline, but of the fine trabecular structure of the bone (such detail is important when examining for the early evidence of neoplasia or of bone infection).

Over-penetration must also be avoided since it may result in complete obliteration of thin areas of bone or hamper simultaneous examination of adjacent soft tissue.

Thus, as a rough guide, correct exposure of a bone radiograph can be judged by the fact that one can clearly perceive both the surrounding soft tissue and the detailed internal structure of the bone in the same film.

(2) Positioning Since many bones are surrounded by a considerable quantity of other tissues and cannot be placed immediately adjacent to the film, considerable enlargement and distortion can occur when radiographing them. Careful and consistent positioning of the patient must always be adopted in order to keep this to a minimum to prevent misdiagnosis and to permit reasonably accurate measurement of bones for orthopaedic purposes.

Radiological Appearance of Normal Bone

In the previous chapter the veterinary radiologist was advised to acquire a familiarity with normal radiological anatomy, both from anatomical specimens and by building up a normal film library. In addition, a number of studies of the radiological anatomy of the skeletal system have been published and many of these are listed at the end of this and subsequent chapters. For this reason, in this work, attention will only be paid to those features of normal anatomy which the authors have found to be of particular significance in the interpretation of clinical radiographs. There are, however, certain general aspects which should be examined more closely at this stage.

(1) The Detailed Structure of Bones

In the accompanying radiograph of an antero-posterior projection of a canine femur the following features can be recognised. These features are of importance in radiological interpretation and most of them are present and can be recognised in any bone.

(a) Calcification It is the deposition of calcium salts within bone which renders it radiopaque. This means that a greater proportion of the X-ray beam is absorbed by bone and, as a consequence, a smaller quantity of X-rays reach and affect the appropriate part of the film, which appears whiter than, and contrasts with, the surrounding soft tissues. Those portions of a bone which are not calcified (i.e., the epiphyses of very young dogs) will not be visualised in a radiograph.

In normal bone, provided comparable exposure factors are employed, the degree of radiopacity recorded on a film will depend on the depth of tissue penetrated and will thus permit recognition of the next two features listed.

(b) Protuberances In the radiograph of the femur the edges of the trochlea groove and the outline of the great trochanter are visible because they represent a greater depth of bony tissue which is penetrated by the X-ray beam. If the patella were present it would be visualised through the lower end of the bone for the same reason.

(c) The Bony Cortex The compact bone of which this is composed is thickest and best seen in the diaphyseal region. It thins out at each end to surround and blend with the cancellous bone of each epiphysis.

(d) The Trabecular Structure of Cancellous Bone Cancellous bone fills the epiphyses and extends into the ends of the medullary cavity. In the living animal, perception of the detailed structure of this portion of the bone may be prevented by movement of the patient, by superimposition of dense areas of tissue or plaster casts, or by poor radiographic technique. It is important to be familiar with the general pattern of this fine detail and to look for it when reading a radiograph, as the first evidence of many pathological changes is seen in the cancellous bone.

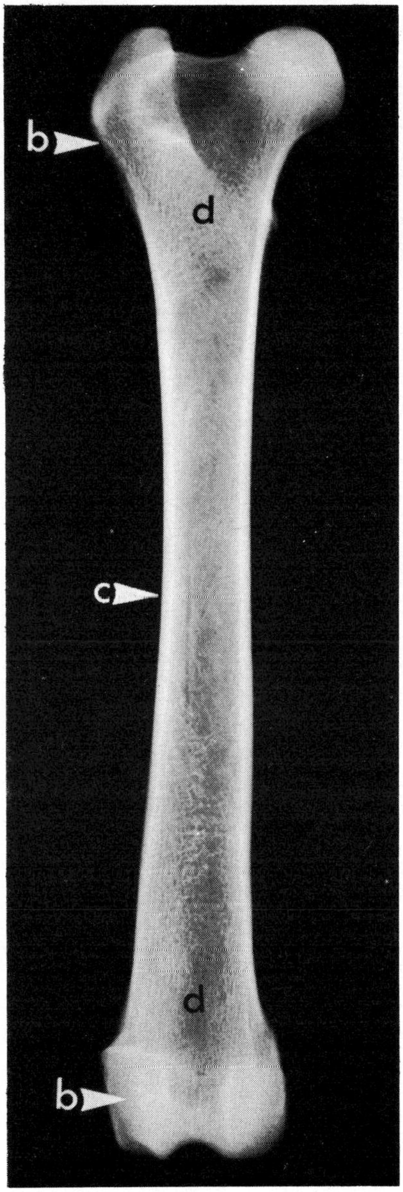

FIG. 3.1.

(e) A feature not visualised in this illustration is the **Nutrient Foramen.** If the presence of this normal structure is not appreciated it can be mistaken for a defect or fracture in the bony cortex.

(2) Bone in the Young Animal

In the young growing animal there will be a variation not only in the size of the bone, but in the amount which is calcified and can therefore be visualised in a radiograph. The majority of the carpal and tarsal bones and the epiphyses of the long bones of the dog and cat are cartilagenous at birth and cannot be demonstrated radiologically (in the larger species of domestic animals these bones are ossified at birth and can be visualised). This fact can make it difficult to provide radiological

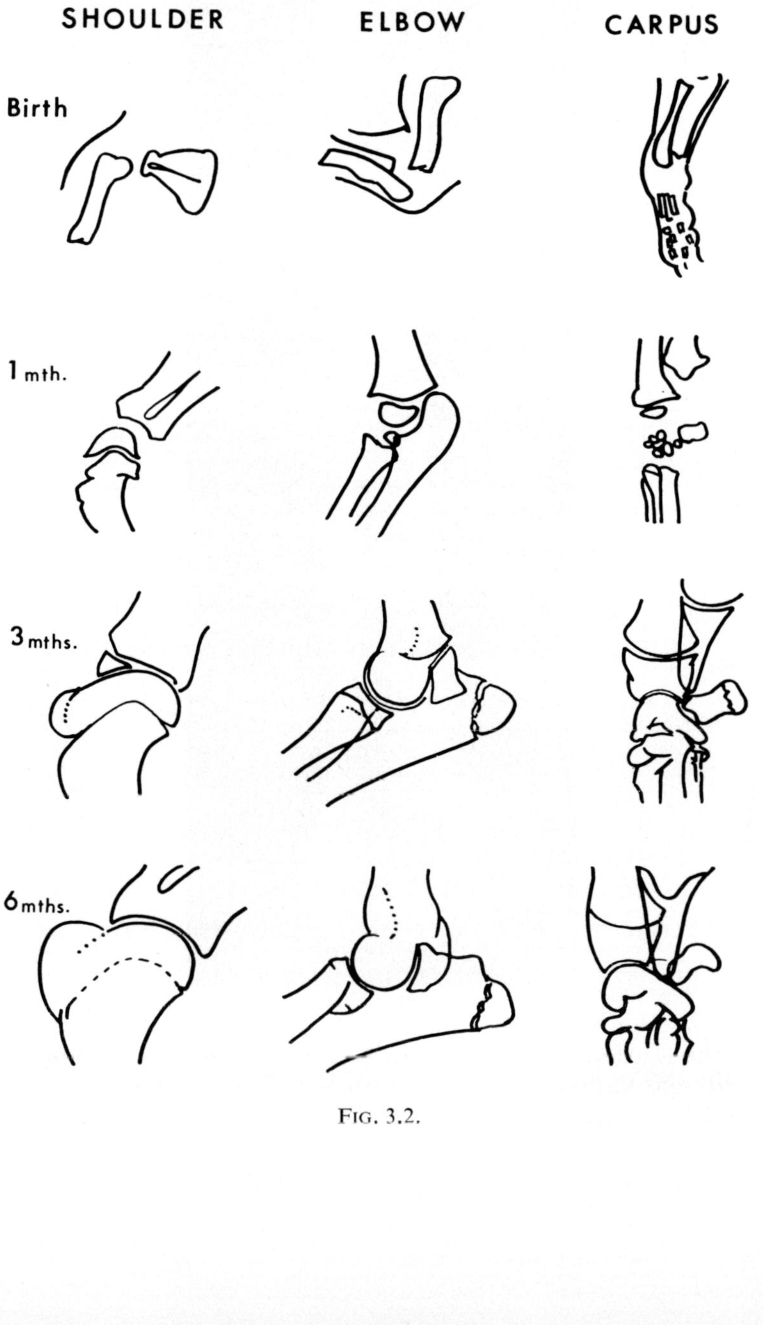

Fig. 3.2.

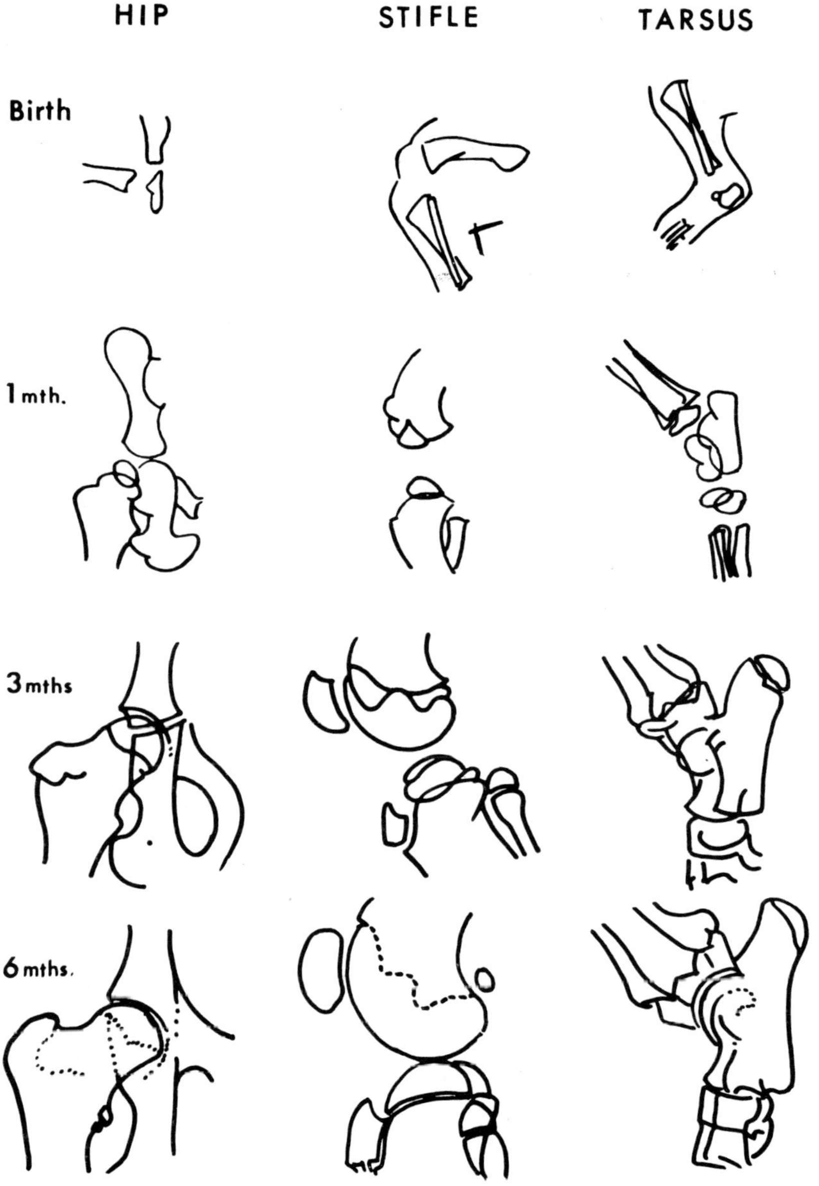

FIGS. 3.2 and 3.3. Tracings to show the development of ossified bone in a young Greyhound.

evidence of congenital dislocations or other joint abnormalities during the first few weeks of life. These bones and the epiphyses become visible as centres of ossification develop, usually during the first 3 months of life, and the process of bone formation extends fairly rapidly through the cartilagenous area.

In man, ossification of the epiphyses and subsequent epiphyseal fusion follows a fairly definite pattern and it is possible to judge the age of a young patient with some accuracy by examining radiographs. It is not possible to do the same with animals, although a number of radiological studies of epiphyseal closure have been carried out. In a paper reviewing the literature on the subject and reporting extensive investigations of his own Sumner-Smith (1966) draws attention to the fact that there can be a variation of several months in the age at which epiphyseal closure occurs in particular bones in the dog. This variation is seen, not only between different breeds, but even between dogs from the same litter. This author does report, however, that in general there is a fairly definite sequence which is followed in the order in which the different epiphyses become fused. The various epiphyses are listed in the accompanying table in the order of epiphyseal fusion reported by Sumner-Smith, together with the lower and upper age limit at which he noted fusion occurring.

Sequence of Epiphyseal Closure in the Dog

Accessory carpal bone	10 weeks— 5 months
Scapular tuberosity	3 months— 5 months
Middle phalanx, fore limb	4 months— 5 months
Proximal phalanx, fore limb	4 months— 5 months
Middle phalanx, hind limb	4 months— 5 months
Proximal phalanx, hind limb	4 months— 7 months
Fibula tarsal bone	11 weeks— 7 months
Metacarpal bones	5 months— 7 months
Metatarsal bones	5 months— 7 months
Proximal ulna	5 months— 8 months
Distal humerus	5 months— 8 months
Proximal radius	5 months— 8 months
Distal tibia	5 months— 8 months
Distal fibula	5 months— 8 months
Distal femur	6 months— 8 months
Distal ulna	6 months— 8 months
Distal radius	6 months— 9 months
Proximal femur	6 months— 9 months
Great trochanter of the femur	6 months— 9 months
Proximal fibula	6 months—10 months
Proximal tibia	6 months—11 months
Lesser trochanter of the femur	9 months—10 months
Proximal humerus	10 months—10 months

It should be noted that Sumner-Smith indicates that minor variations can occur in this sequence, and also that, in a few instances, other authors have reported epiphyseal closure occurring at dates outside the range shown.

The Detailed Structure of Young Bone

The most important features to be observed in radiographs of young bone are illustrated in the accompanying radiograph and diagram of the lower end of the radius of a large dog. These features are:

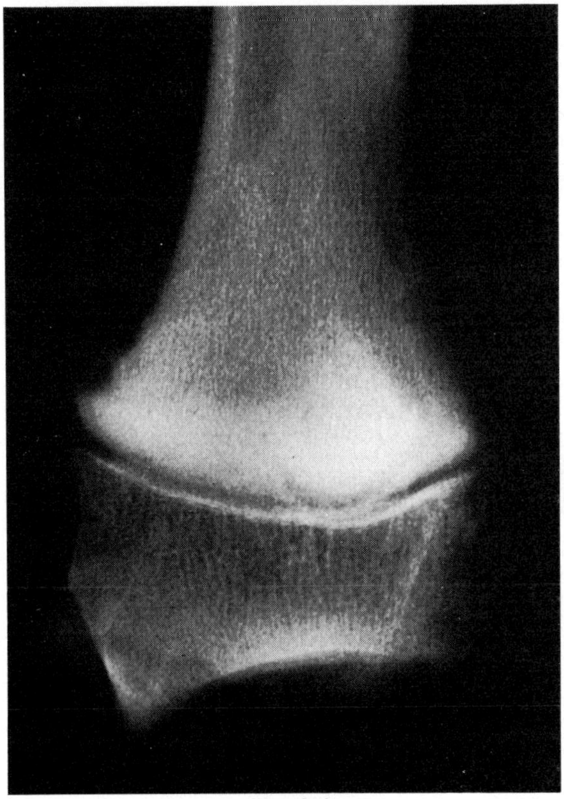

FIG. 3.4.

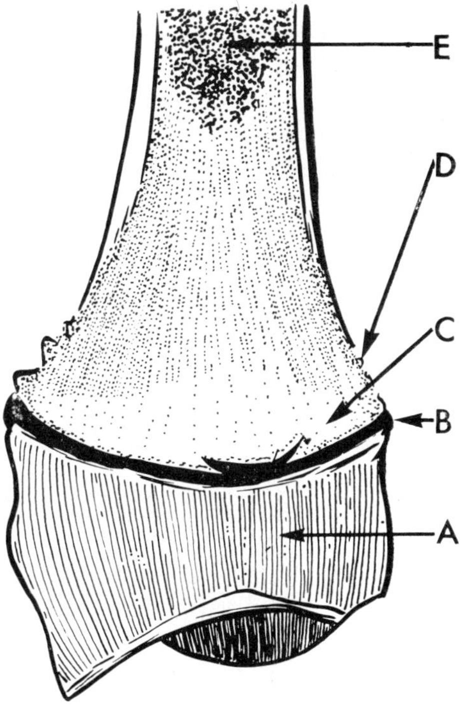

FIG. 3.5.

(A) **The Epiphysis** As already stated, this is normally cartilagenous at birth in dogs and cats and undergoes progressive ossification and radiographic visualisation during the first few months of life. When fully developed the epiphysis shows a particularly narrow and dense periphery and an internal structure made up of fine, somewhat longitudinal trabecular markings.

(B) **The Epiphyseal Line** This line is sometimes spoken of as "The Growth Plate", and indicates the area in which longitudinal growth of bone occurs. It is seen as a narrow radiotranslucent line extending completely across the bone and might be mistaken for a fracture line. Once radiography shows that the bony structure of the epiphysis has merged with that of the metaphysis and obliterated the epiphyseal line no further growth will occur (occasionally this results from an injury to the area and can then occur before normal times of fusion).

(C) **The Metaphysis** This area shows the cancellous bone formed at the epiphyseal line. During the growing period this region undergoes an involved process which results in extension of the shaft of the bone and a reshaping of the bone first laid down. Because of the active proliferation which is occurring, the epiphyseal edge of the metaphysis is wider in the young animal than in the adult and is often poorly visualised (i.e., poorly calcified) at the extreme edge.

(D) **The Cut-Back Zone** This is the area in which the over-expanded bone laid down at the epiphysis is remoulded as growth proceeds, into the denser and narrower bony cortex of the shaft of the bone.

(E) **The Diaphysis** This is the shaft of the bone and shows clearly the dense compact bone of the cortex and the outline of the medullary cavity.

(3) Breed and Individual Variations

The anatomical differences between breeds (e.g., between the skulls of the Greyhound and the Bulldog and between the limb bones of the Dachshund and the Great Dane) are too numerous to describe in detail but must be borne in mind when examining skeletal radiographs.

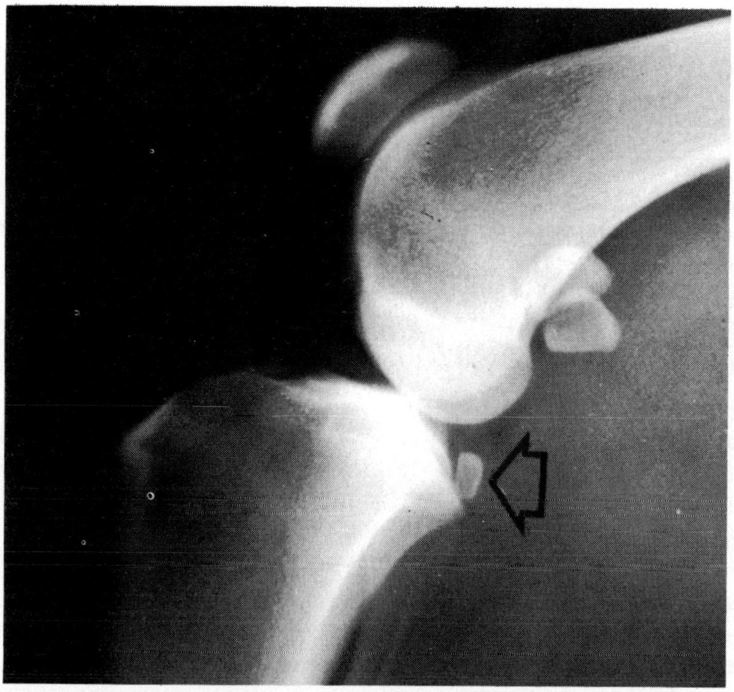

FIG. 3.6. Third fabella of the stifle joint—often overlooked.

Certain supernumerary bones (additional vertebrae, fabellae, etc.) may be encountered in individual animals and not in others and are seldom of clinical significance.

The Vital Properties of Bone

Owing to the obviously inanimate nature of bony specimens, it is easy to forget that in the live animal bone is a living tissue capable not only of growth, but of response to injury and of repair. Radiography permits appreciation of the vital changes occurring within bone, but it must be born in mind that a film obtained at a specific date may only demonstrate a single stage in a protracted process, which can only be fully visualised in a series of radiographs. Furthermore there is always a delay period (often of only a few days' duration) before soft tissues become calcified or (in destructive processes) calcification of existing bony tissue is removed, and can be recognised in a radiograph.

General Evidence of Pathological Changes in Bone

The immediate effects of severe traumatic injury (i.e., fractures and dislocations) are normally easily perceived as a result of a break in the continuity of outline or by obvious displacement of the bones. It is the more subtle and progressive changes in bone structure and density, resulting from a variety of causes, that are more difficult to visualise. Such changes cannot be fully classified and listed, but the following are the commonest manifestation which may be recognised in a radiograph.

(1) Localised Osteoporosis (Osteolysis)

Localised osteoporotic lesions within a bone are usually obvious, since they lack the density and structure which can be seen in normal adjacent bone. While in a few instances they result from failure of ossification of a particular area (e.g., bone cysts), they are usually due to death of a particular portion of bone and its removal by osteolysis. Such osteoporosis occurs in an irregular form in association with malignant neoplasia and osteomyelitis and as a more organised band separating healthy bone from necrotic bone sequestra.

(2) Generalised Osteoporosis (Decalcification)

It should be appreciated that apparent differences in the radiodensity of bone may be due solely to variations in the factors of the radiographic technique (the exposure factors, the thickness and density of the tissue, the use of different kinds of film or intensifying screen, etc.). Caution should be exercised in diagnosing decalcification in a radiograph unless: the feature is very gross and obvious, it is possible to make a comparison with a comparable area (e.g., with the opposite limb) radiographed under identical conditions, or associated changes in the structure of the bone can be appreciated.

When osteoporosis involves the entire skeleton the degree of radiopacity cannot be compared with that of normal bone and the condition will be comparatively advanced before it can be diagnosed with certainty. The fact that the radiopacity is reduced will be shown first by a diffuse grey appearance rather than the normal distinct white. If the condition progresses further practically all evidence of normal bone outline and structure may be lost.

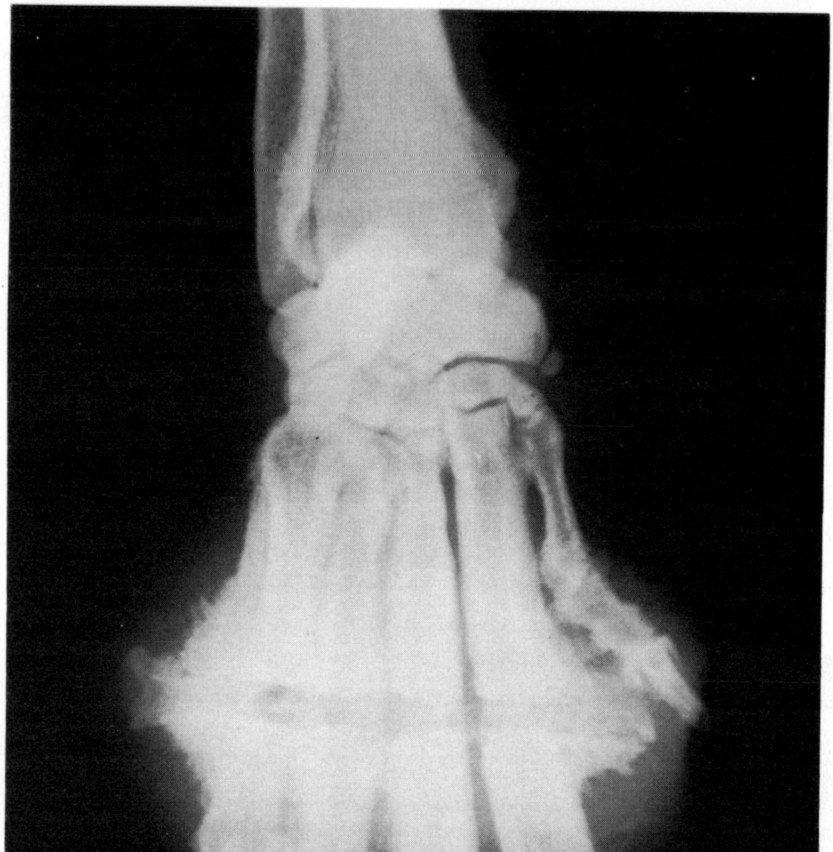

FIG. 3.7. Localised osteoporosis due to necrosis resulting from a constricting elastic band.

Osteoporosis may result from dietetic deficiency or imbalance in the growing animal, or may be associated with removal of calcium from the skeleton of the adult. The condition known as juvenile osteoporosis is usually considered to result from a deficiency of calcium in the diet and is characterised by deficient bone formation with osteoporosis and particularly thin corteces. In rickets some degree of osteoporosis may be apparent but the more typical feature is a failure of calcification of the provisional cartilage forming at the epiphyseal line and the development of a large translucent area in this region. In the adult animal, while decalcification could theoretically be associated with abnormalities of the parathyroid, it has certainly occurred in conjunction with chronic nephritis (renal rickets) and disuse atrophy of a limb. These two manifestations may be confined to a portion of the skeleton (the skull in renal rickets, the bones encased in plaster in disuse atrophy) but there are unlikely to be the changes in bone structure encountered in the younger animal.

(3) New Bone Formation

This may take several forms.

(a) **Callus** Provided that the conditions are suitable, the soft tissue which fills the gap between the portions of a fractured bone becomes ossified and is seen in a radiograph as an irregular mass of calcified tissue. This mass undergoes a gradual process of remodelling and is replaced by bone showing a more regular outline and normal internal structure. In cases in which there has been little displacement remodelling may be so complete that the site of the fracture becomes almost imperceptible.

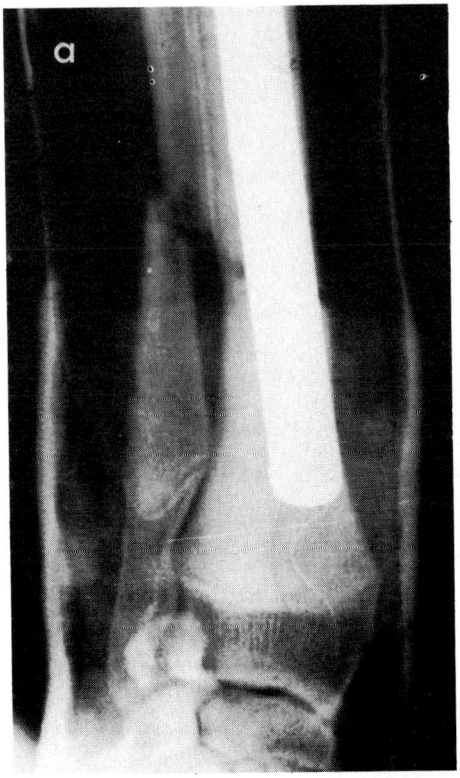

FIG. 3.8.

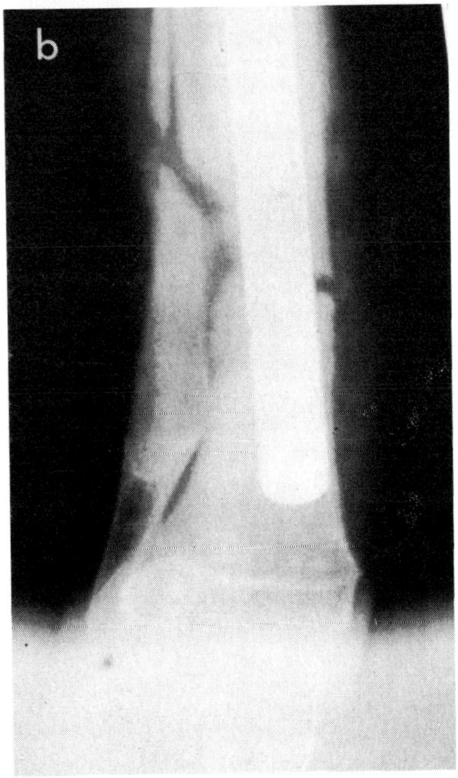

FIG. 3.9.

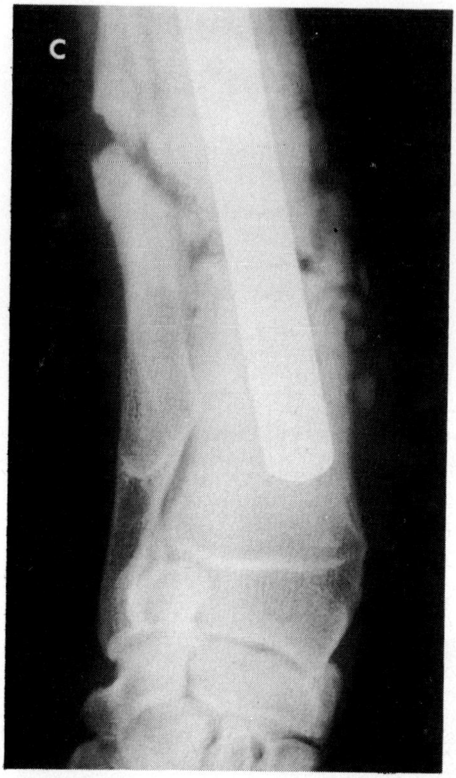

FIG. 3.10.

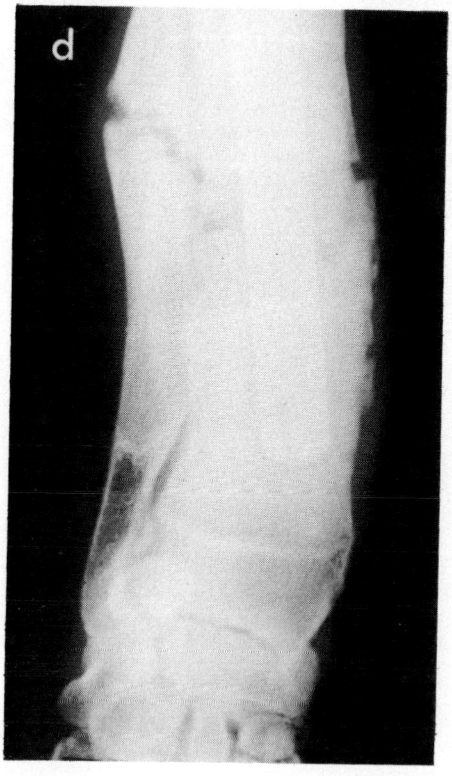

FIG. 3.11.

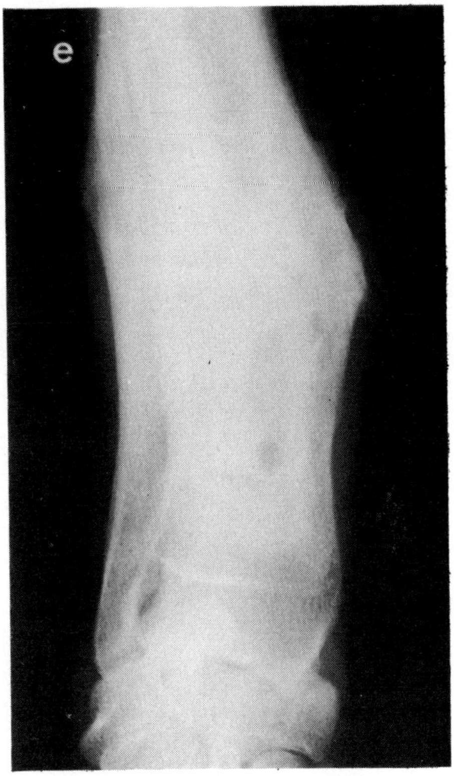

FIG. 3.12.

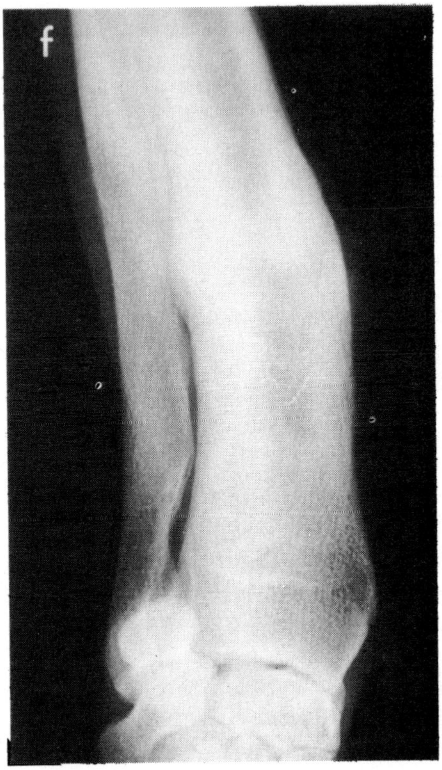

FIGS. 3.8 to 3.13. Healing and remodelling of a fracture over a period of a year.

FIG. 3.13.

It is of considerable importance to be able to judge from a radiograph when bony union has occurred, and that it is therefore safe to remove splints or bone plates. In most instances the union by calcified tissue will be obvious, but care must be exercised in recognising those cases (usually in which there is some movement at the fracture site) in which large masses of callus form at the two fractured ends and overlie each other but do not unite.

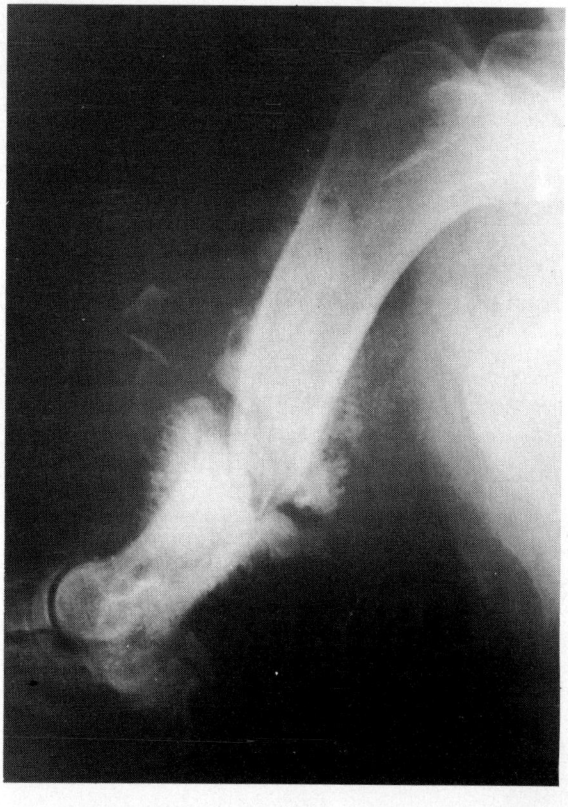

FIG. 3.14. Non-union of a fracture, despite considerable callus formation.

(b) **Osteophytes** This term is used to describe areas of new bone formation (usually small, but occasionally large) arising from the cortical region and protruding out into soft tissues. Such outgrowths occur in association with inflammatory processes (traumatic and infective), are encountered around joints in osteoarthritis and also arise from the periosteal region of the lower limb bones of horses (e.g., ringbone). When such osteophytes are small their presence may easily be missed if too much penetration is employed or if insufficient projections are obtained. From a close examination of such outgrowths it may be possible to judge if the underlying inflammatory process is still active (the edge of the lesion is ill-defined and tends to merge with soft tissues) or has subsided (the edge of the protrusion is likely to be more clearly demarcated).

(c) **Subperiosteal bone formation** Any process which raises the periosteum from the cortical bone will stimulate new bone formation in the gap. This is seen around fracture sites and areas of malignant bone neoplasia and also occurs as a result of pulling of tendinous insertions into bone. In these circumstances the new bone will arise separately from the cortical bone but will tend to merge with it before long.

(d) **Sclerosis** This term is used to describe an area of increased radiopacity within existing bone structure and probably comprises both increased calcification and greater bone density. It is seen in those situations in which bone tissue has reacted to various types of injury. Thus, evidence of sclerosis may occur immediately beneath eroded lesions in joint cartilages or around areas of osteomyelitis. Similarly a narrow sclerotic band may develop in a bone at the site of a previous "hair line" fracture which, because it was not associated with any displacement, may not have been radiologically perceptible at the time of its occurrence.

(e) **Neoplasia** Comparatively regular formation of new bone will be seen in benign neoplasia but this appears to be a rare condition in animals. In the more frequently occurring malignant bone neoplasia there is usually evidence of the simultaneous occurrence of osteolysis and of new bone formation. The whole subject of bone neoplasia will be considered in greater detail later in this chapter.

Specific Pathological Conditions

Fractures

While most fractures are obvious in a radiograph, overlap of bone can mask the break if only a single film is taken, and it is always advisable to have at least two projections to demonstrate the full extent of the injury.

Another possible source of error is that the uncalcified epiphyseal region in the young animal can be mistaken for a fracture. When injuries do occur in the region of the epiphyseal line it must be borne in mind that subsequent healing can result in epiphyseal closure and cessation of bone growth.

Neoplasia

This is probably best considered under four headings:

(1) *Benign Bone Neoplasms*

Simple tumours of bone (osteomata) are rare in animals. The typical radiological findings are likely to comprise a localised region of new bone formation in which the bone is comparatively uniform and regular in structure, and which does not involve other bones or adjacent soft tissues. Evidence of extension of the lesion should be seen in subsequent radiographs.

(2) *Malignant Bone Neoplasms*

Malignant tumours of bone are relatively common in dogs and are seen less frequently in other species. Accurate diagnosis of this condition is very largely

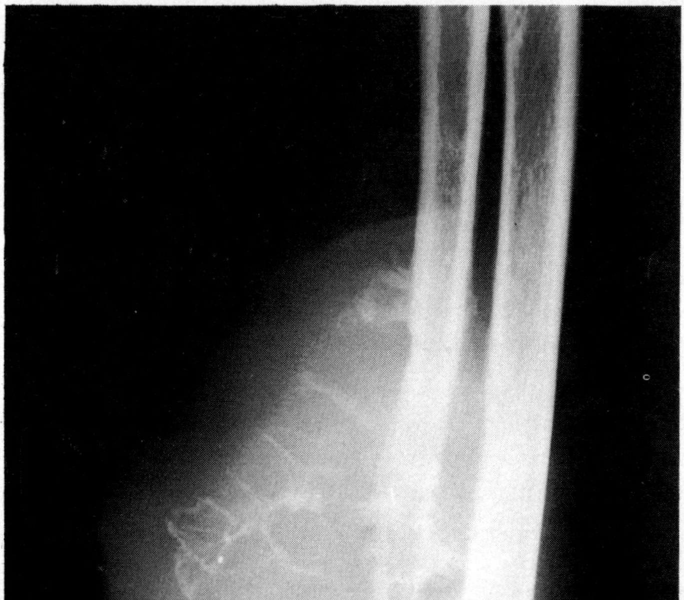

FIG. 3.15. Fibrosarcoma arising in the ulna and involving the radius.

dependent on the radiological findings, but it should be stressed that it can be difficult to differentiate this from other bone conditions (e.g., osteomyelitis) and even more difficult (and often impossible) to identify the precise type of malignant tumour, by radiography alone.

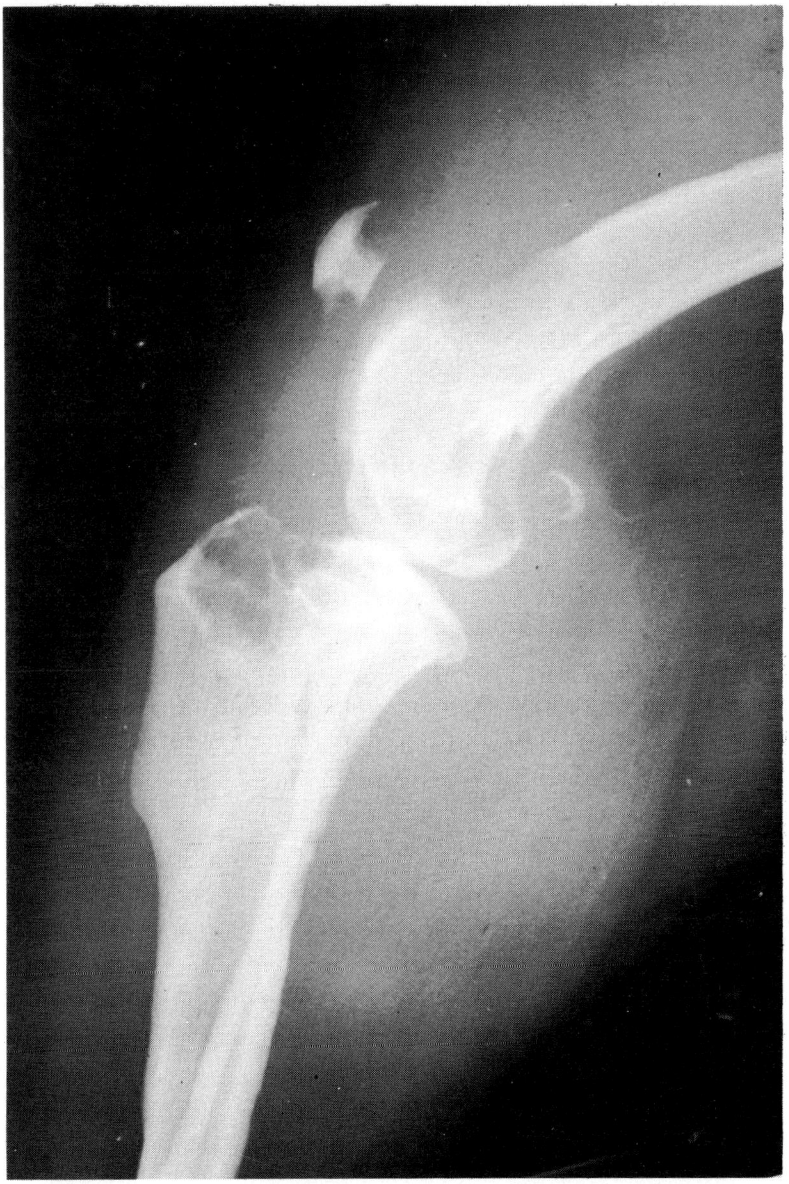

FIG. 3.16. Fibrosarcoma involving all the bones of the stifle joint.

The principal radiological features of malignant bone neoplasia may be considered as follows:

(*a*) *Site* The condition is seen most frequently affecting the larger breeds of dog, where it is normally confined to the ends of certain limb bones (the upper end of the humerus, the lower end of the radius and ulna, and both ends of the femur and tibia—but it is extremely rare for the bones around the elbow joint to be involved). However, any other bone can occasionally be affected, particularly in cats and the smaller dogs, and malignant neoplasms involving the skull, the vertebrae, the scapula, the pelvis and the metacarpals and metatarsals have occurred.

The lesion is usually confined to a single bone and while advanced cases may occasionally spread to adjacent bones (e.g., a neoplasm of the radius may extend into the ulna), it is most unusual for the process to extend across a joint space, although this too has been seen on rare occasions (Figs. 3.15 and 3.16).

(*b*) *Changes within the bone* If the lesion is examined early enough the first change is likely to be a small area of osteolysis or, less frequently, of osteosclerosis. This will be succeeded in later radiographs, by further disorganisation of bone structure and the simultaneous appearance of areas of dense bone formation and areas of bone absorption. In particular tumours one or other of these processes may predominate and the neoplasm be "osteogenic" (Fig. 3.19) with a dense irregular appearance; or "osteolytic" (Fig. 3.20) with loss of large areas of bony tissue (this type is frequently associated with pathological fractures of the bone).

The affected area of bone merges with the surrounding normal bone and is not clearly demarcated from it.

(*c*) *Changes external to the bone* The above changes cause some distortion of, and usually break right through, the cortex of the bone. At the same time new bone is laid down in the surrounding soft tissue, either as irregular poorly defined areas or, more frequently, as spicules extending outwards at right angles to the shaft of the bone. In many instances, a small triangular tuft of new bone formation will be seen just external to the cortex at the edge of the lesion. This consists of relatively normal bone which develops as a result of elevation of the periosteum by the tumour. This is known as Codman's Triangle and is considered to be typical of malignant bone neoplasia (Fig 3.21).

(*d*) *Metastases* Indirect radiological evidence of malignancy can be obtained by demonstrating secondary spread of the original tumour. This is most likely to be recognised in the lungs but may occasionally be seen in other bones or in the liver or kidneys.

(*e*) *Progress of the condition* A characteristic feature of malignant neoplasia is that the typical changes can be seen in subsequent radiographs to be extending through the adjacent bone with no evidence of the development of a

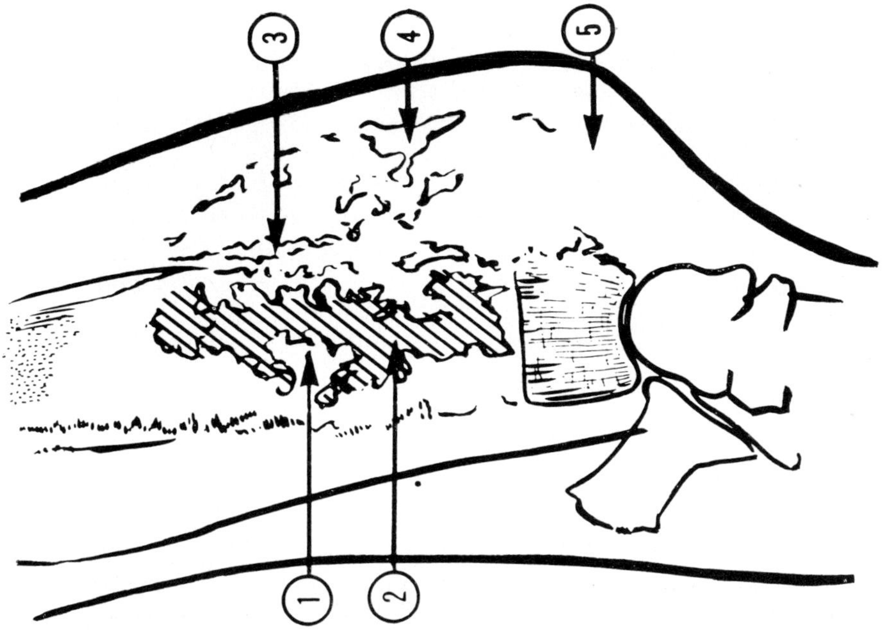

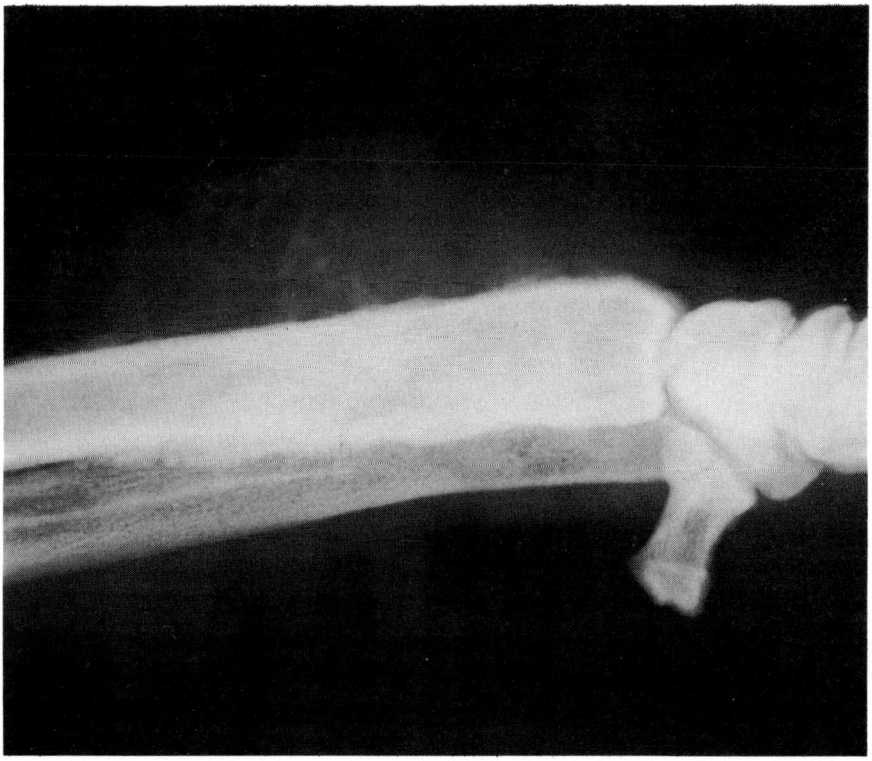

FIGS. 3.17 and 3.18. A typical osteosarcoma. (1) osteosclerotic area. (2) osteolytic area (shaded). (3) periosteal bone formation. (4) new bone forming within the soft tissue extension of the tumour. (5) soft tissue swelling.

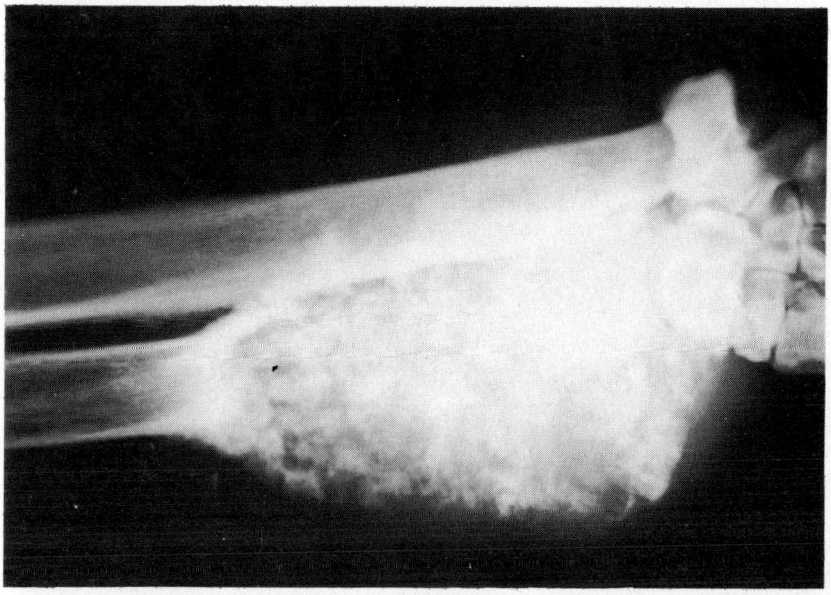

FIG. 3.19. A primarily osteogenic sarcoma.

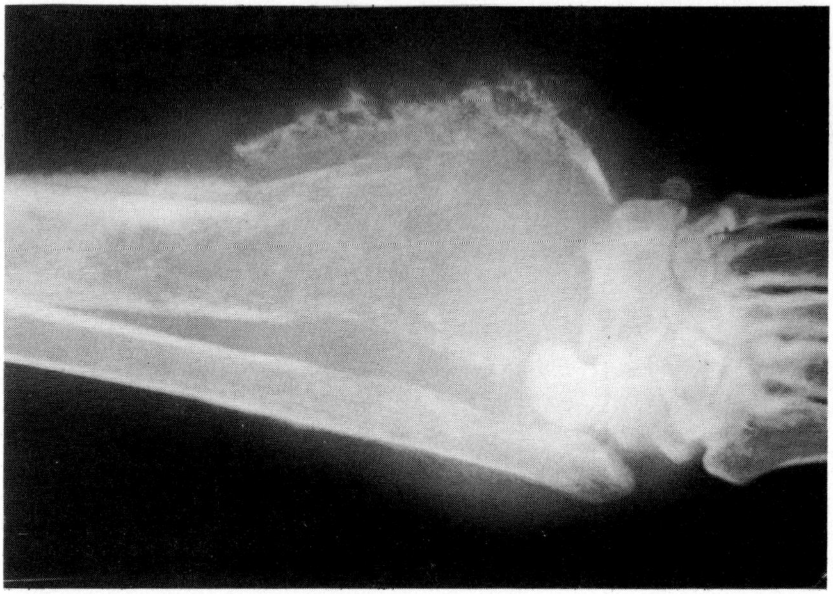

FIG. 3.20. A primarily osteolytic sarcoma.

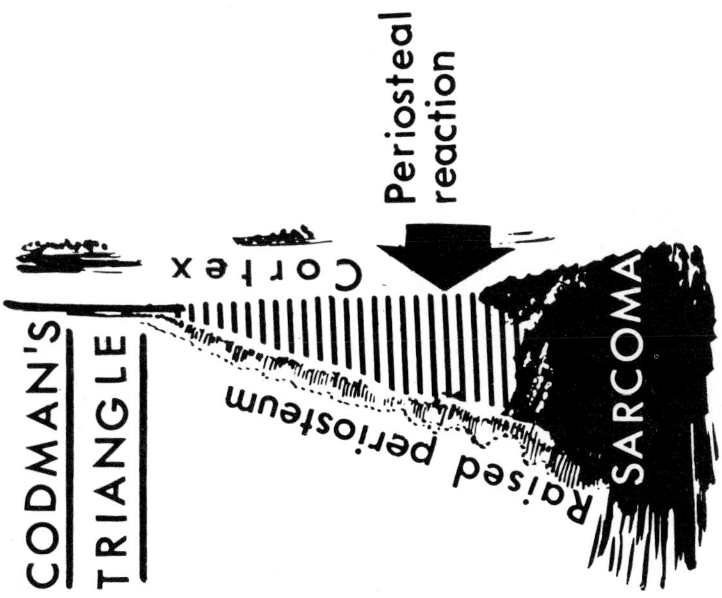

FIG. 3.21.

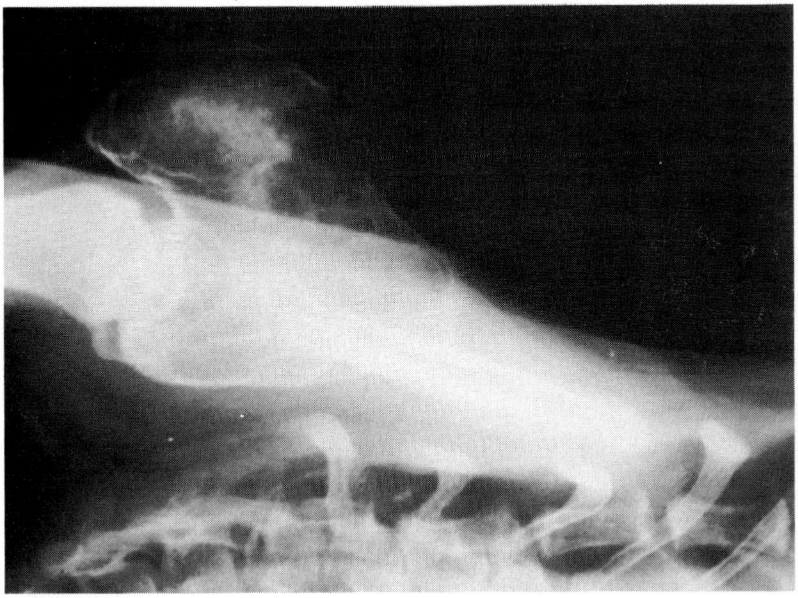

FIG. 3.22. Osteoclastoma of the scapula of a cat.

sclerotic barrier (as often occurs in response to osteomyelitis) in the surrounding healthy bone. The rate at which this process extends will vary greatly—the interval necessary to show changes in later films can vary from days to weeks.

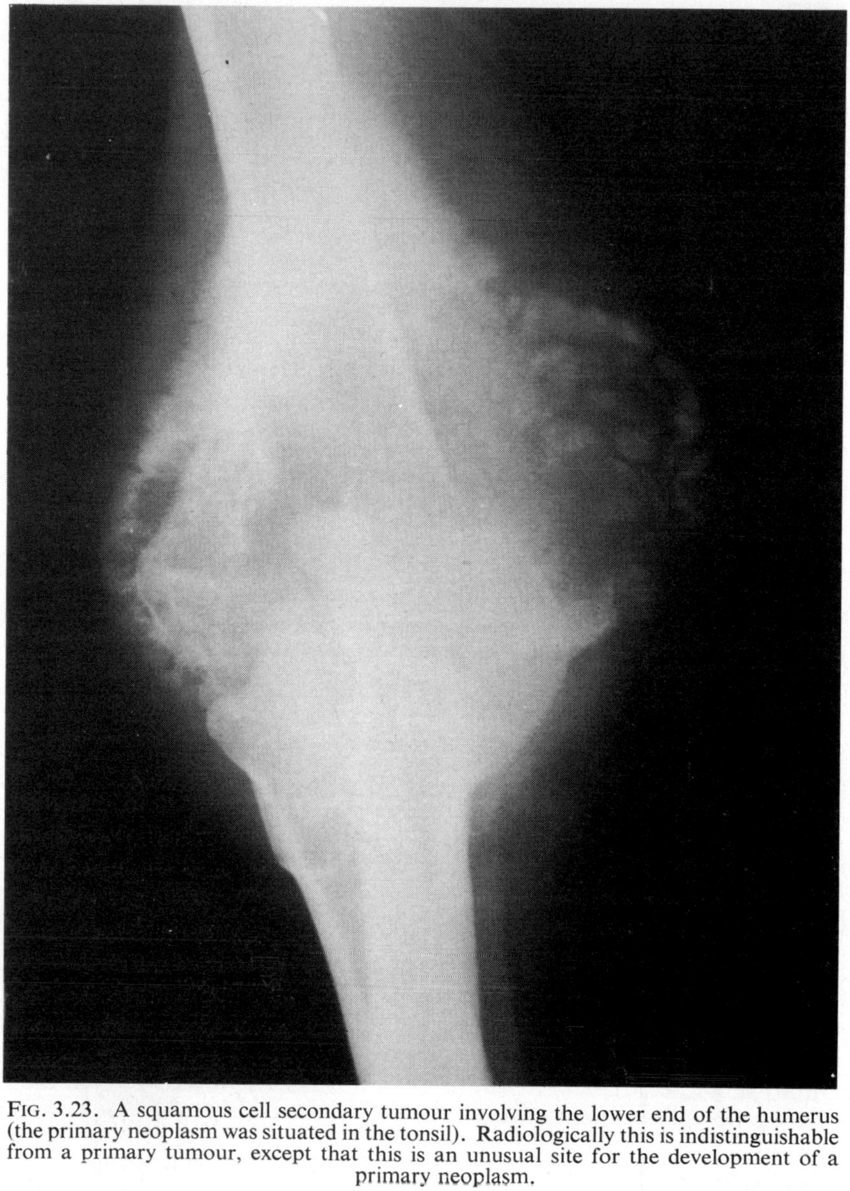

FIG. 3.23. A squamous cell secondary tumour involving the lower end of the humerus (the primary neoplasm was situated in the tonsil). Radiologically this is indistinguishable from a primary tumour, except that this is an unusual site for the development of a primary neoplasm.

Certain specific bone tumours can show characteristic features which may permit their precise identification from a radiograph. These include the chondrosarcoma which typically shows extensive osteolsis and disappearance of large areas of bone, and the osteoclastoma (Fig. 3.22) which is characterised by an expanded and thinned cortex ("egg shell" or "soap bubble" effect). However, there can be so much variation in individual cases that it is seldom possible to distinguish between these and other types of malignant neoplasia on their radiological appearance alone.

For those wishing to pursue the subject in greater detail suggestions for further reading are listed at the end of the chapter.

(3) *Secondary Bone Neoplasms*

There is seldom any radiological difference between primary and secondary malignant bone neoplasms. The main features suggesting that such lesions were secondary would be the fact that they were multiple and that they occurred in less typical situations (e.g., in the vertebrae).

(4) *Invasion of Bone by Neoplasia arising in Soft Tissues*

Neoplasms arising in soft tissues immediately adjacent to bone do occasionally invade the bony tissue. The most frequent and typical example of this is fibrosarcomata developing in the gum and extending into the jaw. In the early stages radiography will show erosion of the bony cortex and an osteolytic process extending into the underlying bone. In some more advanced cases bone formation commences within the tumour and the radiological appearance becomes indistinguishable from that of osteosarcoma.

Osteomyelitis

This term is used here to describe any form of infective process occurring within bone. The condition is comparatively rare in dogs, but it also occurs in farm animals where it may assume a particularly severe form.

There is likely to be a delay of some days after the introduction of infection before the inflammatory process results in bone changes which can be demonstrated radiologically. The first evidence will be seen as a hazy appearance of the bone structure and some roughening of the trabecular outline. As the condition progresses the affected area becomes disorganised and there will be evidence of bone absorption and some reactionary bone formation occurring simultaneously. As a result of lifting of the periosteum some of the new bone formation may be external to the bone. Where infection is associated with the presence of a foreign body (e.g., a bone screw) this will be shown by the development of an area of osteolysis around the offending object (a somewhat similar appearance is seen when infection develops around tooth roots).

As already indicated, the radiological appearance of this condition can closely resemble that of malignant bone neoplasia. An important point in the differential diagnosis is the fact that osteomyelitis may occur anywhere in a bone and anywhere in the skeletal system and there are no predilection sites. Furthermore if osteomyelitis occurs in the end of a bone it tends to spread across the joint and into adjacent bones.

Another difference is the fact that this is essentially a destructive process and osteolysis is the predominant feature. However, while the extensive new bone formation seen in osteogenic bone tumours does not occur, there can be considerable inflammatory sclerosis and new bone formation—both within the adjacent bone and in the periosteal region.

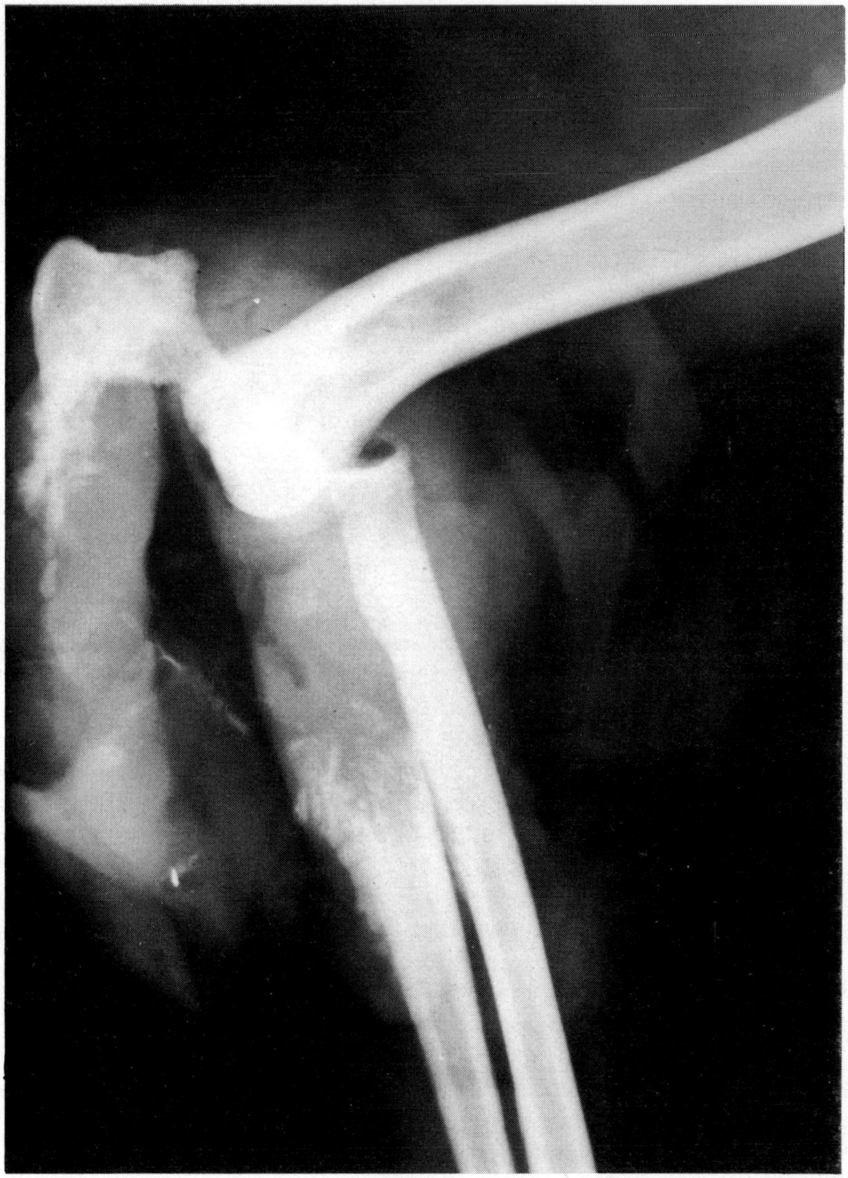

FIG. 3.24. Severe osteomyelitis with a pathological fracture.

In some cases films will show the reaction of the surrounding healthy bone to the presence of infection by the development of a band of sclerosis around the lesion.

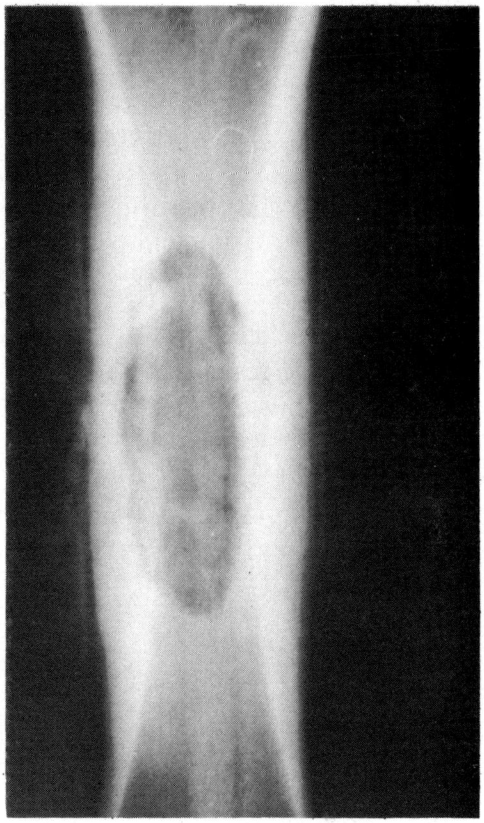

FIG. 3.25.

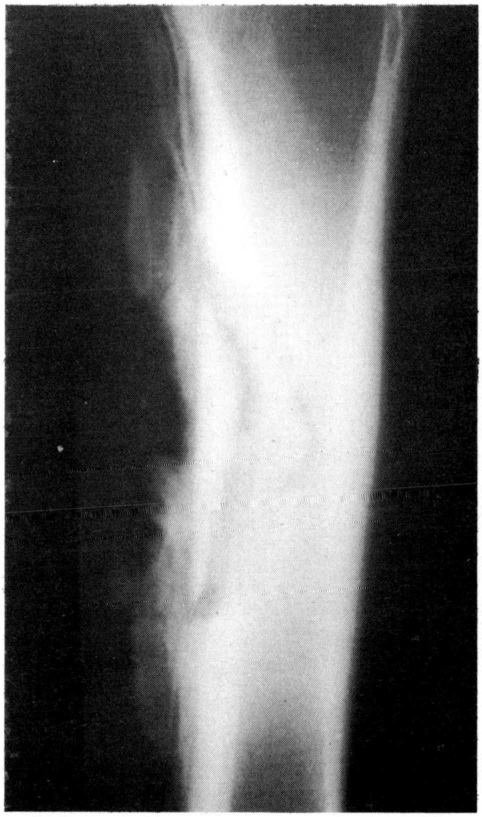

FIGS. 3.25 and 3.26. Lateral and antero-posterior projections of the metacarpal bone of a calf showing osteomyelitis and sequestrum formation.

FIG. 3.26.

Response to treatment will be shown by cessation of osteolysis and by the development of a more distinct appearance of bone outline and structure. With time there will be a gradual redevelopment of normal bone structure.

During the pathological or reparative process *bone sequestra* (Figs. 3.25 and 3.26) may become apparent. They are recognised as areas of bone, possibly with a slightly less distinct structure, which becomes separated from the adjoining bone by a zone of non-bony tissue and often also by an outer sclerotic band situated in the healthy bone. The fact that the sequestum is necrotic is demonstrated by the complete absence of any change in its structure in subsequent radiographs.

Hypertrophic Pulmonary Osteoarthropathy (Marie's Disease)

This condition is characterised by the widespread development of new bone along the shafts of most of the long bones. This new tissue arises immediately external to the cortex and remains completely distinct from it. Typically it has a palisade-like appearance with closely packed spicules of bone extending outwards at right angles to the long axis of the bone. The condition is encountered as a complication of

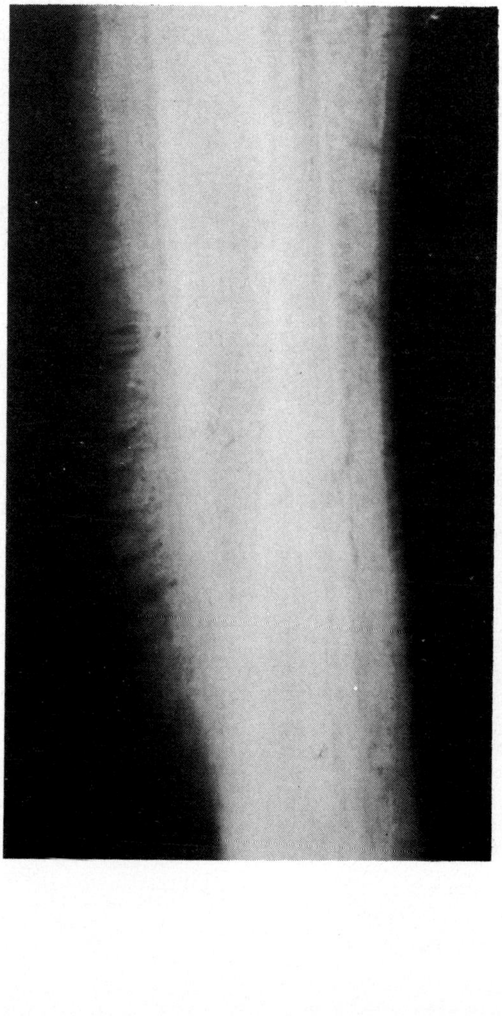

FIG. 3.27. Hypertrophic pulmonary osteoarthropathy.

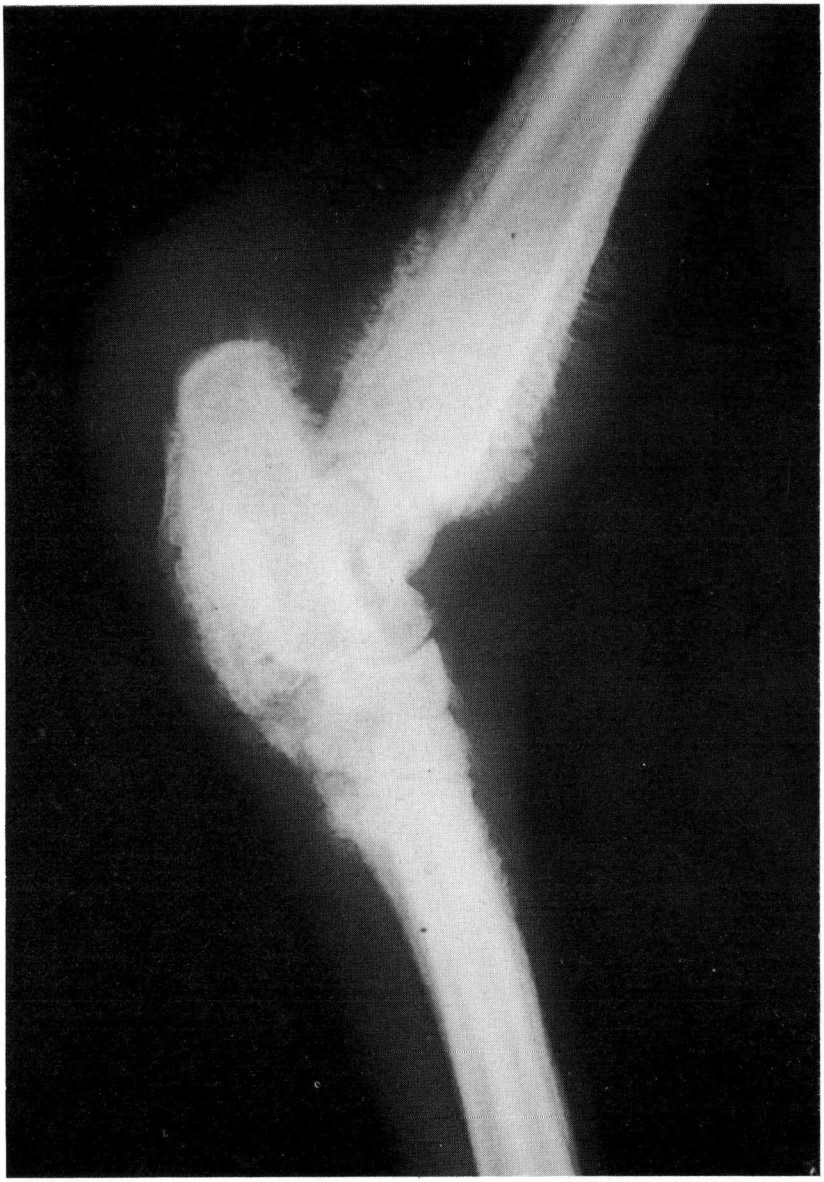

FIG. 3.28. Some regression of lesions of Marie's Disease following removal of a chest neoplasm.

chronic pulmonary disease (usually tuberculosis or neoplasia) and even if respiratory symptoms are not already apparent, radiographic examination of the chest should always be undertaken. Should it prove possible to correct the chest lesion (Rex, 1959) subsequent radiographs will demonstrate a "smoothing off" of the irregular edge of the new tissue and its gradual absorption. While the condition has been reported most frequently in the dog, it has been encountered in the lion (Nielsen and Bishop, 1953; Hall, 1957) and its likely association with tuberculosis should be borne in mind when dealing with circus or zoo animals.

Bone Conditions associated with Dietetic Deficiencies

Radiology can play an important part in the recognition of those deficiency diseases which are associated with bony changes.

The term "rickets" is used clinically for a variety of conditions affecting the bones of young dogs and associated with a number of symptoms such as lameness, pain, swelling around the joints, and various deformities. Many such cases are treated with mineral and vitamin supplements and, as the symptoms often improve with age, are not radiographed. When radiography is employed it may not be used until minor injuries have become aggravated into gross deformities, and by then the underlying osteodystrophy may be resolving spontaneously. There is now clinical, laboratory, and radiological evidence available that at least three (and possibly more) clinical entities, associated with dietetic and other causal factors, have to be considered under this heading.

If radiography is to be of real assistance in the investigation of such conditions it is important that it should be undertaken as soon as bone disease is suspected and that the films should be of high quality so that the degree of calcification and the detailed bone structure (particularly of the epiphysis) can be appreciated.

The clinical entities mentioned above will now be considered.

Rickets

While rickets is commonly diagnosed clinically in the large growing dog it is now rare for this to be confirmed radiologically. The cause of this misdiagnosis is the

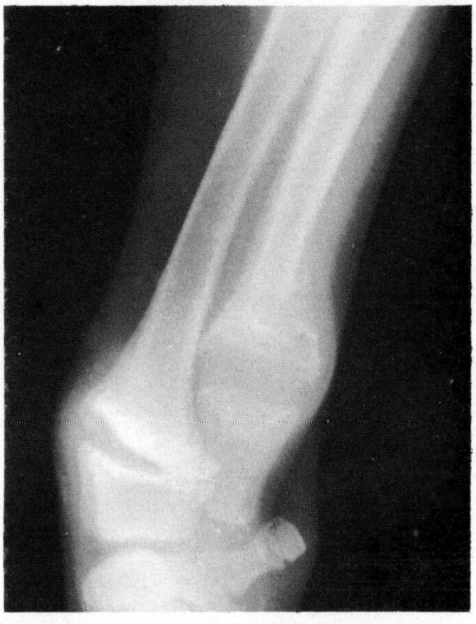

FIG. 3.29a. Marked widening of the ephiphyseal line associated with rickets in a 9 week old Setter.

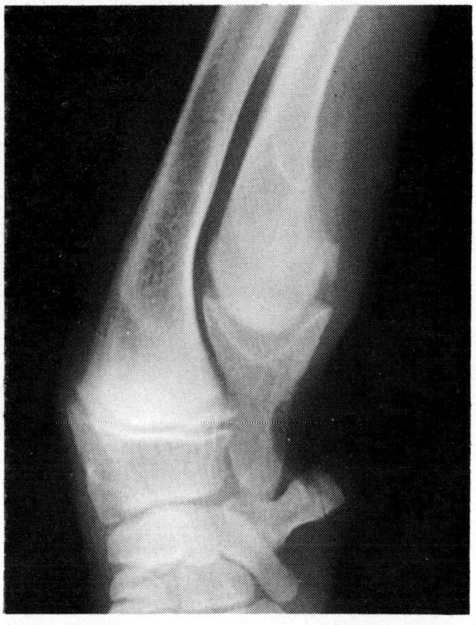

FIG. 3.29b. Considerable improvement shown 4 weeks later after correction of the diet.

fact that in the larger breeds of dog, during the period of maximum epiphyseal bone growth, the diameter of the epiphyseal and metaphyseal region of the long bones is considerably enlarged in relation to the diameter of the diaphysis. As growth ceases, remodelling of the region occurs and the relative enlargement subsides.

The radiological evidence of true rickets comprises:

(1) Gross widening of the non-calcified band comprising the epiphyseal line (this is the most characteristic feature).
(2) Widening of the epiphyseal and metaphyseal borders of the epiphyseal line with a poorly defined lipping of the latter edge.
(3) Poor calcification of the skeletal system in general with a tendency to bowing of the long bones.

Radiographs showing the characteristic features have been published by Campbell (1964) and Riser (1964).

Juvenile Osteoporosis

In addition to the above, a number of other titles—Nutritional Osteoporosis, Feline Osteodystrophy, Osteogenesis Imperfecta—have been used for what appears

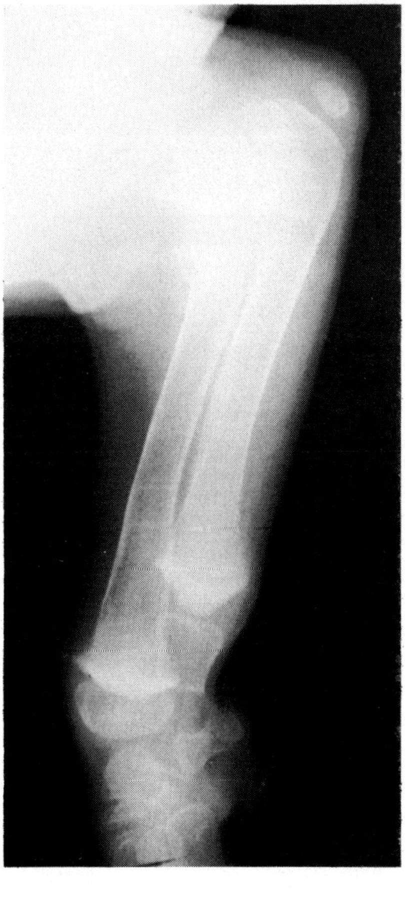

FIG. 3.30. Juvenile osteoporosis in an Alsatian puppy.

to be an identical condition occurring in both dogs and cats. The last title was used because the radiological appearances closely correspond with human Osteogenesis Imperfecta which is due to inherited causes. However, in animals there is evidence (Campbell, 1962; Riser, 1962; Jackson and Jackson, 1967) that it is associated with diets deficient in calcium and that this deficiency may be aggravated during the period of maximum growth or by administration of excessive amounts of vitamin D.

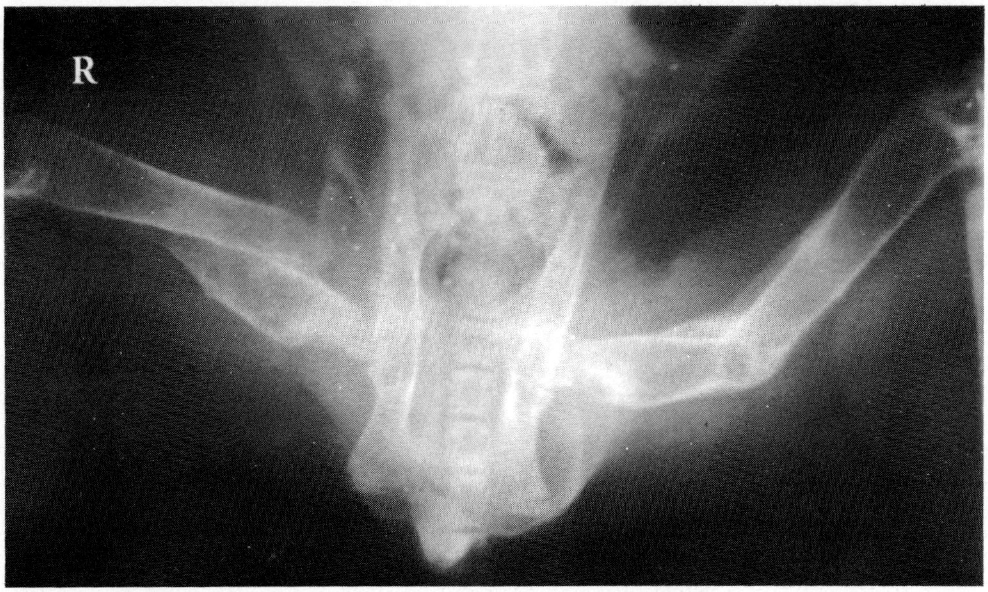

FIG. 3.31. Juvenile osteoporosis in a cat.

The typical radiological findings are:

(1) Marked osteoporosis of the entire skeletal system (where this condition is suspected the exposure factors should be considerably reduced or the bone will be overpenetrated and all detail lost.
(2) Loss of cancellous and cortical bone—the corteces becoming almost "paper thin".
(3) A zone of increased radio-density immediately on the metaphyseal side of the epiphyseal line.
(4) A tendency to spontaneous fractures occurring anywhere in the skeleton. These fractures may show compression of a vertebra, distortion of a long bone, or merely a sclerotic line indicating the site of a hair line fracture. A characteristic feature of the fractures is that there is seldom much separation of the fractured ends and the injury comprises a "buckling" of the bone.

This condition will often clear spontaneously, or as a result of administration of calcium, in the course of a month or two. Radiography at this stage may only show deformities or "stress marks" at the site of previous minor injuries.

Skeletal Scurvy

This term is used for a definite, but not very common, clinical entity reported by Meir, Clark, Schnelle and Will (1957) and others, and considered to result from a failure in Vitamin C utilisation. The typical radiological features are first noted in the epiphyseal region with the development of a line of increased density on the metaphyseal side of the epiphysis together with an adjacent line showing loss of density, thus producing the effect of a double epiphyseal line. This is followed by the appearance of irregular calcified areas around the shafts of the bones. These lesions, which are calcifying subperiosteal haematomata, may be small and barely perceptible or large and comparatively extensive. All these changes appear to be confined to the long bones.

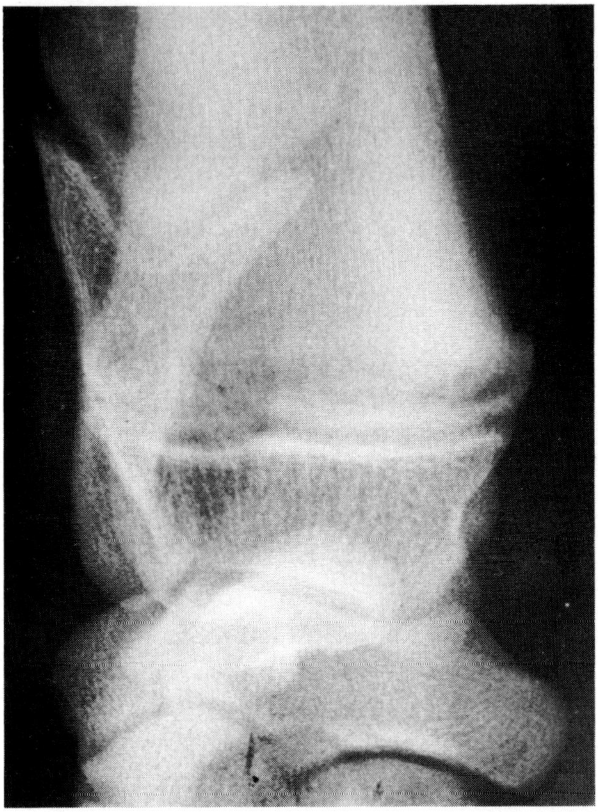

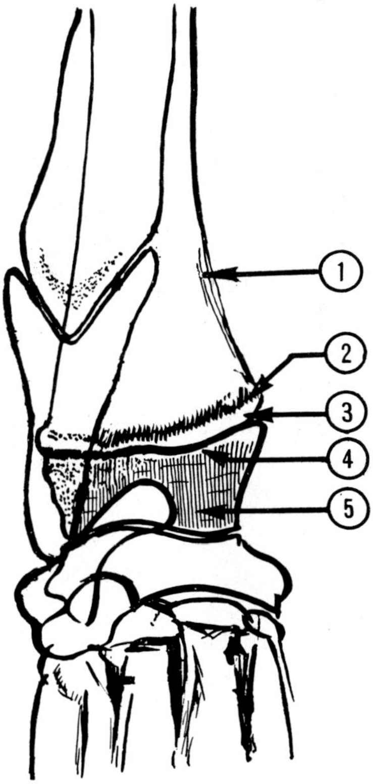

FIGS. 3.32 and 3.33. The essential features of skeletal scurvy. (1) Calcifying subperiosteal haematoma. (2) Radiotransparent band. (3) Area of increased density or scorbutic lattice. (4) Epiphyseal line. (5) Epiphysis.

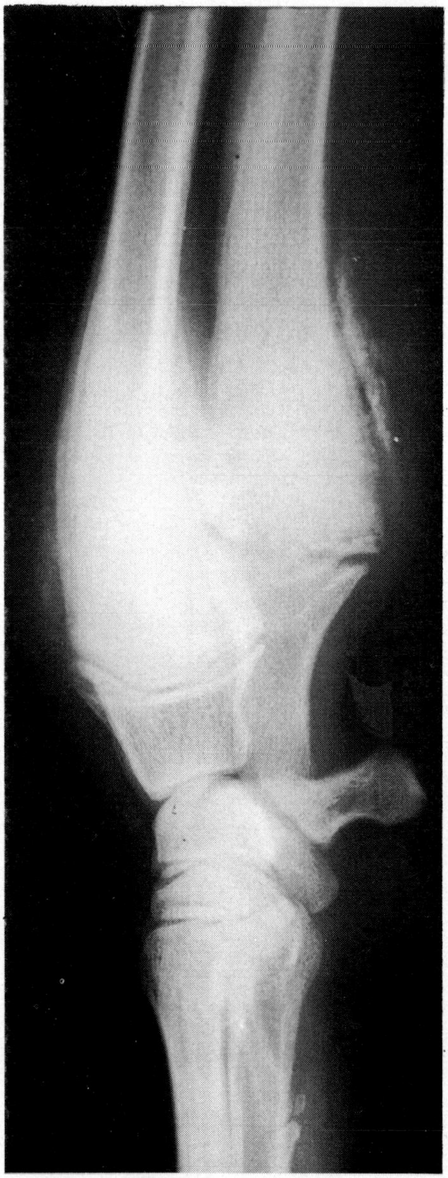

FIG. 3.34. An early case of skeletal scurvy.

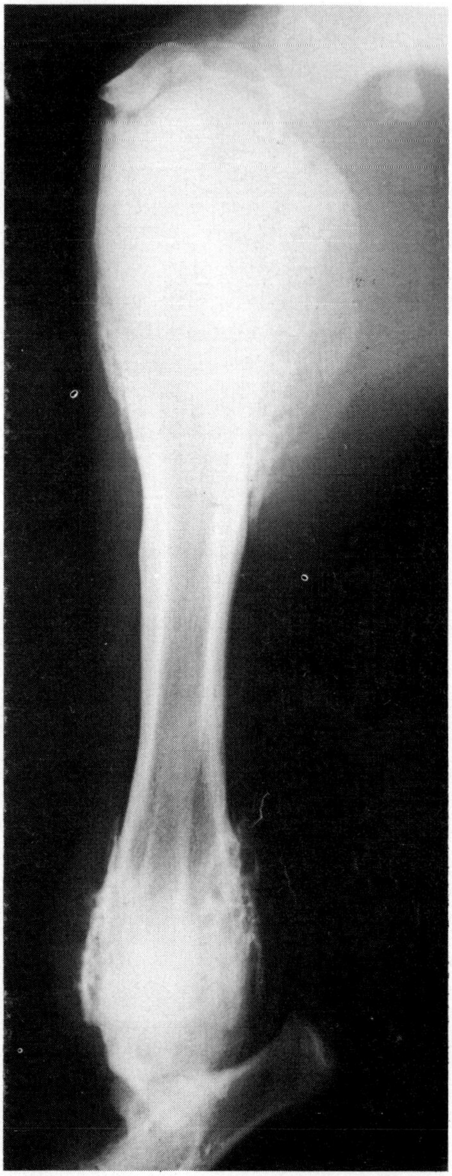

FIG. 3.35. An advanced case of skeletal scurvy showing some evidence of regression.

JOINTS

Radiography

One of the most important purposes in radiographing a joint is to demonstrate the joint space. The apparent size of this space can be easily altered if the X-ray beam is directed obliquely or if the bones comprising the joint are moved in relation to each other. It is therefore important to adopt precise and consistent positioning.

Contrast media techniques have been employed for the demonstration of the joint space but it is seldom that such methods will produce any more information than can be obtained from carefully produced plain radiographs.

When radiographing joints for suspected dislocations or subluxations it is important to remember that positioning may temporarily correct the displacement, and to take at least one film in such a way as to demonstrate the malalignment.

Radiology

The essential components of a joint, the articular cartilage, the ligaments and the joint capsule, cannot normally be identified in a radiograph. Usually, however, the position of the joint and of these structures can be estimated from an examination of the outline of the bones comprising the joint. In the young dog and cat such estimation will be hindered until calcification of the epiphyses is complete.

Radiologically the non-calcified area between the ends of the bones is usually referred to as the **joint space,** although it very largely consists of the articular cartilages, and the space is a potential one. Provided that positioning errors can be eliminated the apparent size of the normal joint space varies in different regions. Some joints show a comparatively wide space (e.g., the stifle joint) while elsewhere no definite space can be identified (e.g., the intercarpal joint). The most important feature is that the space should be of uniform width.

General Evidence of Pathology

(1) Alteration in the Joint Space

Widening Enlargement of the joint space occurs as the result of the introduction of infection and may be seen in septic arthritis.

Narrowing Injuries to a joint which are associated with erosion of the articular cartilage are likely to show thinning of the space.

Distortion An irregular width to a joint space is a feature of congenital malformations and of traumatic injuries to joint ligaments.

(2) Alteration in the Adjacent Bones

Malalignment The gross displacement of one bone in relation to another which occurs in dislocations is usually obvious but can be missed if only one projection is obtained (e.g., luxation of the elbow may not be clearly shown if only a lateral view is obtained). The slight displacement which occurs as a result of injuries to joint ligaments is more subtle and difficult to demonstrate (e.g., displacement of the femur on the tibia following rupture of the cruciate ligaments, lateral angulation of the phalanges as a result of tearing of the medial collateral ligaments). Where this latter type of injury is suspected positioning should be directed towards emphasising the displacement rather than correcting it.

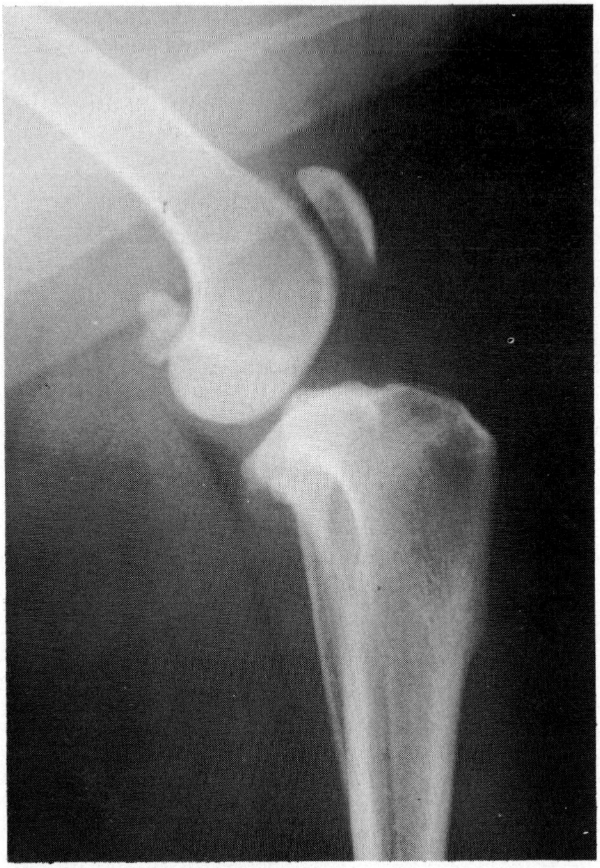

FIG. 3.36. Malalignment of the femur on the tibia, associated with rupture of the cruciate ligaments.

Malformation Deformities of the bones comprising a joint can occur if the articular surfaces are subjected to abnormal stress or wear during the period of bone growth. This may arise from injuries or congenital abnormalities. The term "Dysplasia" is usually reserved for specific congenital malformations of particular joints (e.g., the hip, elbow and shoulder joints).

(3) Localised Changes

Osteoporosis Small areas of bone absorption on the articular surface usually indicate extension of inflammatory processes through the cartilage into the underlying bone. Similar areas around the joint may show the site of damage to ligamentous insertions into the bone.

Sclerosis Areas of increased bone density may be seen in association with the osteoporotic lesions mentioned above and represent the inflammatory response of the bone tissue to such injuries.

Osteophyte Formation The development of small spurs of new bone is a common accompaniment of chronic inflammatory conditions of joints in animals.

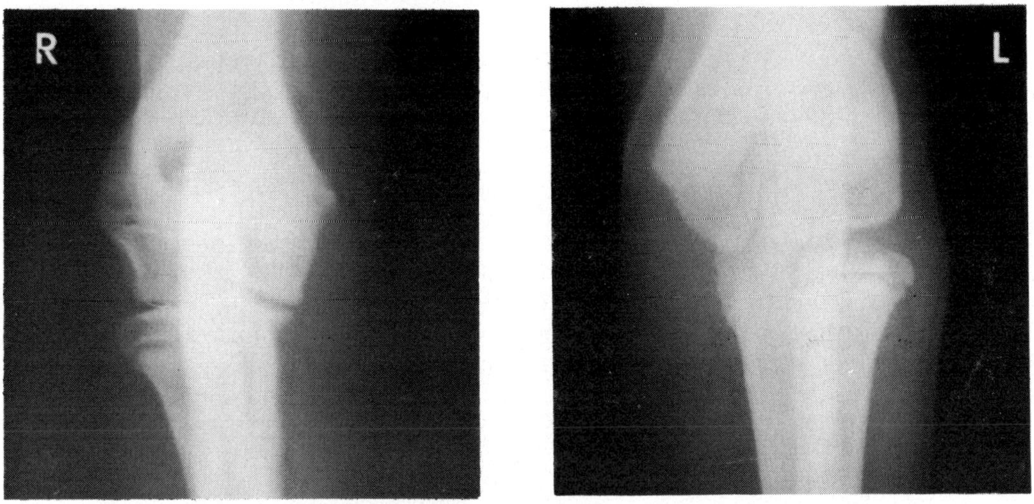

FIGS. 3.37 and 3.38. Malformation of the articular surfaces of the left humerus and radius consequent upon a congenital subluxation of the joint. The unaffected opposite joint is shown for comparison.

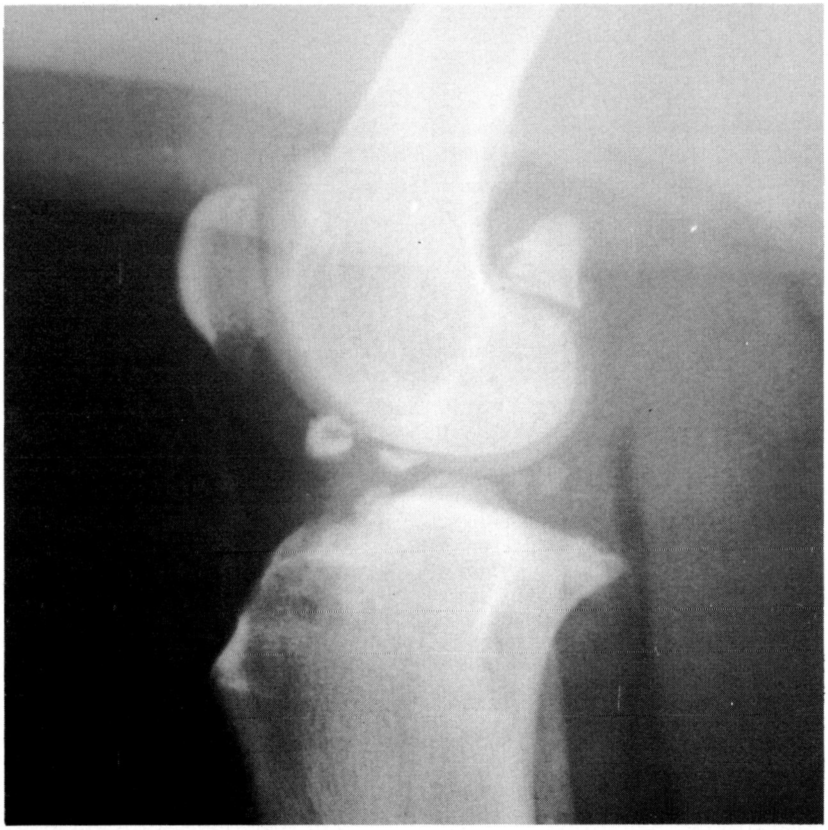

FIG. 3.39. An example of "joint mice" associated with severe osteoarthritis of the stifle joint.

"Joint Mice" This term is used for small fragments of bone found free within the joint space. They are not often encountered and indicate destructive involvement of the bone beneath the cartilage (Fig.3.39).

Specific Conditions

Osteoarthritis

This is the common form of arthritis encountered in animals and is considered to be due to chronic trauma, with destructive injuries to the articular and underlying bone and compensatory fibrosis and bone formation around the joint. It is important to remember that the early changes are confined to the soft tissues and that the

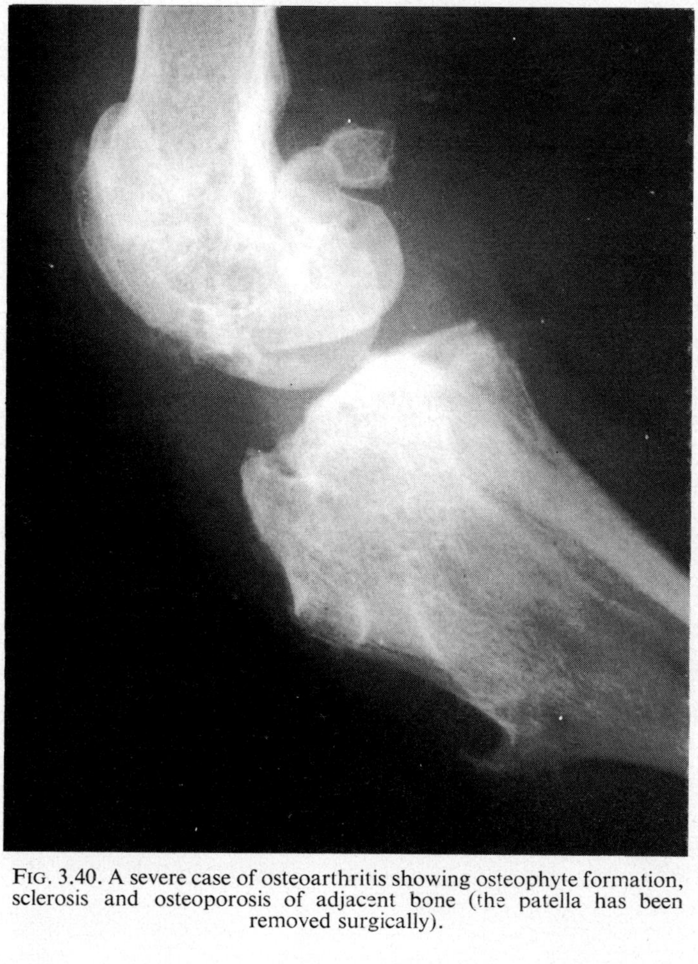

FIG. 3.40. A severe case of osteoarthritis showing osteophyte formation, sclerosis and osteoporosis of adjacent bone (the patella has been removed surgically).

condition has usually been in existence for a long period before radiological changes can be demonstrated. The usual and most typical of these changes is the development of osteophytes around the edge of the joint surface, but narrowing of the joint space and the occurrence of sclerotic and, less frequently, osteoporotic areas under the articular surface may be encountered.

Septic Arthritis

This is not a common condition and is seen more frequently in farm animals than in dogs and cats. When pus accumulates within the joint cavity radiography may demonstrate enlargement and increased density of the joint space. The more typical feature is evidence of osteomyelitis in the epiphysis of one or more of the bones forming the joint, and rapid extension of this process across the joint to involve any unaffected bones.

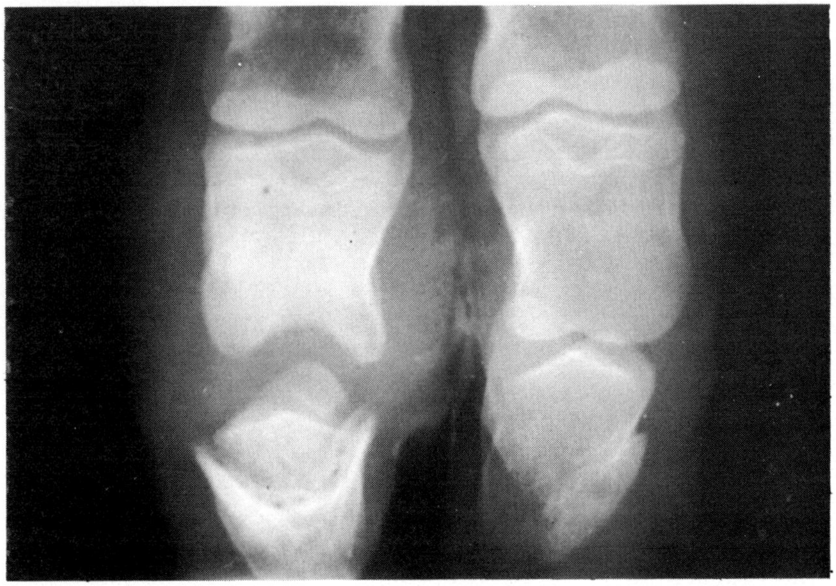

FIG. 3.41. Marked enlargement of an interdigital joint space associated with septic arthritis in a calf.

Osteochondritis Dissecans

This condition which is recognised in human radiology has been reported in the dog affecting the femur (Carlson, 1961) and the humerus (Craig and Riser, 1965; Vaughan and Jones, 1968). It is seen in joints showing no other evidence of osteochondritis, as a small localised area of osteoporosis extending into the subchondral bone. There may be a small bone sequestrum in the centre of the lesion or loose in the joint space as a "joint mouse". The affected part of the bone is often surrounded by a narrow band of sclerosis.

REFERENCES

Campbell, J. R. (1962), Vet. Rec., **74**, 1340.
Campbell, J. R. (1964), J. small Anim. Pract., **5**, 229.
Carlson, W. D. (1961), Veterinary Radiology, Philadelphia: Lea and Febiger.

Craig, P. H., and Riser, W. H. (1965), J. Am. vet. Radiol. Soc., **6**, 40.
Hall, L. W. (1957), personal communication.
Jackson, O. F., and Jackson, E. K. M. (1967) J. small Anim. Pract., **8**, 3.
Meier, H., Clark, S. T., Schnelle, G. B., and Will, D. H. (1957), J. Am. vet. med. Ass., **130**, 483.
Nielsen, S. W., and Bishop, E. J. (1953), N. Am. Vet., **34**, 867.
Rex, M. A. E. (1959), Vet. Rec., **71**, 409.
Riser, W. H. (1962), J. Am vet. Radiol. Soc., **3**, 50.
Riser, W. H. (1964), J. Am. vet. Radiol. Soc., **5**, 15.
Sumner-Smith, G. (1966), J. small Anim. Pract., **7**, 303.
Vaughan, L. G., and Jones, D. G. C. (1968), J. small Anim. Pract., **9**, 283.

The following articles, concerned with various aspects of bone neoplasia, are suggested for additional reading.

A Clinical and Radiological Study of Canine Bone Neoplasms. Brodey, R. S., McGrath, J. T., and Reynolds, H. (1959), J. Am. vet. med. Ass., **134**, 53.
Metastatic Bone Neoplasms in the Dog. Brodey, R. S., Reid, C. F., and Sauer, R. M. (1966), J. Am. vet. med. Ass., **148**, 29.
Observations on Canine Osteosarcoma. Owen, L. N. (1961), Res. vet. Sci., **2**, 117.
Differential Diagnosis of Bone Tumours in the Dog. Owen, L. N. (1962), Vet. Rec., **74**, 439.
Multiple Osteosarcoma having Multicentric or Metastatic Origin. Owen, L. N. (1965), Br. J. Radiol., **38**, 520.

The following work is recommended as a reference book for normal radiological anatomy.

Schebitz, H., and Wilkens, H. (1968), Atlas of Radiographic Anatomy of Dog and Horse, Berlin, Paul Parey.

CHAPTER 4

THE SKULL

Radiography

The skull is the most difficult portion of the skeletal system to examine radiologically. There are a number of factors which complicate its investigation:

(a) The marked variation in the shape of the skull between different breeds of dog.

(b) The difficulty of immobilising and accurately positioning this region in the conscious patient.

(c) The superimposition which occurs in radiographs taken in either the dorso-ventral (or ventro-dorsal) or lateral projections.

(d) The fact that the skull is a complex structure containing a number of parts (teeth, nasal passages, cranial cavity, etc.) any of which can require detailed investigation.

Therefore, if the maximum information is to be obtained from skull radiographs, it is important that considerable care and thought should be given to the radiographic technique. In many instances this will necessitate anaesthetisation of the patient so that the skull may be positioned accurately and, where necessary, intra-oral radiographs may be obtained.

The requirements of a good radiograph with regard to both positioning and exposure factors will vary with the part being examined.

Radiology

The radiologist must be familiar with the appearance of the skull as a whole (and with breed variations) in the usual projections. However, it would obviously be impracticable to illustrate all the variations of position, breed or species; and while a number of illustrations of the radiological anatomy of this region have been published, the veterinary radiologist would be well advised to produce his own reference films from a carcase or skull.

In attempting to give a detailed description of the skull it is proposed to consider the component parts separately and to describe the normal and pathological appearance of each, rather than to attempt the confusing problem of dealing with them collectively.

The whole of the bones of the skull are ossified at birth, although not united with each other, and should be demonstrable in a radiograph. At the same time it must be remembered that most of the bony structure of the skull in a young puppy is extremely thin, and it will be difficult to obtain good detail and contrast in a film.

THE LOWER JAW

The Horizontal Ramus The general outline of this region can be recognised in precisely placed dorso-ventral and lateral views and gross changes in contour will be noted. However, superimposition will frequently mask less obvious lesions (osteomyelitis around teeth, fractures with little or no displacement, etc.). The general shape of each ramus will vary from the long narrow outline of the dolicocephalic breeds to the relatively thick curved contour of the brachycephalic types.

Ventro-dorsal projections, with the film placed in the mouth, will obviate overlapping but the plate can seldom be placed further back than the fourth premolar region. This view demonstrates the fact that there is no bony union between the rami at the symphysis—a feature which can lead to confusion when investigating suspected fractures at this site.

Oblique views provide another method of partly overcoming the problem of superimposition. When using this technique particular care must be taken in labelling the radiographs, so that the right and left rami may be differentiated.

The Vertical Ramus The coronoid process, being thin and also overlying the skull, may be barely perceptible in lateral views. Dorso-ventral views will show this region "end on" as an apparent thickening on the outer aspect of the horizontal ramus.

The Articulation The position of this joint is indicated by recognition of the comparatively dense condyle.

However, in accurately placed lateral views the two joints will overlap, while in dorso-ventral views they are obscured by the posterior region of the zygomatic arch. This region is best demonstrated by 45° oblique views. Each of these films will show what is, in effect, a lateral projection of the joint placed lowermost and a dorso-ventral projection of the upper joint.

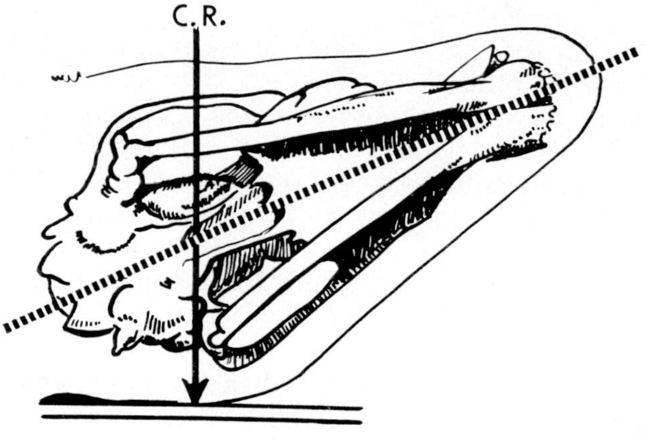

FIG. 4.1. Positioning of the anaesthetised dog to permit demonstration of the tempero-mandibular joint.

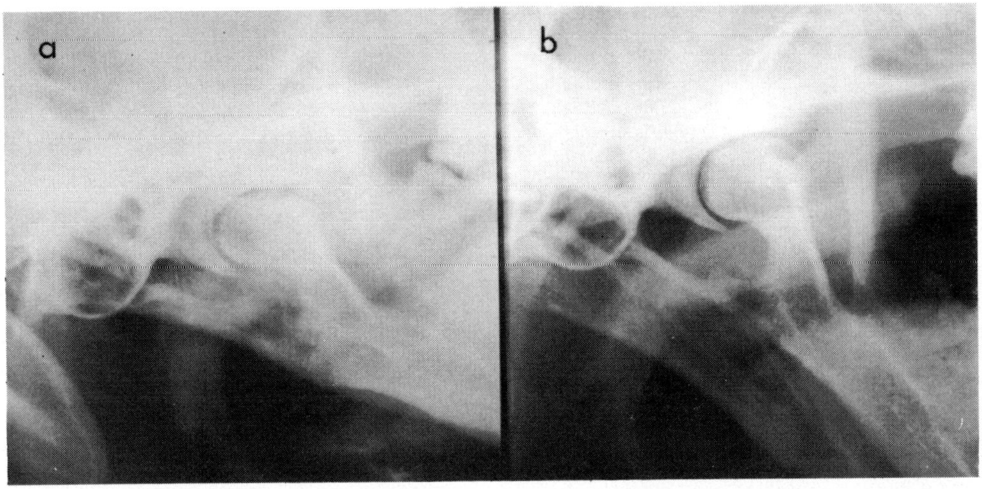

FIG. 4.2. Radiographs showing demonstration of the joint in the normal animal by the technique illustrated above. (a) with the mouth closed. (b) with the mouth open.

Another method of demonstrating these joints, which is only practicable in the anaesthetized animal, is to position the dog in lateral recumbency and then to bend the head sideways (upwards from the horizontal) until the upper joint no longer overlies the lower one (the exact angle necessary will vary with the shape of the skull). The central ray is directed vertically through the lower mandibular condyle and two films are taken (with the mouth closed and fully open) and, if necessary, repeated after turning the dog over.

Pathological Conditions

Fractures While fractures with marked displacement should be easily demonstrated, less obvious injuries which are obscured by overlapping bone can easily be missed. The radiologist must endeavour to identify and examine the entire contour of the mandible before he can definitely eliminate the presence of any fracture.

Dislocation of the Tempero-Mandibular Joint While evidence of displacement of a ramus in relation to the rest of the skull may provide an indication of this lesion, a clear reproduction of both joints in both planes is usually necessary for diagnosis. This will necessitate precise positioning and immobilization.

Neoplasia Comparatively benign tumours (epuli, etc.) of the gum are of comparatively common occurrence and may involve adjacent bone. This will be shown in radiographs as localised areas of bone absorption or, more frequently, new bone formation.

This is not a common situation for malignant bone neoplasms but they may be encountered.

Osteomyelitis Small lesions around infected teeth are common and will be described subsequently. More extensive spread may occur, and the general appearance of this condition has already been considered (page 41).

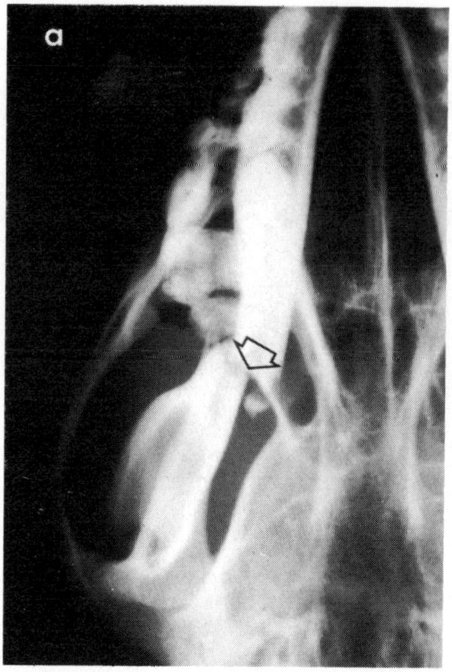

FIG. 4.3. Fracture of the horizontal ramus.

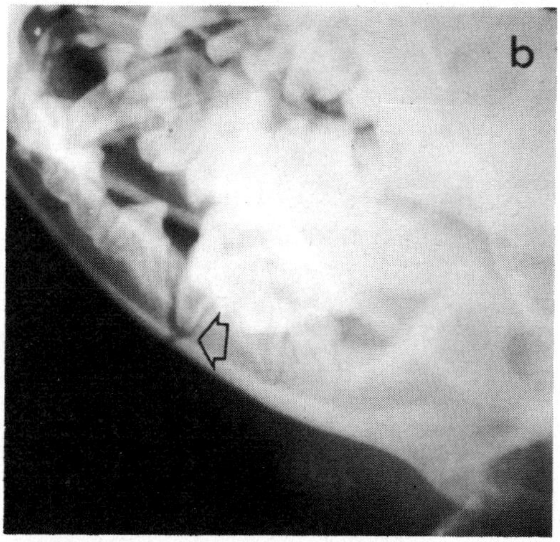

FIG. 4.4. Pathological fracture through an infected tooth socket.

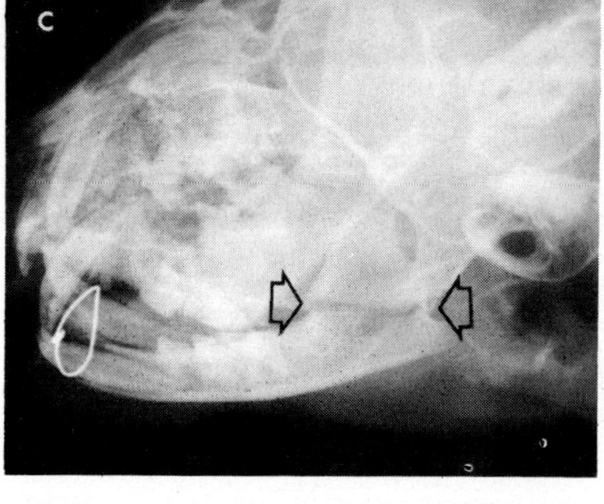

FIG. 4.5. Fracture of the vertical ramus in a cat.

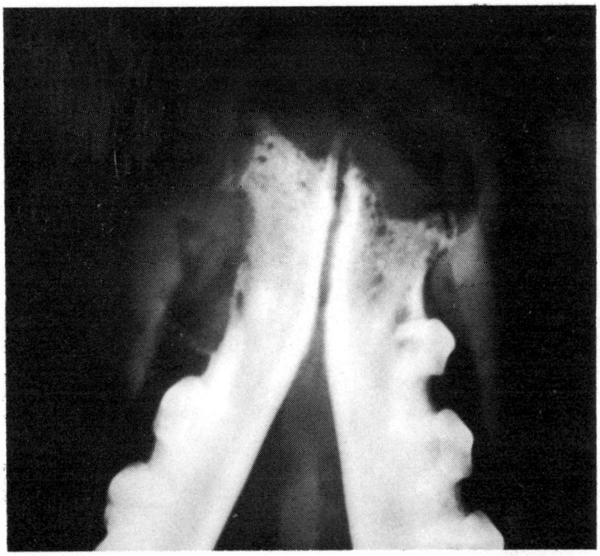

FIG. 4.6. Invasion of the bone of the lower jaw by a malignant neoplasm (melanoma).

Bone Cysts Cysts, while not common, do occur in this region and may contain a tooth which has failed to erupt. Radiologically these lesions are recognised as a particularly well defined translucent area within bone, which usually contains a

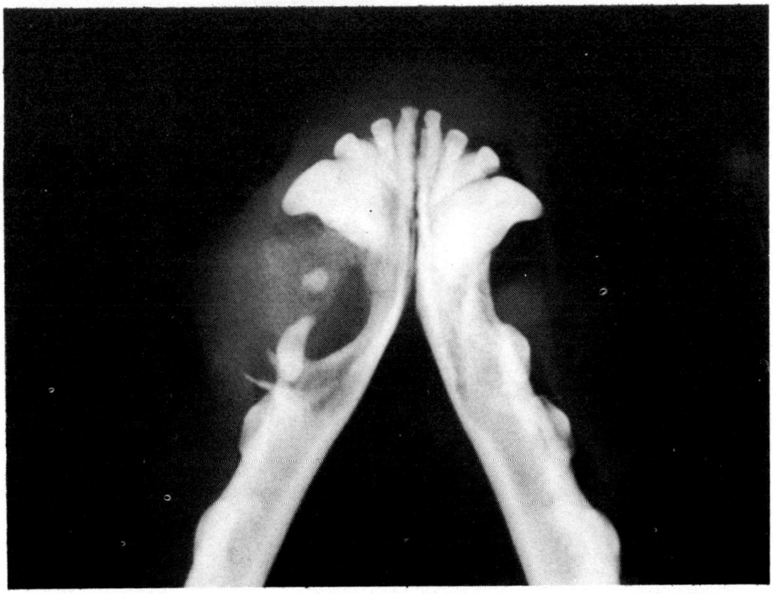

FIG. 4.7. Bone cyst containing a partly developed tooth.

toothlike structure. The surrounding bone is likely to show some increased density and, if thin, may be distorted by pressure from the cyst.

Renal Rickets (Rubber Jaw, Renal Osteodystrophy) While not necessarily confined to the lower jaw, the condition is first seen there and it affects this area more severely than the rest of the skull. The first radiographic evidence of this condition is likely to be a generalised increase in the width of the alveolar membrane of all the teeth. As the condition progresses the more obvious changes of decalcification and

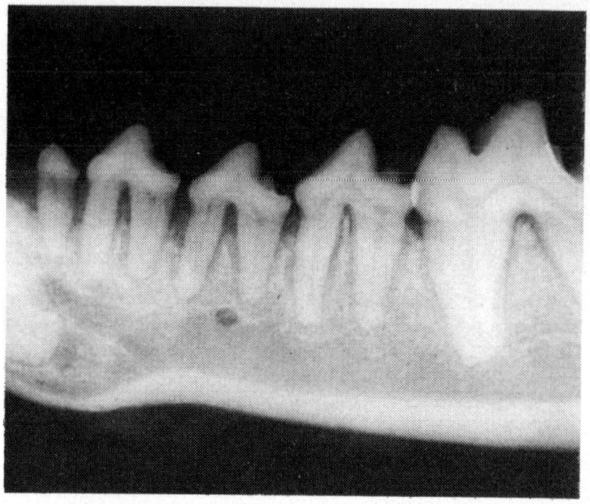

FIG. 4.8. Increased width of the alveolar membrane in an early case of renal rickets.

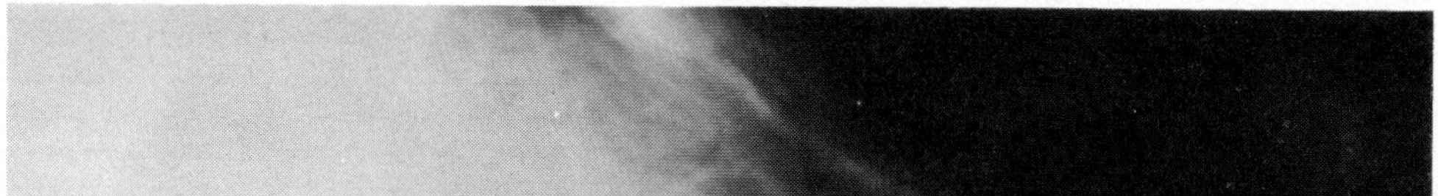

FIG. 4.9. Extensive decalcification associated with renal rickets.

loss of density become apparent but there is little appreciable change in the shape or structure of the bone. If normal exposure factors are employed the teeth show up in marked contrast to the barely perceptible bone substance.

Cranio-Mandibular Osteoarthropathy This condition, which is of unknown etiology, occurs most frequently in West Highland White Terriers (occasionally in

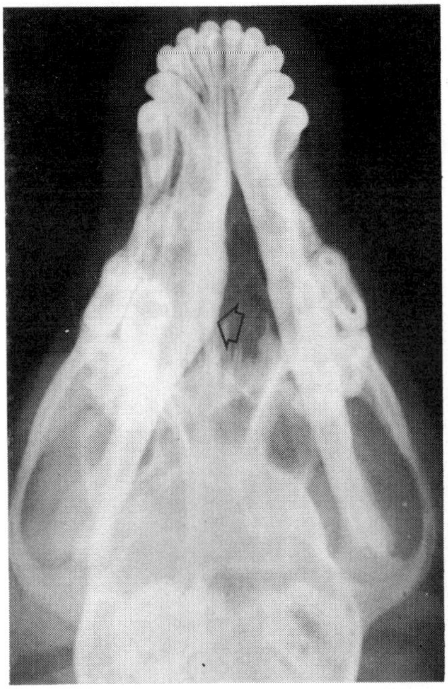

FIG. 4.10. Cranio-mandibular osteoarthropathy. Thickening of the lower jaw of a 6 month old West Highland White Terrier.

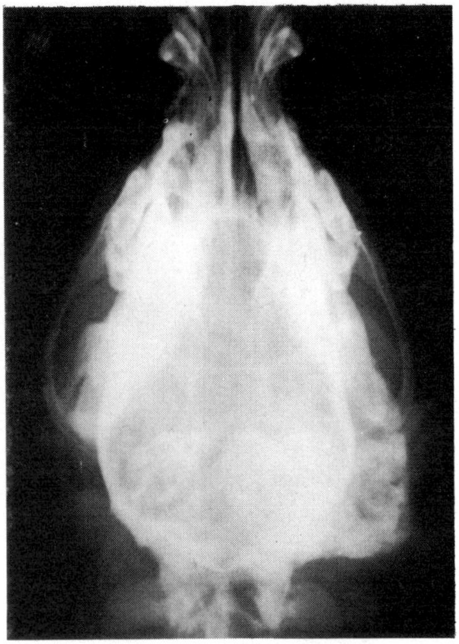

FIG. 4.11.

FIG. 4.12.

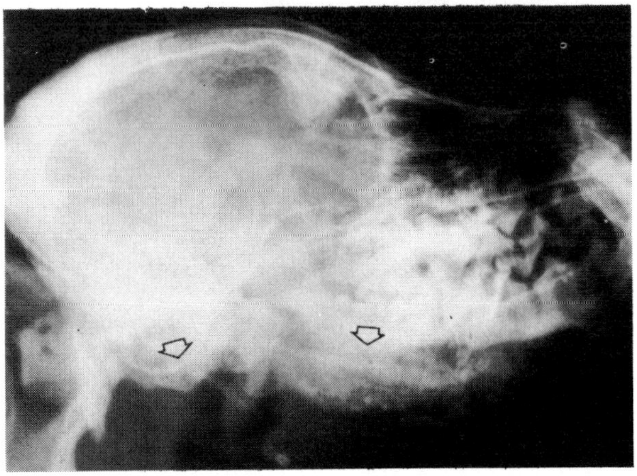

FIGS. 4.11 and 4.12. An advanced case of cranio-mandibular osteoarthropathy affecting a 6 month old West Highland White Terrier.

Cairn Terriers). Littlewort (1958) drew attention to the abnormality and has suggested the above descriptive designation. The radiological changes commence in the petrous temporal and occipital bones but usually spread to the lower jaw, and consist of an irregular laying down of new bone around the angle of the jaw and extending along the horizontal ramus. In most instances both rami are affected.

THE UPPER JAW

If the upper jaw is considered to consist solely of the premaxilla and maxilla most of the comments on the lower jaw can be applied to this region.

THE NASAL PASSAGES

The nasal passages are outlined by the air which they contain and will be visualised in accurately positioned dorso-ventral views. However, if there is any obliquity in positioning, the mandibles will obscure the region and, for a full examination of

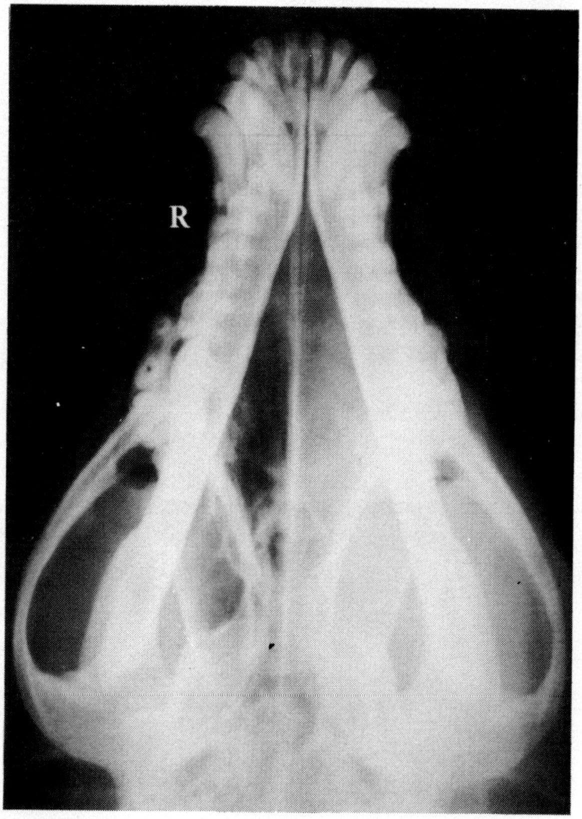

FIG. 4.13. Opacity of the left nasal chamber due to the presence of chronic infection.

the area, ventro-dorsal projections through the mouth of the anaesthetised patient are necessary. Care must be taken not to over-expose, or the typical fine bony structure of the region will be lost.

Evidence of Pathology

The main reason for radiographing this area is in the investigation of chronic nasal discharge, which may be associated with foreign bodies, infection or neoplasia. Foreign bodies will be obvious if they are radio-opaque but grass seeds, thorns or splinters of wood are unlikely to be demonstrated.

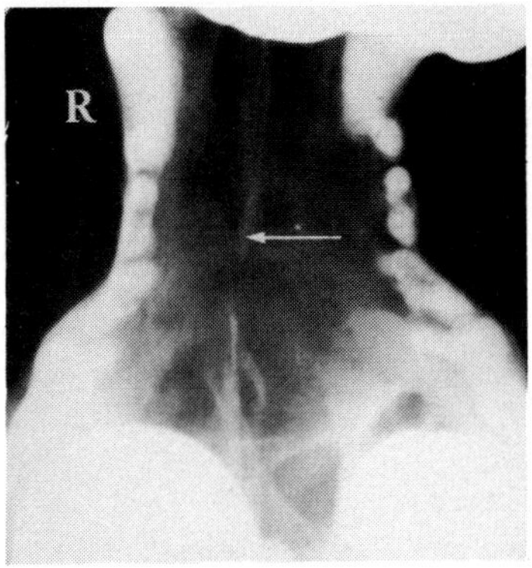

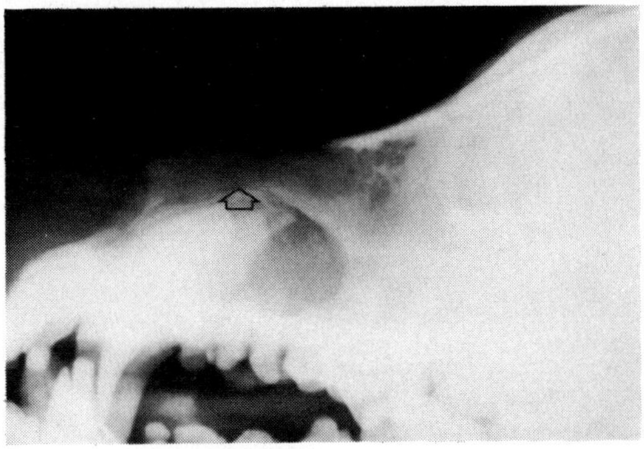

FIGS. 4.14 and 4.15. Malignant neoplasm producing erosion of the nasal bone and of the nasal septum.

In all instances of nasal discharge, radiography is likely to reveal increased density of the affected nasal chamber, and in the unilateral case it will be helpful to compare the structure of the normal aerated side with the increased density and loss of detail on the affected side. If only soft tissues are involved, it will not be possible on purely radiological grounds to differentiate between nasal catarrh and neoplasia. However, in most instances neoplasia in this region arises in bone and shows a typical appearance, with loss of the fine bony structure of the region and its replacement by a homogenous mass—the whole process spreading through the nasal septum and into adjacent denser bone. In contrast, chronic infections of the nasal passages will show increased soft tissue density but are less likely to involve bone (although this may occur in old-standing cases) but changes will often extend into the frontal sinuses.

THE FRONTAL SINUS

The frontal sinus is similarly outlined by the air which it contains and is most clearly visualised in a lateral view. Dorso-ventral or ventro-dorsal views will separate the two frontal sinuses and permit their individual examination but they will be superimposed on the posterior region of the nasal chambers and unless special angulation of the tube is employed, the lateral extension of the sinus will be obscured by the body of the mandible.

Pathology

The chronic nasal infections and neoplastic conditions already considered may spread into the frontal sinuses. This spread would be shown by the substitution of a diffuse opacity for the normal air-filled appearance.

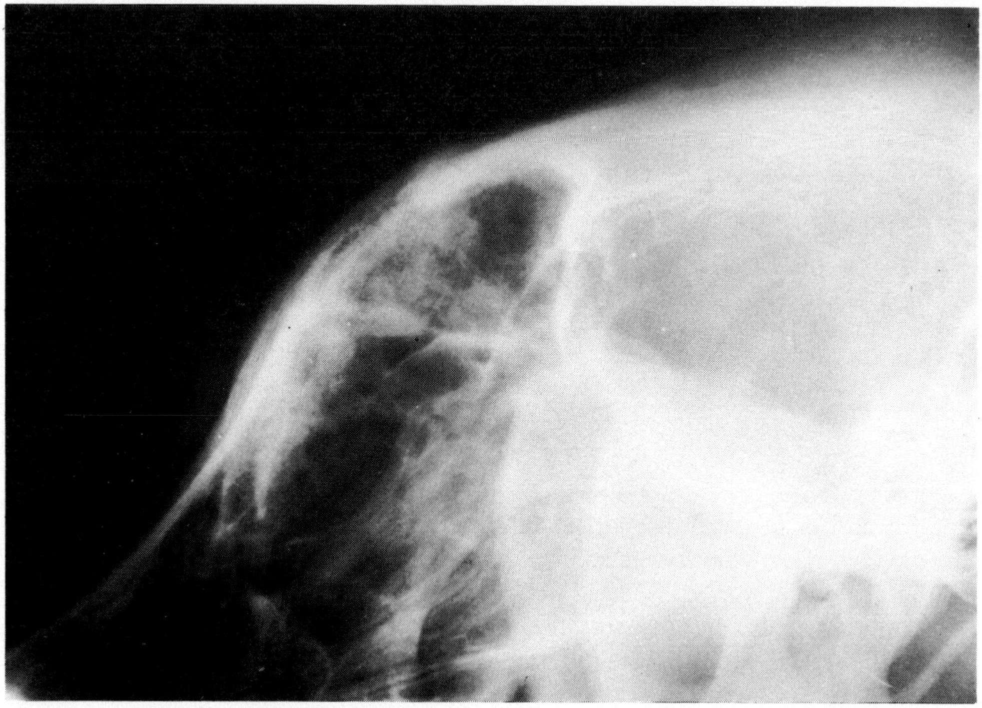

FIG. 4.16. Opacity of the frontal sinus due to invasion by malignant neoplasia.

THE TEETH

Radiography has only been employed to a limited extent in the examination of the teeth of animals. It is also true that caries is not of common occurrence in animals and can usually be recognised on a detailed examination of the teeth. However, radiography can reveal unsuspected alveolar infection in non-carious teeth and, when dealing with some chronic mouth infections, radiography may be the only accurate method of distinguishing between infected and sound teeth.

In a radiograph of a normal tooth it should be possible to recognise the following structures (Fig. 4.18):

(1) A narrow, almost linear, pulp cavity.
(2) The dentine, surrounding the pulp cavity and forming the largest part of the tooth substance.

(3) The alveolar membrane, which is seen as a narrow non-opaque band immediately surrounding the dentine (this area is barely perceptible in the normal tooth and any localised increase in the amount of non-calcified tissue suggests the presence of infection).
(4) A thin plate of dense bone, which outlines the alveolus and merges into adjacent bone.

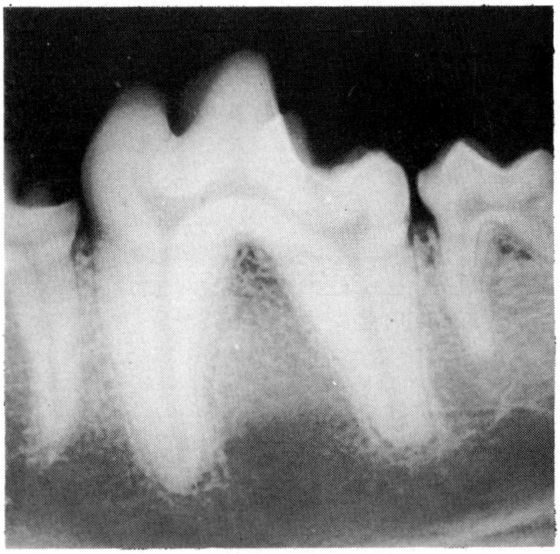

FIG. 4.17.

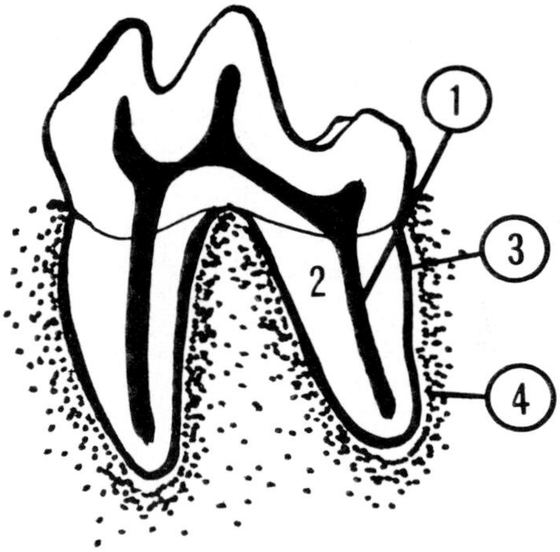

FIG. 4.18.

The presence of infection involving a tooth will be indicated by areas of rarifaction. This usually commences at the base of the pulp cavity, extends into the region of the alveolar membrane and then into surrounding bone. In old standing cases there may be evidence of extensive osteomyelitis around the area.

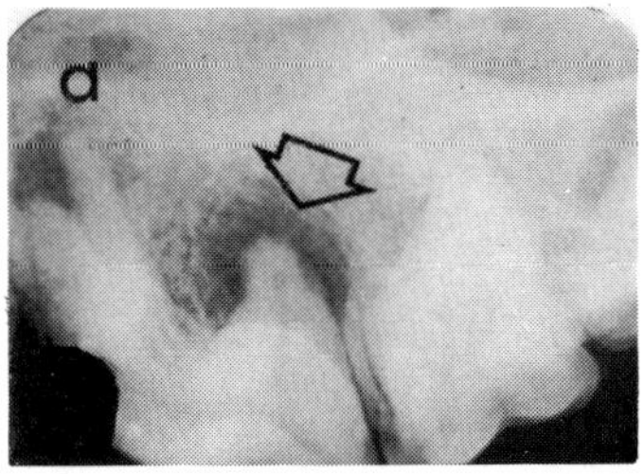

FIG. 4.19. Abscess around the root of the first upper molar tooth.

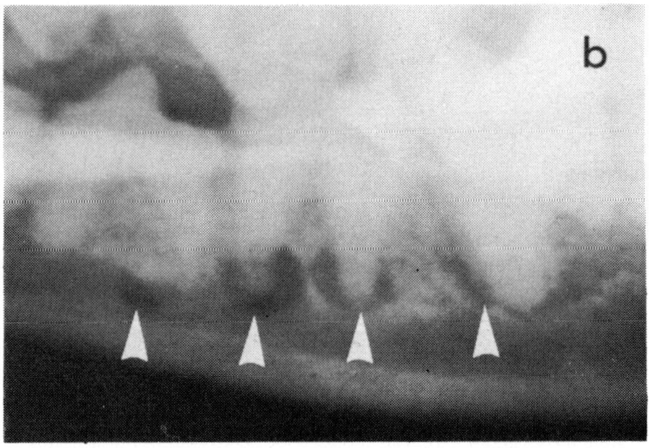

FIG. 4.20. Evidence of infection involving several molar roots in the lower jaw.

Radiography may also be employed to locate tooth roots left in situation after previous extractions.

THE CRANIUM

See Chapter 14 (The Nervous System).

THE AUDITORY APPARATUS

The External Ear is shown most clearly in underexposed skull films and may be barely perceptible when normal exposure factors are used. The column of air in the canal acts as a contrast agent and helps to visualise the vertical and horizontal canals and the external auditory meatus.

Chronic inflammatory conditions will result in increased opacity of the external ear and in particularly neglected cases radiography may demonstrate new bone formation extending out from the external auditory meatus and around the horizontal canal. This radiological evidence of the extent and severity of the inflammatory changes can be of assistance in formulating a prognosis.

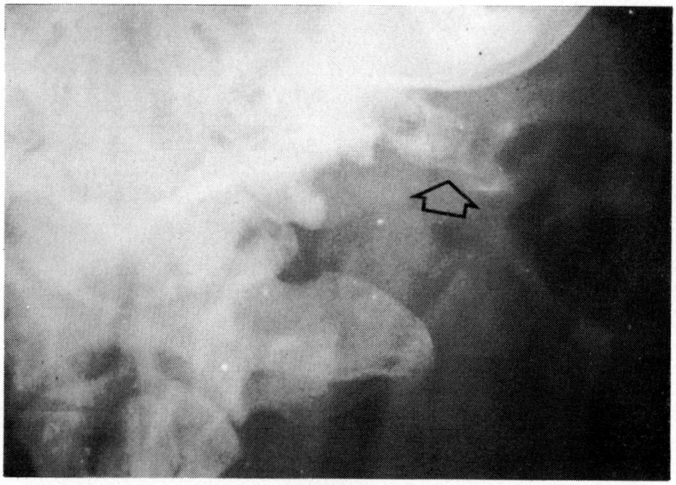

FIG. 4.21. Calcification of the external ear associated with chronic otitis.

The Middle Ear and Tympanic Bulla are also outlined by the air which they contain. Since any pathological changes in this region will be small and not easily perceived, it is helpful to compare films taken in the three skull projections which may be employed to examine this area. These are:

(a) ventro-dorsal,
(b) latero-oblique,
(c) antero-posterior (as described by Barone and Guelfi, 1966).

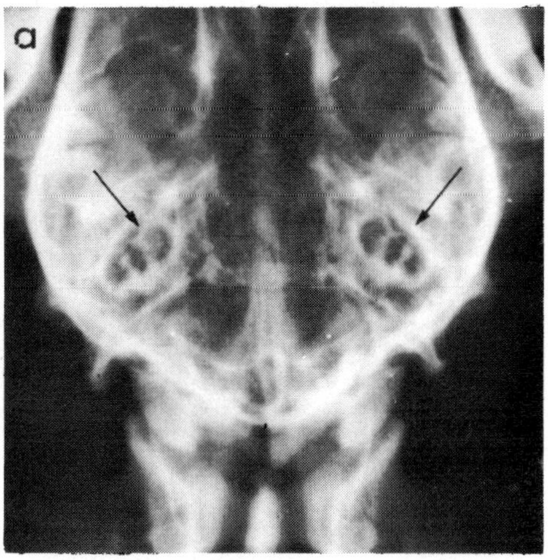

FIG. 4.22.

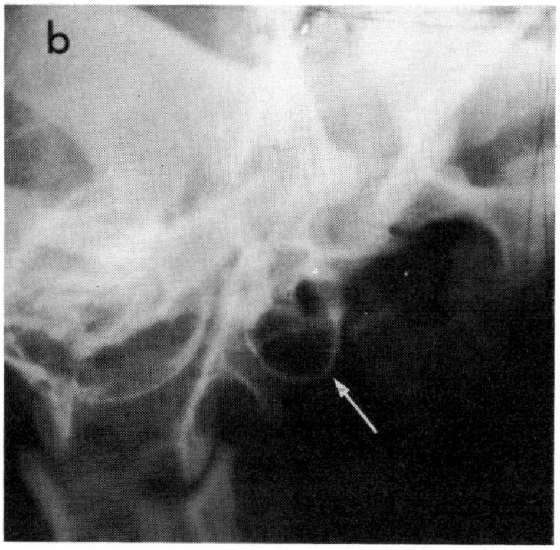

FIG. 4.23.

FIGS. 4.22 to 4.24. Visualisation of the normal tympanic bulla by each of the projections mentioned above.

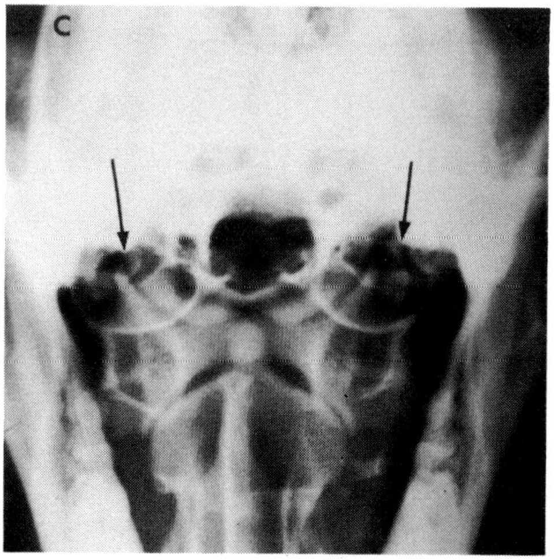

FIG. 4.24.

THE ORBIT

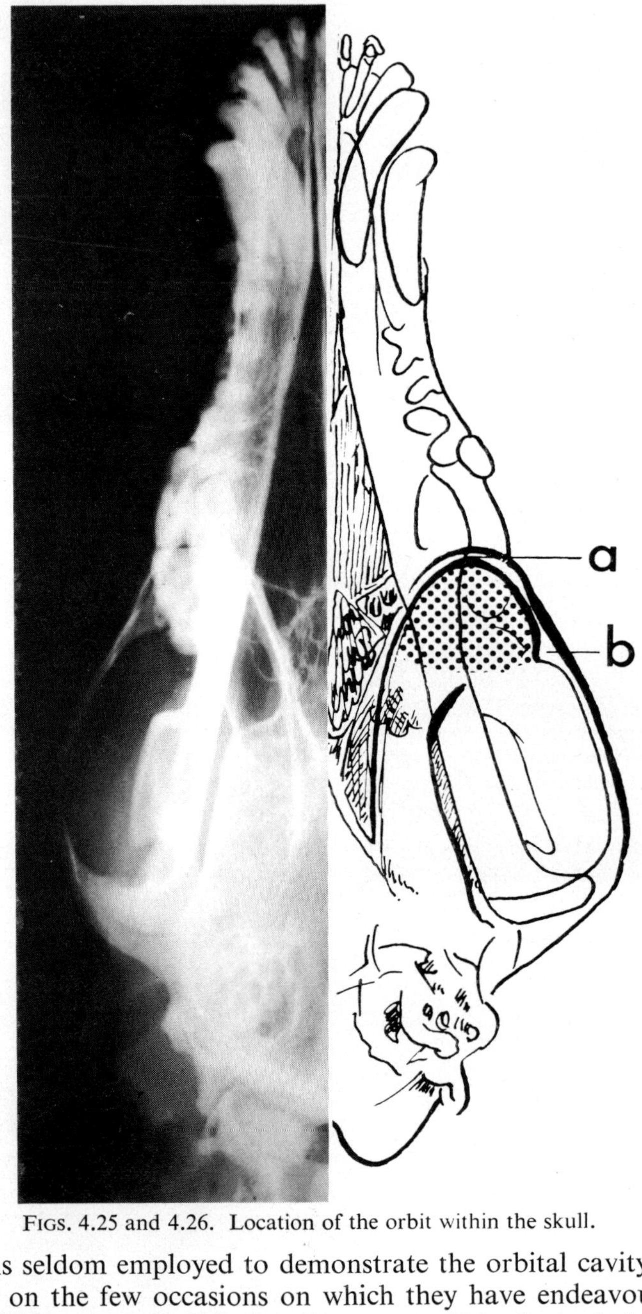

Figs. 4.25 and 4.26. Location of the orbit within the skull.

Radiography is seldom employed to demonstrate the orbital cavity. The authors have found that on the few occasions on which they have endeavoured to do this (e.g., when attempting to show if lead pellets were within the eye) they have experienced difficulty in locating the exact position and extent of the orbital cavity in a radiograph of the skull. From the examination of a limited number of radiographs, it would appear that in dorso-ventral projections the anterior edge of the eyeball corresponds roughly with the arch formed by the orbital part of the frontal bone, the lachrymal bone and the malar portion of the zygomatic arch (a), and that the posterior edge is shown by the processus frontalis of the zygomatic process of the malar bone (b). However, these identification points only give an approximate position and it is probable that variation occurs with different types of skull.

It should also be borne in mind that the zygomatic arch is a fairly common site for fracture. As this bone is small and there may not be much displacement, such injuries can be easily overlooked.

REFERENCES

Littlewort, M. C. G. (1958), Vet. Rec., **70,** 977.
Barone, R., and Guelfi, J. (1966), Cah. Med. vet., **3,** 1.

Annotated radiographs and diagrams of the skull:

Barone, R., and Guelfi, J. (1966), Cah. Med. vet., **3,** 1.
Carlson, W. D. (1967), Veterinary Radiology, Second Edition. London: Bailliere, Tindall and Cassell.
Douglas, S. W., and Williamson, H. D. (1963), Principles of Veterinary Radiography. Bailliere, Tindall and Cox, London.
Hare, W. C. D. (1958), J. Am. vet. med. Ass., **133,** 149.
Schebitz, H., and Wilkens, H. (1968), Atlas of Radiographic Anatomy of Dog and Horse, Berlin, Paul Parey.

CHAPTER 5

THE VERTEBRAL COLUMN AND RIB CAGE

While the vertebral column is commonly regarded as a whole, it is made up of a large number of bones each of which shows some anatomical variation and which, at different levels of the spine, can require modification of the radiographic technique necessary for its demonstration. For this reason, only a superficial examination, or the recognition of gross lesions, should be attempted from radiographs covering large areas of the vertebral column. For a precise and detailed examination the field covered should be restricted to about half a dozen vertebrae.

It is proposed to discuss general aspects of the vertebral column, and then to consider particular regions of the spine and to describe anatomical and other features peculiar to that region. Finally, pathological conditions (which usually involve more than one region) will be considered.

GENERAL CONSIDERATIONS

Radiography

The comparative mobility of portions of the vertebral column (particularly the cervical region) make careful positioning essential and may necessitate the use of general anaesthesia in order to achieve this.

The usual projections are those in the lateral and ventro-dorsal planes. Oblique views may, in certain circumstances, provide additional information, but such projections have not been fully studied and unless the radiologist is familiar with the normal appearance of such views, they may prove more confusing than of assistance.

Radiology

In examining radiographs of the vertebral column the radiologist will obviously note the general line and contour of the whole column (in order to locate gross fractures or dislocations), but he should also make a detailed examination of each vertebra on the film and endeavour to note and identify the following:

(1) The alignment of the vertebra in relation to those adjacent to it.
(2) The general outline of the neural canal and any evidence of compression or irregularity.
(3) The following portions of each bone:

The vertebral bodies.
The articulations.
The spinous processes.
The transverse processes.

Intervertebral Discs

The normal intervertebral disc is not radio-opaque and cannot be visualised in a radiograph. Its size and shape has to be assumed after demonstration of the intervertebral space between adjacent vertebral bodies. This space will be clearly shown only if the X-ray beam traverses it precisely at right angles. Those discs which are "off centre" in the radiograph will be projected obliquely, and, if it is necessary to examine them in detail, further radiographs, centred over such areas, will be required.

The centre of a disc (the nucleus pulposus) may become calcified and demonstrable on radiography. While this provides evidence that degenerative changes are occurring, it is unlikely, in the otherwise normal disc, to be of clinical significance.

Prolapse or protrusion of an intervertebral disc usually results in nervous symptoms, and the pathological aspects of these structures will be considered in Chapter 14.

REGIONAL CONSIDERATIONS

The Cervical Region

Radiography

As already mentioned, this is a very mobile region of the vertebral column and, in particular, movement of the atlas on the axis can lead to an erroneous diagnosis of dislocation by those not familiar with the amount of movement possible between these two bones.

A pad should be placed under the neck and a certain amount of traction applied to the head during radiography of this region, provided that the patient will tolerate it.

The posterior cervical vertebrae can be obscured by the shoulder region of the fore limbs, and these should be drawn as far backwards as possible.

Anatomical Features

The general anatomy of this region must be kept in mind, particularly the marked difference between the first cervical vertebra (the atlas) and the rest of the cervical vertebrae. The atlas has no vertebral body and there are no intervertebral discs on either side of it. This bone slightly overlaps the occipital region of the skull and the occipito-atlantal joint cannot be clearly demonstrated. In lateral projections the wings of the atlas will be shown as a dense oblique line but in ventro-dorsal projections the wings, being particularly thin, can be obliterated by over-exposure.

The first intervertebral disc is situated between the second and third cervical vertebrae. It must be appreciated that the cervical intervertebral discs are not precisely at right angles to the cervical spine, and that, for their demonstration in the ventro-dorsal plane, the x-ray beam must be directed at a slight angle towards the head.

The transverse and spinous processes of these vertebrae are thin and, in the posterior part of the region may be difficult to distinguish from the surrounding muscle, unless a careful radiographic technique is employed.

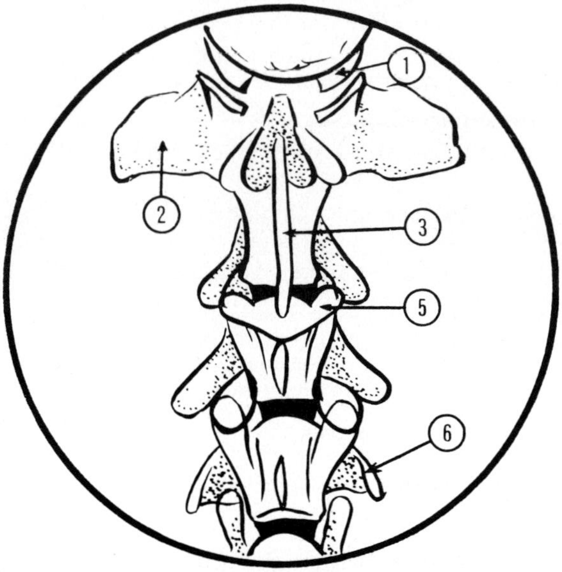

THE CERVICAL REGION

FIG. 5.1.

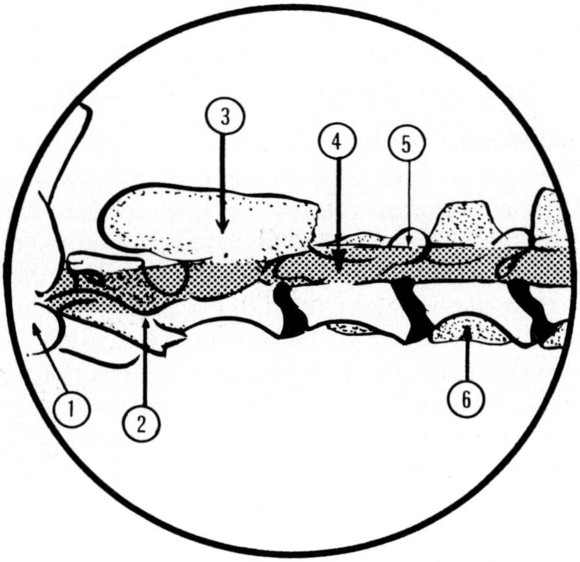

FIGS. 5.1 and 5.2.
(1) Occipital condyle
(2) Wing of atlas
(3) Spinous process of axis
(4) Neural canal
(5) Articular facets
(6) Transverse process

FIG. 5.2.

It is unusual to find any variation in the number of vertebrae in this area, but fusion of two vertebrae (usually the second and third) is said to occur occasionally in Dachshunds and not to be of clinical significance (Olsson, 1964).

The Thoracic Region
(Including the Ribs and Sternum)

Radiography

While there is far less mobility of this portion of the vertebral column, precise positioning in the ventro-dorsal and lateral planes is not easy, but is important if the part is to be accurately demonstrated. Even then, there will be superimposition of the sternum, heart and mediastinum in ventro-dorsal projections, and of the upper end of the ribs in lateral views. Precise positioning in these planes is also essential for accurate visualisation of the ribs and dorso-ventral views will inevitably give a "doubled up" foreshortened impression of the ribs.

Anatomical Features

The Thoracic Vertebrae are, on the whole, uniform in shape and comparable with each other, except for the dorsal spine. The angle of the dorsal spine is progressively more acute in each succeeding vertebra and the last 3 thoracic spines are small and comparatively insignificant. In ventro-dorsal projections, because of the angulation, the "end on" view of the dorsal spines will be superimposed on the next vertebra.

The intervertebral spaces are set at right angles to the line of the vertebral column, but are often obscured in lateral views by the head of the ribs—particularly if there is any obliquity in positioning.

The articulation with the ribs is most clearly seen in ventro-dorsal views, while that between the vertebrae is best demonstrated in lateral projections.

Variation in the total number of thoracic vertebrae occurs and a manifestation of this is the presence of a fourteenth vertebra (commonly associated with an additional pair of rudimentary ribs).

Antero-posterior compression of the bodies of the thoracic vertebrae is common in certain breeds (e.g., Bulldogs). While this will be considered further under Pathological Conditions, this malformation is not necessarily associated with clinical symptoms and could be considered as a "normal variation".

The Ribs. Exact identification of a particular rib requires comparison of the two standard projections and careful numbering of each rib. The ribs arise from the anterior aspect of each thoracic vertebra, and the articular head and the neck will only be visualised in a ventro-dorsal projection. The shaft of each rib extends uniformly downwards to the costro-chondral junction, where it is continued by the narrower band of cartilage to the sternum. With age this cartilage becomes increasingly calcified—often giving rise to an irregular blotchy appearance.

The Sternum In a correctly positioned dorso-ventral projection of this region the sternum will be hardly perceptible, and a lateral view (with the fore limbs drawn forward and upward) is the only satisfactory method of demonstrating this bone.

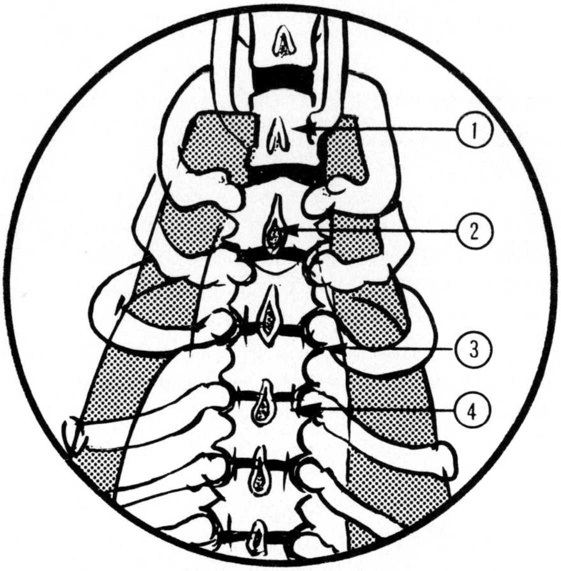

THE THORACIC REGION

FIG. 5.3.

FIGS. 5.3 and 5.4.
(1) Vertebral body
(2) Spinous process
(3) Rib articulation
(4) Articular facets
(Stippling represents lung tissue)

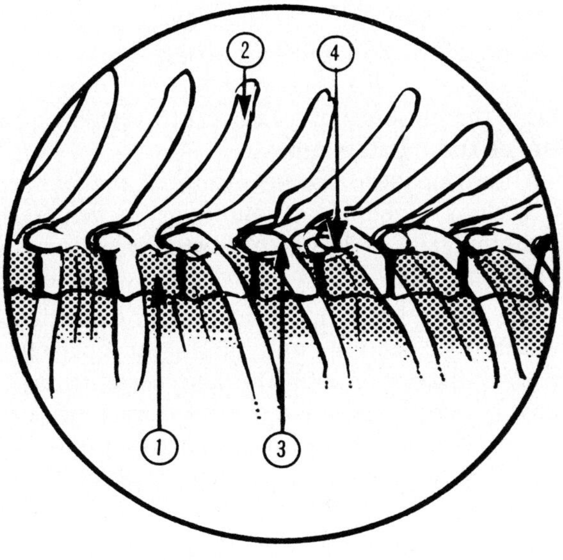

FIG. 5.4.

THE LUMBAR REGION

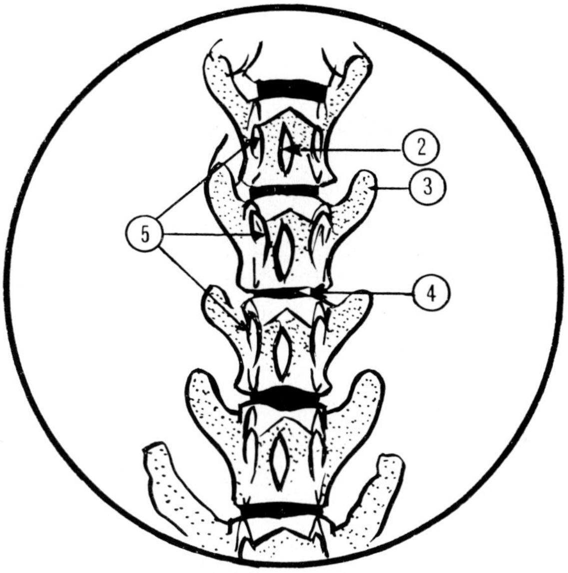

FIG. 5.5.

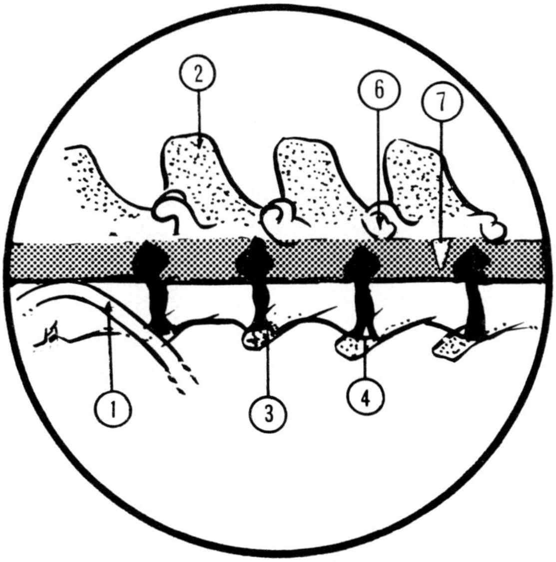

FIGS. 5.5 and 5.6.
(1) Last rib
(2) Spinous process
(3) Transverse process
(4) Intervertebral disc
(5) Pedicle of neural arch
(6) Articular facets
(7) Neural canal

FIG. 5.6.

In such a projection the sternum will be visualised as a chain of eight small bones. Some displacement of the posterior two or three bones is a common feature.

The Lumbar Region

Radiography

There are no great problems with regard to the positioning of this region but it is essential to check that the axis of the spine is parallel with the film at the time of radiography. This may be difficult to achieve in ventro-dorsal projections of dogs showing marked kyphosis in association with painful lesions of the spine, or in lateral views of dogs possessing a broad thorax but narrow abdomen. Obviously, ventro-dorsal projections will be employed in preference to dorso-ventral exposures.

In heavily muscled dogs scatter can result in significant loss of detail and it is advisable to use a grid.

Anatomical Features

The lumbar vertebrae show little individual variation and it is comparatively easy to demonstrate and recognise the principal anatomical features. However, since radiography of this area requires the use of comparatively penetrating exposure

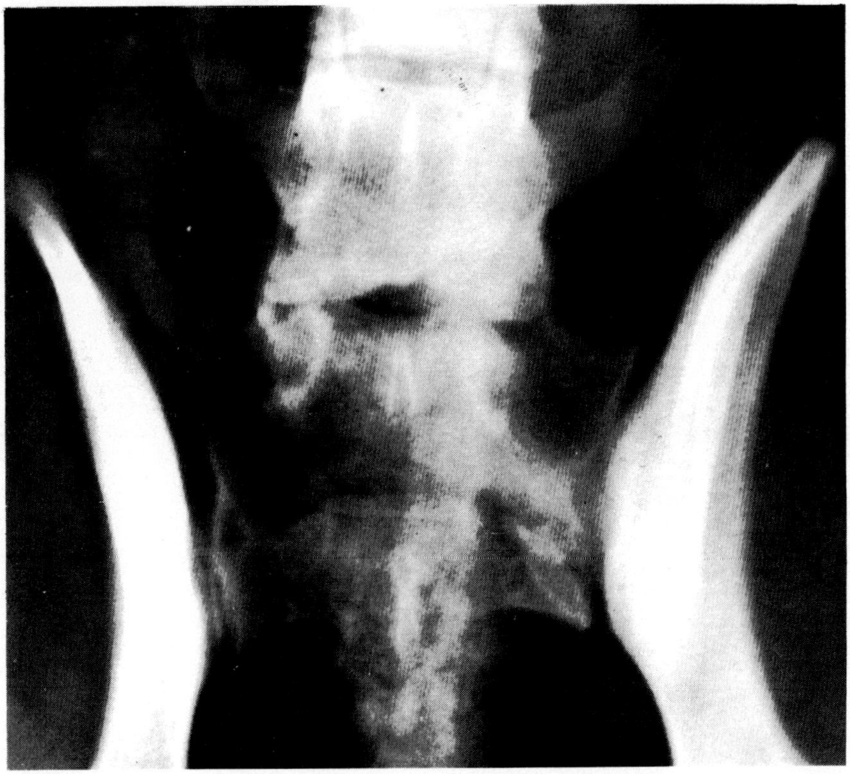

FIG. 5.7. Partial sacralisation of the 7th lumbar vertebra.

THE SACRAL REGION

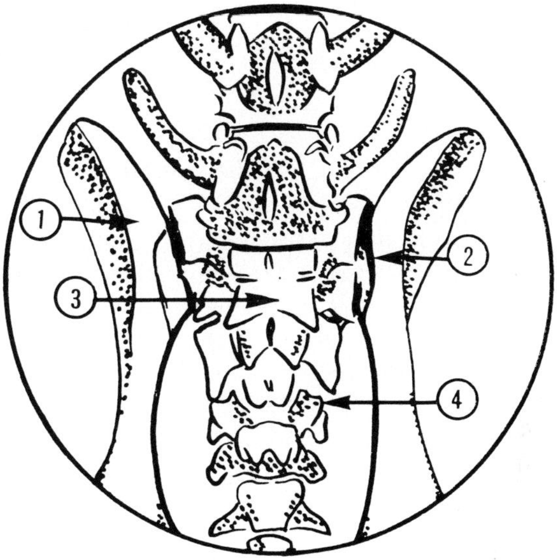

Fig. 5.8.

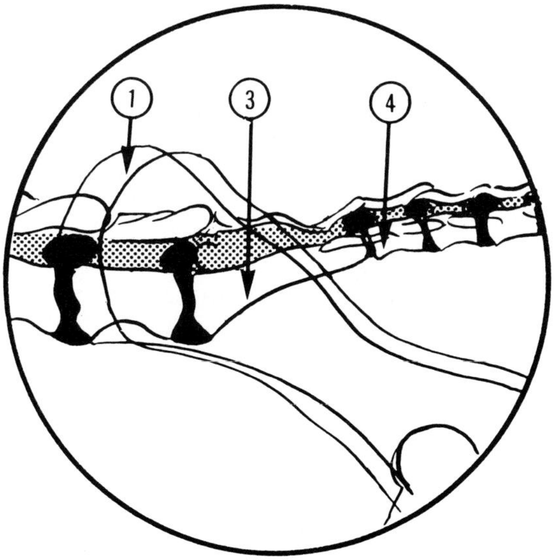

Fig. 5.9.

Figs. 5.8. and 5.9.
(1) Wing of ileum
(2) Sacro-iliac junction
(3) Sacrum
(4) First coccygeal vertebra

factors, the dorsal spines and lateral processes are frequently over-penetrated and poorly visualised.

Sacralisation or fusion with the sacrum, involving the seventh or an additional lumbar vertebra is a common feature and must be regarded as a normal variant.

Compared with the dog, the lumbar vertebrae of the cat are relatively long and narrow.

The Sacral Region and the Tail

Radiography

The sacrum is set at a variable angle to the lumbar vertebrae, and ventro-dorsal projections of this bone will give a foreshortened view, unless the primary beam is angled to compensate for this effect. Particularly precise positioning in this plane is essential if the sacro-iliac junction is to be demonstrated. Dense faeces within the rectum can obscure the area, and preparation of the patient to remove this may be necessary in some circumstances. In lateral projections the two ilia will be superimposed on the sacrum but the outline of the latter bone is usually still sufficiently visible.

Anatomical Features

The Sacrum does not show any very unusual anatomical features. The sacro-iliac junction normally reveals a definite gap between the two bones, but with age bony union may occur. Partial or complete fusion with the last lumbar or first coccygeal vertebra does occur and is not normally of clinical significance.

The Tail should be extended as far as practicable for radiography and the exposure factors will require considerable reduction. In this region non-screen film can be used if fine detail is required.

Only the first few coccygeal vertebrae have a neural arch, the remainder comprise little beyond the vertebral body.

PATHOLOGICAL CONDITIONS

The Vertebral Column

Lesions of this region usually also involve the spinal cord and result in nervous symptoms. Therefore there will be some overlap between the conditions described here and those listed in Chapter 14.

In general, those abnormalities which are confined to the bony vertebral column will be discussed on the succeeding pages, and those involving the associated non-bony structures will be dealt with in the penultimate chapter.

Fractures

Fracture of the vertebral body is a common feature of severe injuries (e.g., motor car accidents) in this region. Such lesions are usually easily demonstrable by radiography, which will show marked displacement of the bony fragments and a definite

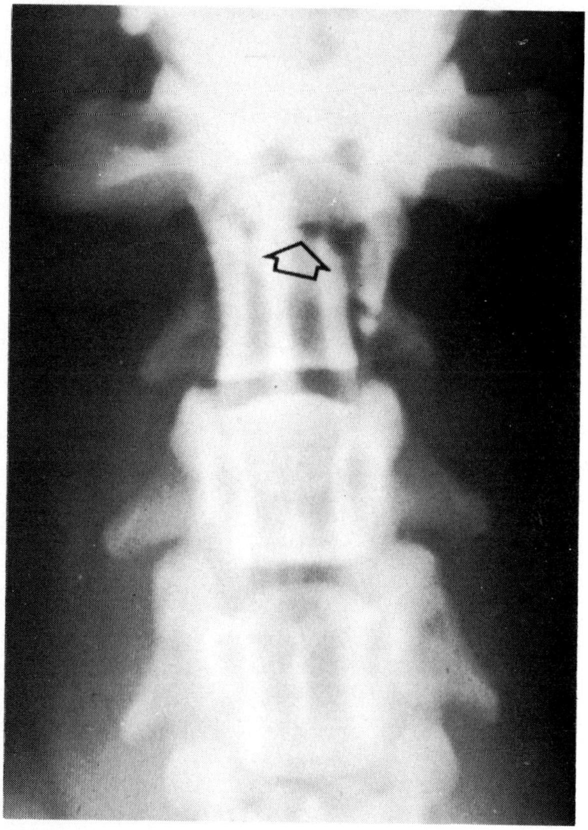

FIG. 5.10.

FIGS. 5.10 and 5.11. Fracture of 2nd cervical vertebra.

FIG. 5.11.

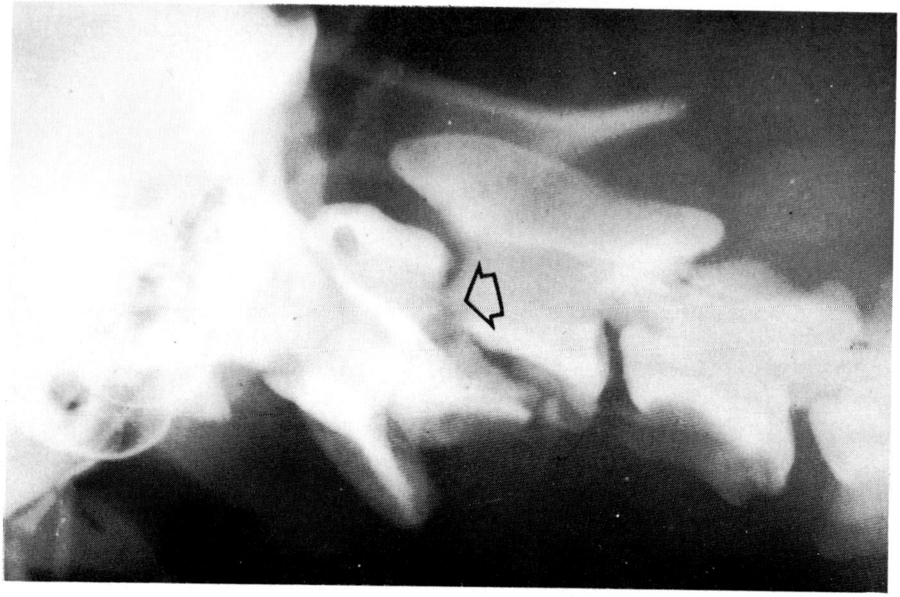

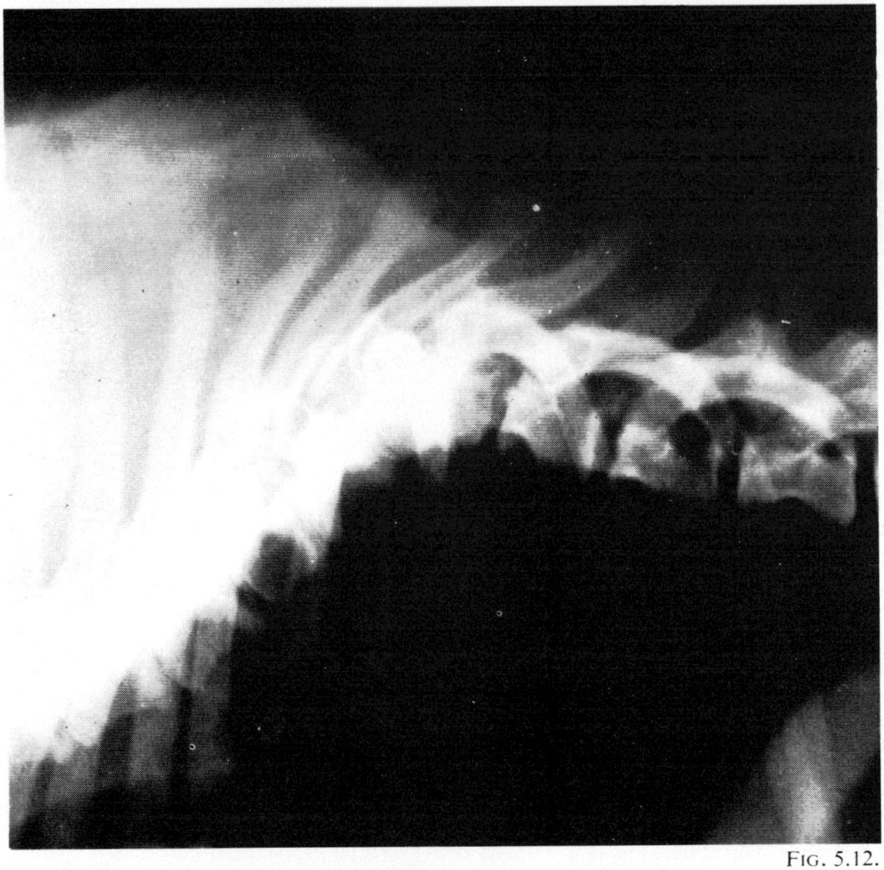

FIG. 5.12.

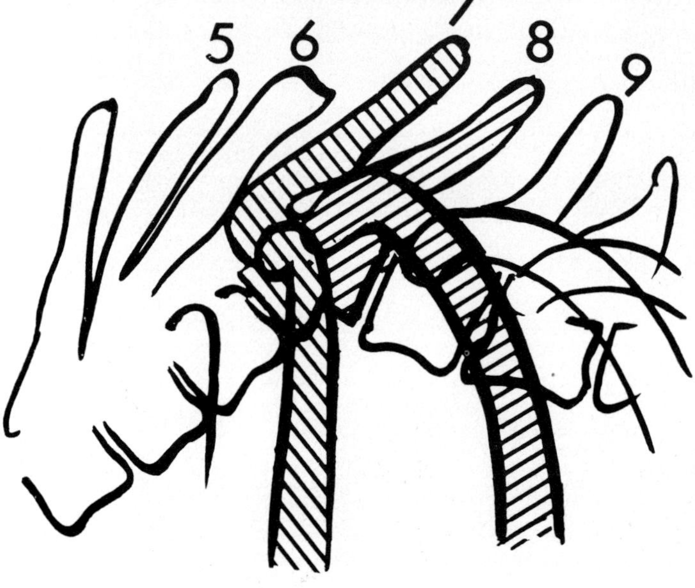

FIGS. 5.12 and 5.13. Compression of the bodies of the 7th and 8th thoracic vertebrae.

"step" in the line of the neural canal. However, the portions of the vertebral body tend to overlap and such injuries can be overlooked if radiography is confined to one plane (this is most likely to occur if only ventro-dorsal projections are obtained).

Suspected fractures of the atlas and of the odontoid process of the axis can be a source of confusion because of the mobility of the atlas. To investigate such a problem it is usually necessary to anaesthetise the patient and to extend the neck, while undertaking precise radiography in at least two planes.

Fractures of vertebral spines or processes can occur, but are seldom associated with clinical symptoms and for this reason are not often radiographed.

Compression Injuries

Collapse of a vertebra is usually the result of pathological bone weakness rather than of traumatic injury. Such lesions are seen in the young animal as a result of deficiency diseases (e.g., "juvenile osteoporosis") and as a comparatively "normal" occurrence in certain breeds of dog (e.g., Bulldogs) where they may be associated with developmental abnormalities. This lesion is shown radiologically by a definite shortening and bending of the vertebral body (in severe cases this may result in a V-shaped contour). The normal trabecular structure of the body will be lost and replaced by irregular dense bone, The angulation of the vertebra may be sufficiently severe to result in obvious kyphosis of the spine.

Dislocations

Dislocation of one vertebra from another, without an associated fracture, is not common but appears to occur more frequently in those breeds subject to degeneration of the intervertebral disc (Dachshunds, Spaniels, etc.). Complete dislocation with displacement of the vertebral column should be obvious radiologically, but in other instances the evidence of this injury may only be seen as narrowing of the inter-vertebral space, a slight break in the line of the neural canal, and separation of the articular facets.

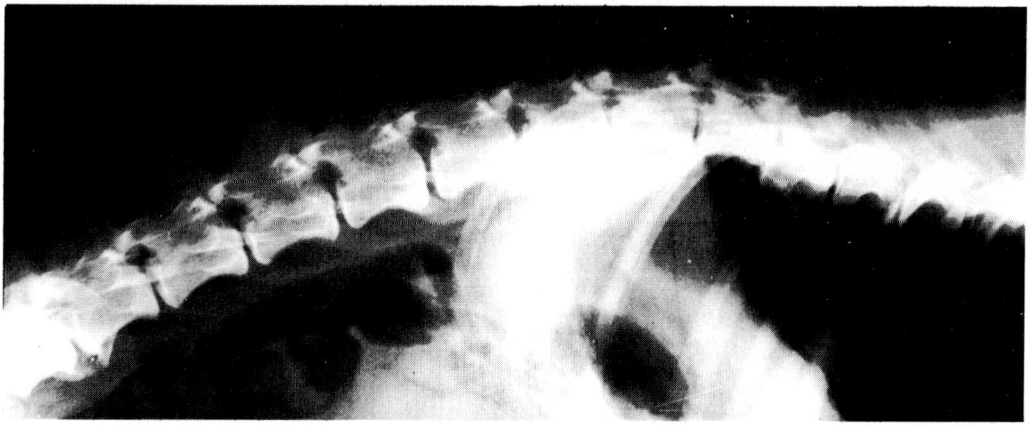

FIG. 5.14. Dislocation of thoracic vertebrae.

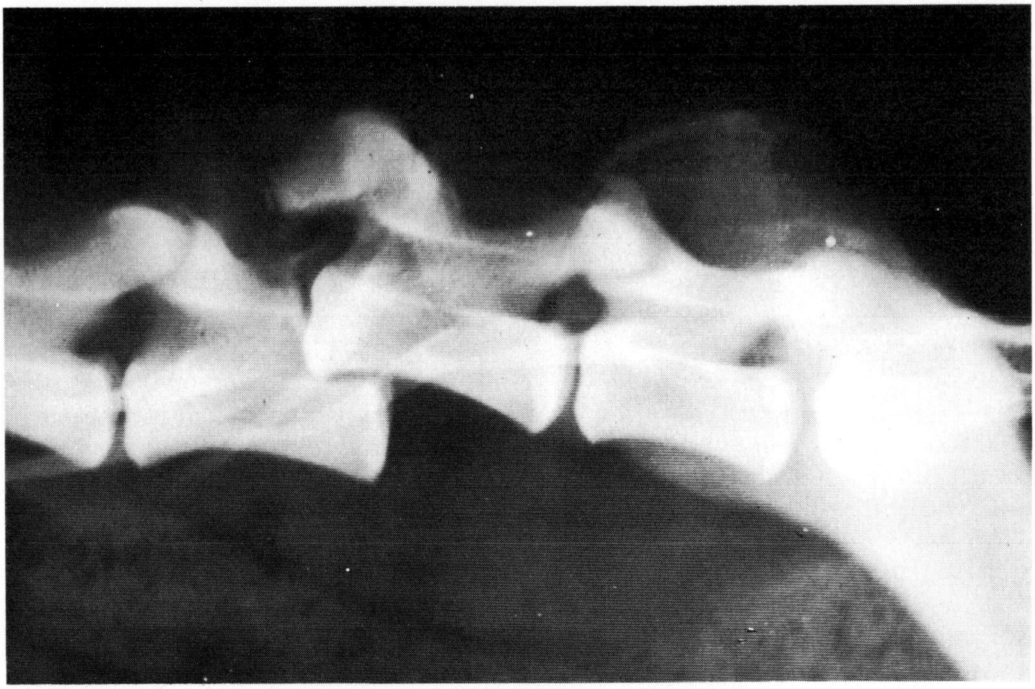

FIG. 5.15. Fracture-dislocation of lumbar vertebrae.

Ossifying Spondylosis

This term is used for a condition seen frequently on radiography of the vertebral column in which there is a progressive lipping and ankylosis of the bodies of adjacent vertebral bodies. The condition has also been described as "hypertrophic degenerative arthritis" (Carlson 1967). Radiologically the first evidence of the lesion is seen as a

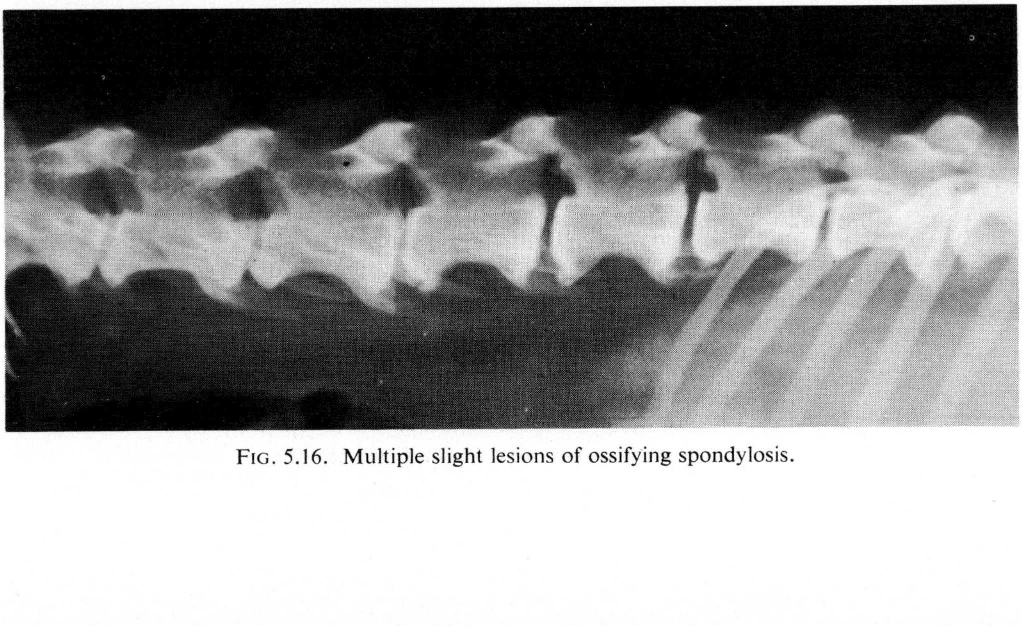

FIG. 5.16. Multiple slight lesions of ossifying spondylosis.

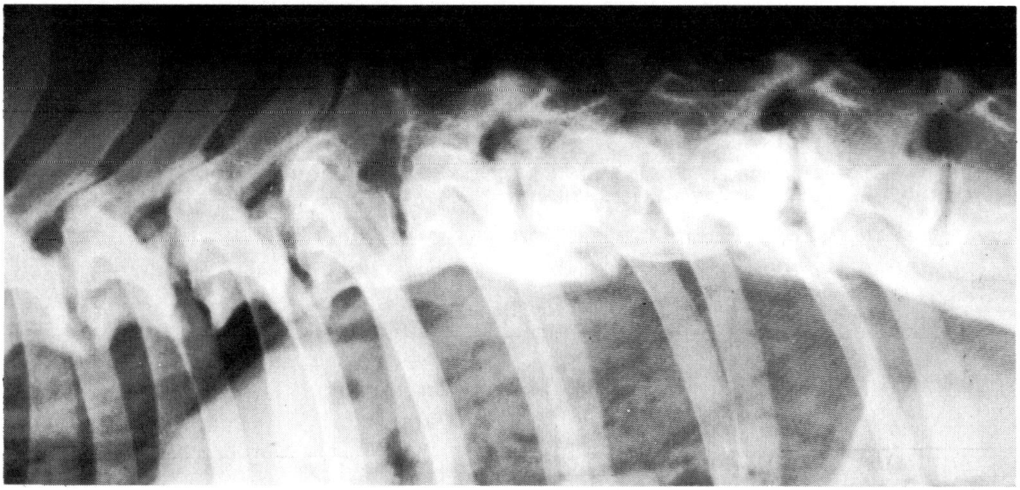

FIG. 5.17. Extensive ankylosis of the vertebral column as a result of ossifying spondylosis.

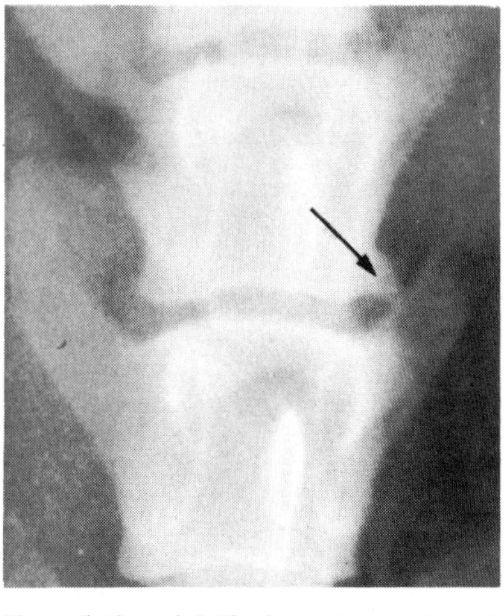

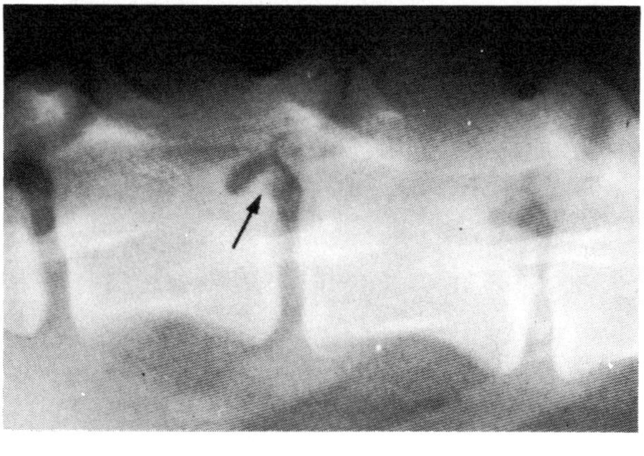

FIGS. 5.18 and 5.19. Localised lesion of ossifying spondylosis situated on the dorsal aspect of the vertebral body.

slight protrusion of the ventral bony contour at the posterior and anterior ends of adjacent vertebrae. In more advanced cases the protrusions will be seen to be extending in a hook-like fashion until they meet and unite ventral to the intervertebral disc. In particularly severe cases there may be a large irregular mass of new bone formed ventrally which unites several vertebrae. While the condition is normally best demonstrated in lateral views of the vertebral column, it should be appreciated that the process of new bone formation can extend laterally around the vertebral bodies (and occasionally involves the neural arches) and ventro-dorsal projections may be required to permit visualisation of the full extent of the lesion.

The condition rarely involves the cervical vertebrae and occurs most frequently in the regions of the thoracic-lumbar and lumbar-sacral junctions. It is seen most commonly in the larger breeds of dog and is encountered less frequently in cats.

The clinical significance of this radiological finding is open to considerable differences of opinion. Certainly the lesion is frequently demonstrated in dogs radiographed for other purposes and showing no associated symptoms, while at the other extreme, the significance of severe extensive lesions in causing complete rigidity of portions of the spinal column or of compression of spinal nerves can be shown by radiography. It is the intervening cases in which lesions of ossifying spondylosis are demonstrated in dogs showing mild symptoms of lumbar pain which can lead to varying opinions as to whether the radiological findings are of significance.

Neoplasia

The vertebral column is not a common site for bony neoplasia but the authors have encountered both primary and secondary malignant neoplasms involving this

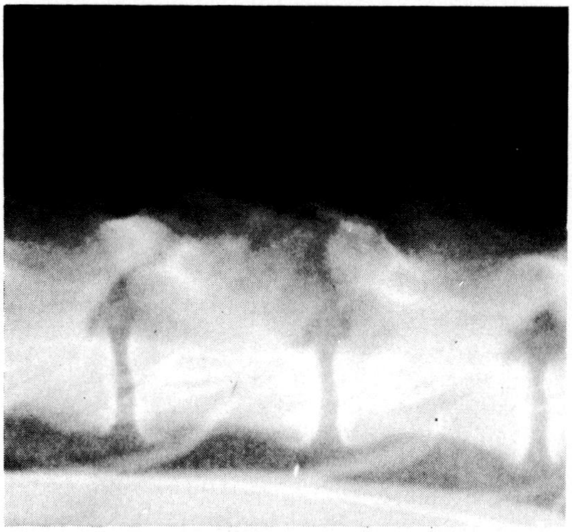

FIG. 5.20.

FIGS. 5.20 and 5.21. Osteosarcoma arising from the neural arch of a lumbar vertebra.

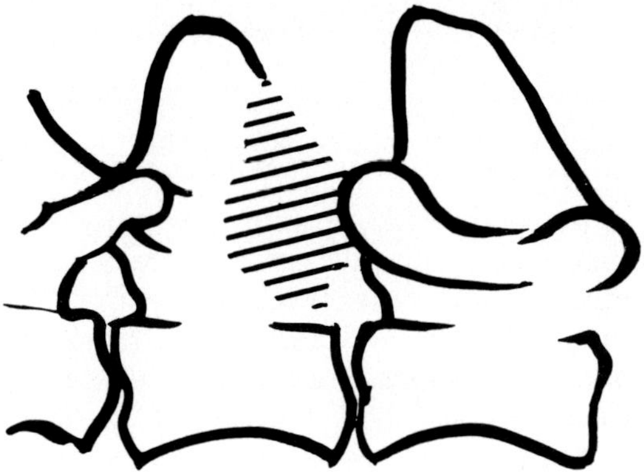

FIG. 5.21.

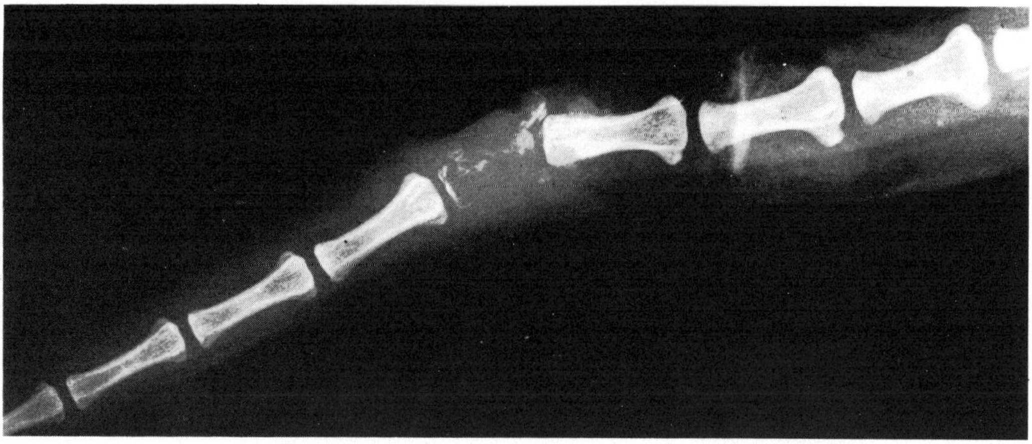

FIG. 5.22. Secondary neoplasia resulting in the destruction of a coccygeal vertebra (the primary was a mammary carcinoma)

region. The radiological evidence of neoplasia has been discussed earlier (page 33) but its occurrence in this area can be overlooked because of its comparative rarity and the need for particularly careful radiography and detailed examination of each individual vertebra.

Osteomyelitis

The radiological features of this disease have also been described previously (page 41). The condition occurs as a result of wounds and bites and by spread from adjacent foci of infection. As with neoplasia, the condition can be overlooked unless

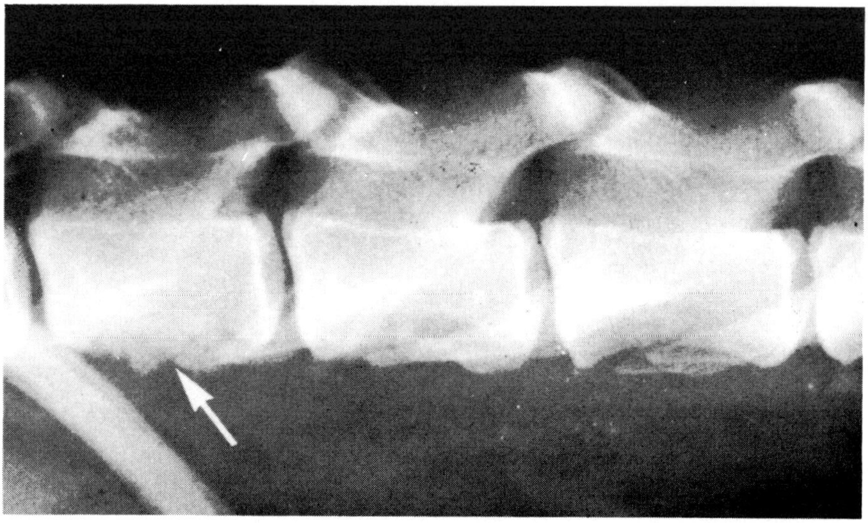

FIG. 5.23. A chronic form of osteomyelitis due to Nocardial infection.

maximum definition and detail is obtained in the film. With dogs of any size the use of a grid would be essential.

The Ribs

Fractures

Rib fractures are comparatively common as a result of traumatic chest injuries, but their presence is easily missed on examination of radiographs. This is due to the fact that separation of the ends of the bones is usually slight and may be obscured

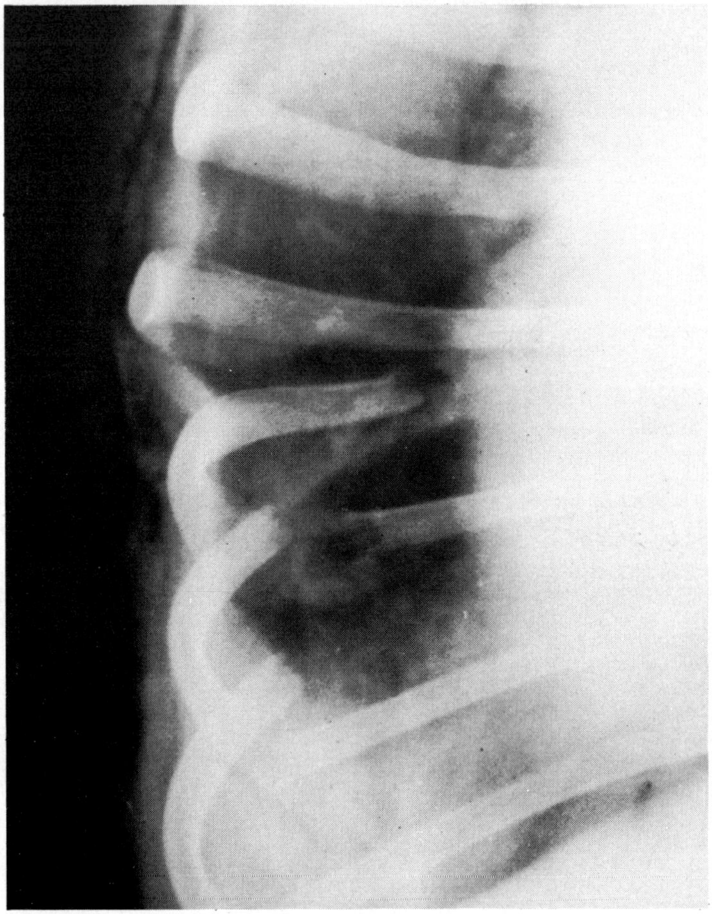

FIG. 5.24. Fractured ribs showing considerable displacement and subcutaneous emphysema associated with the injury.

by superimposition of other ribs. If such injuries are to be noted it is necessary to make a systematic examination of the contour of each rib in turn—preferably in both planes.

Neoplasia

Neoplasia of the ribs is encountered more frequently than tumours of the vertebrae. It is seen both as primary tumours and as involvement of ribs in adjacent malignant soft tissue tumours. In general, costal tumours tend to contain less bone and more soft tissue than bony neoplasia occurring elsewhere.

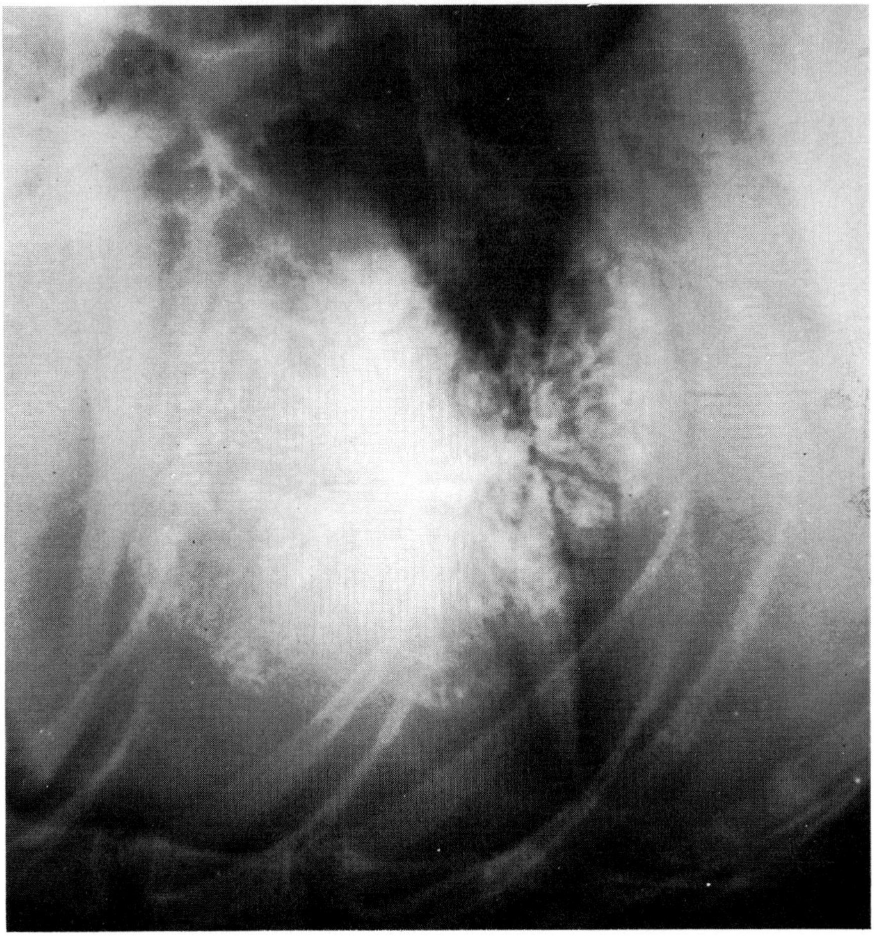

FIG. 5.25. Osteosarcoma involving a rib.

Rickets

The presence of a "rickety rosary" is always considered to be a typical manifestation of this condition. However, as mentioned in Chapter 3 true rickets is now considered to be rare in the dog. Nevertheless, radiography of the larger breeds of dog at about 4–5 months of age frequently reveals some enlargement of the lower end of the ribs. This swelling usually resolves spontaneously during the succeeding few months, but may well represent a mild manifestation of rickets during the period of maximum mineral and vitamin requirements.

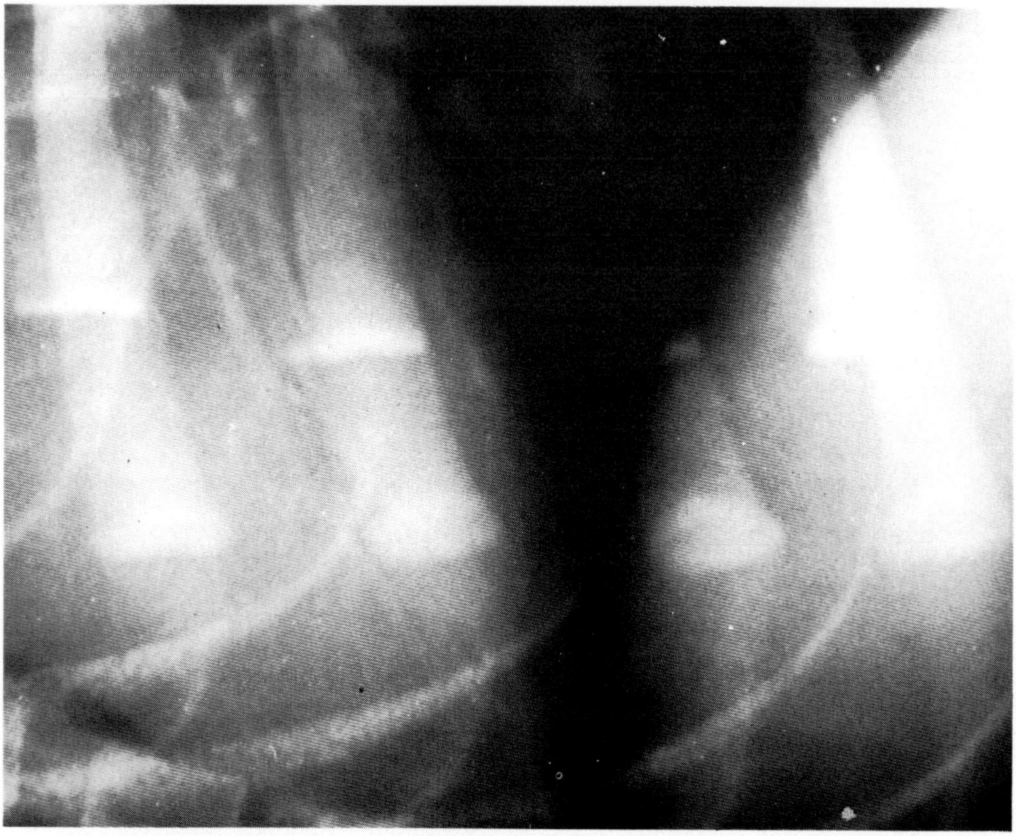

FIG. 5.26. Enlargement of the lower ends of the ribs in a 5 month old Alsatian.

REFERENCES

Carlson, W. D. (1967), Veterinary Radiology, Second Edition. London: Bailliere, Tindall and Cassell.
Olsson, S.-E. (1964), Personal communication.

CHAPTER 6

THE LIMB BONES AND JOINTS

Introduction

The reader is reminded that in Chapter 3 a number of general radiological features concerning the normal and pathological anatomy of the skeletal system were discussed. These features, which include:

(a) The structure of bone in both the young and the adult animal.
(b) The significance of the epiphyseal line.
(c) The evidence of local pathological conditions of bone and joints (neoplasia, osteomyelitis, arthritis, etc.).
(d) The evidence of more generalised bone pathology (juvenile osteoporosis, hypertrophic pulmonary osteoarthropathy, etc.)

are of particular importance in relation to the radiology of the limb bones and joints and should be borne in mind throughout this chapter.

Since these general matters have already been dealt with, the individual bones and joints will now be listed and only those radiological features of normal or pathological significance which are typical of, or peculiar to, these structures will be studied.

Scapula

Owing to its relative thinness and its superimposition on the chest and rib cage, this bone is not easy to visualise and evidence of fractures or of neoplasia can easily be overlooked. Provided the patient can be suitably positioned, postero-anterior projections are likely to be the most informative. In lateral views the edge of the bone may be barely perceptible but any break in the continuity of the denser line of the spine of the scapula would suggest a fracture.

Shoulder

Since this is a ball-and-socket joint, the bones comprising it can be moved in more than one plane. Therefore care must be taken to adopt standard positioning, or rotation of the humerus will alter the appearance of the joint and render comparison with the opposite joint difficult.

The shoulder joint is not a common site of radiological lesions but complete dislocation and "loose joint" or subluxation may be demonstrated. Chronic arthritic conditions associated with new bone formation are extremely rare.

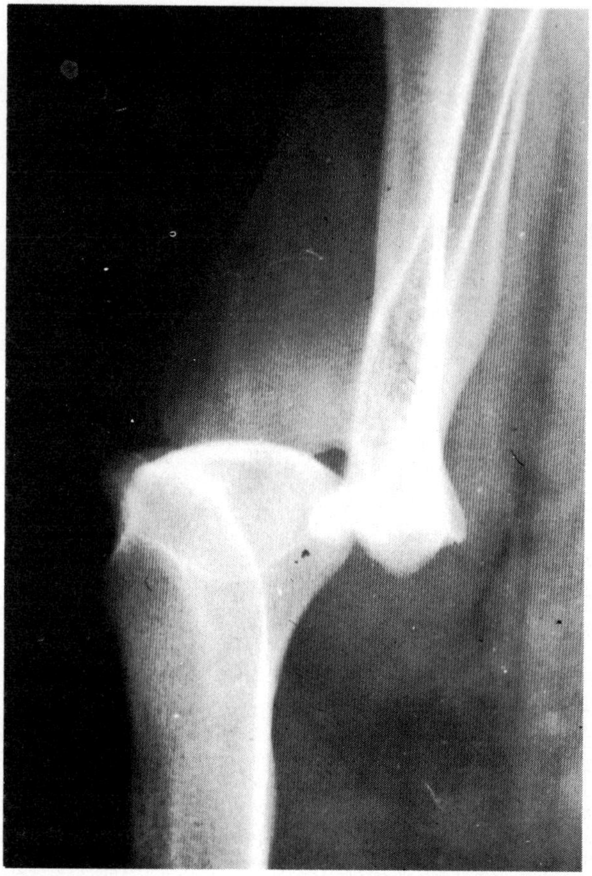

FIG. 6.1. Dislocation of the shoulder joint.

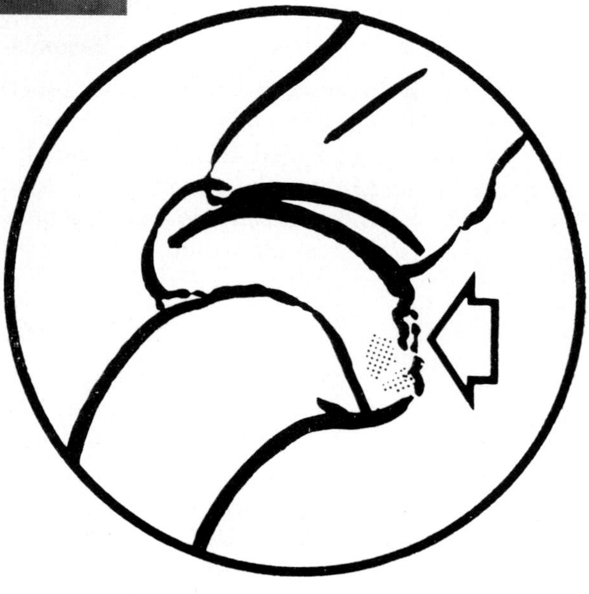

FIG. 6.2. Diagram illustrating the essential features of osteochondritis dissecans of the shoulder joint.

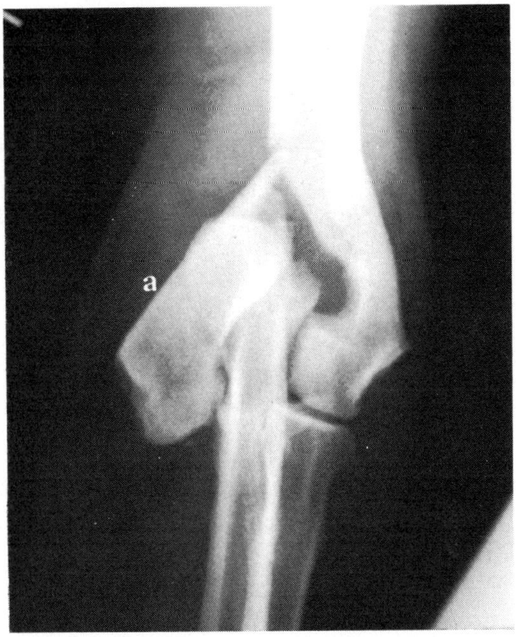

FIG. 6.4. Separation of the medial condyle of the humerus.

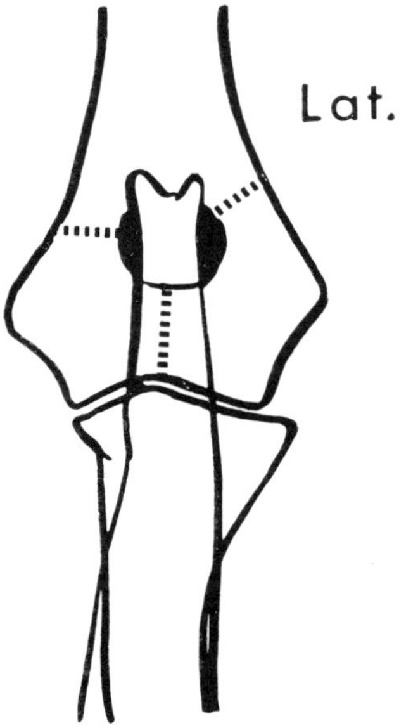

FIG. 6.3. Common sites of condylar fracture of the humerus.

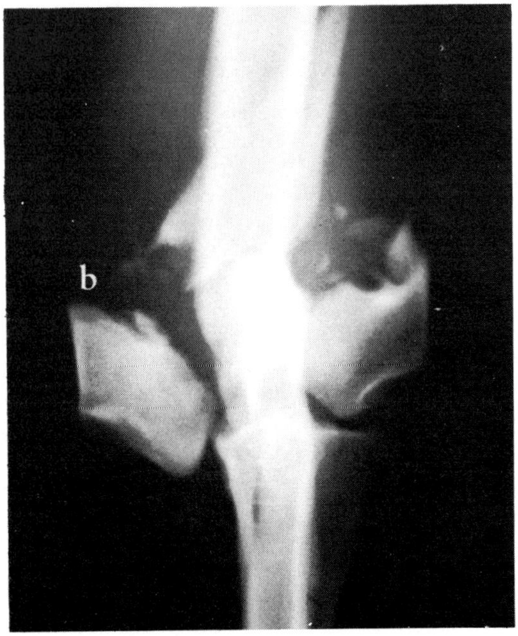

FIG. 6.5. "Y" fracture with separation of both condyles.

Craig and Riser (1965) have drawn attention to the occurrence, in the larger breeds of dog, of a lesion within this joint which they consider to be identical with osteochondritis dissecans of man. However, these authors indicate that it is only the more severe manifestations of this condition which can be demonstrated radiologically during life. Such lesions will be recognised as a defect in the posterior third of the articular outline of the upper end of the humerus. In some instances the defect, or area of bone absorption, extends into the depth of the articular head and is surrounded by a zone of increased bone density. This condition may be accompanied by the presence of a small bone sequestrum within the joint space.

Dysplastic changes affecting this joint are rare, but have been reported (Evans, 1968).

The fact that in the cat the presence of the clavicle could be mistaken for a foreign body, is probably too well known to need stressing here.

Humerus

The marked difference in the amount of soft tissue surrounding the upper and lower ends of this bone is likely, in thick muscled dogs, to result in under-exposure of the upper half or over-exposure of the lower half, if the bone is radiographed as a whole. For good detail it is advisable to concentrate on a particular portion of the bone and to adjust the exposure factors accordingly.

When investigating injuries of the lower end of the humerus it is important to demonstrate clearly the full extent of any condylar fractures so that the surgeon may be able to decide on the most suitable method of fixation, and radiography in both planes is essential. The usual sites of such fractures are shown in the accompanying diagram (Fig. 6.3). In those cases in which little or no displacement occurs the injury can be difficult to recognise—particularly a fracture between the condyles which can be masked by superimposition of the ulna.

Elbow

It is again important to be able to compare radiographs taken in the usual two planes when making a radiological investigation of the joint. In addition, lateral views of the completely flexed joint are essential if injuries of the olecranon process are suspected. The following conditions of this joint require further comment:

Dislocation Both complete dislocation and various forms of subluxation can occur and the use of radiography is essential to permit their differentiation. In the former, the radius and ulna remain united, but are completely displaced from the humerus. Whereas, in the latter, separation of the ulna from the radius or the occurrence of an ulna fracture, can result in displacement of the radius while the ulna remains in normal apposition with the humerus.

In the young animal subluxation of the radius on the humerus may be difficult to demonstrate radiologically until the epiphyses are fully calcified (approximately 3 months). If such an abnormality is congenital or occurs at an early age, radiography may show subsequent malformation of the upper end of the radius.

Elbow Dysplasia This term is used for a congenital condition of the joint occurring most frequently in Alsatians in which there is a partial or, more commonly, complete failure of union of the aconal process of the ulna. Since the lesion is small and easily masked by the humerus, it will require radiography of the fully flexed joint for its demonstration. In old standing cases there may be evidence of an associated osteo-arthritis of the joint.

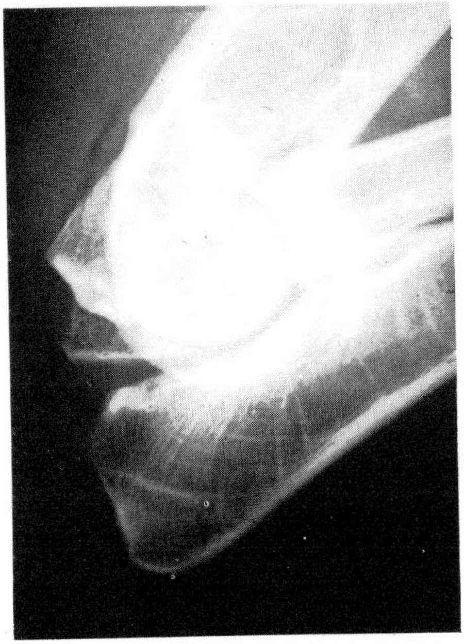

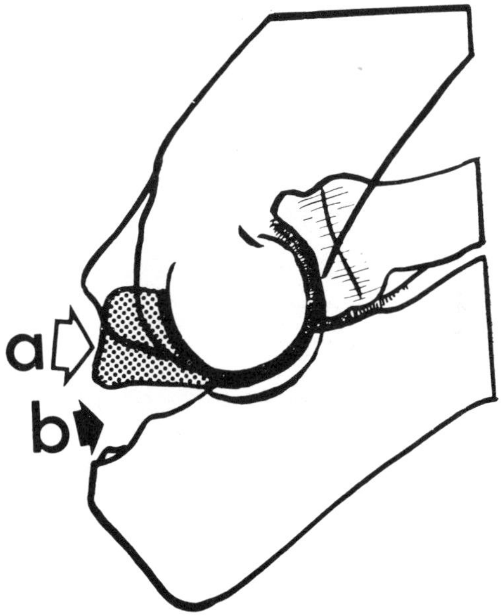

FIGS. 6.6 and 6.7. Elbow dysplasia in an 8 month old Alsatian dog. (a) Aconal process (b) Area separating the aconal process from the ulna.

Radius and Ulna

It is not always appreciated that there are a number of factors which can have a marked effect on the radiological anatomy of these bones during the growing period. These are:

(a) Considerable remodelling occurs and results in variation in the ratio of the transverse measurements of these bones. This is most marked in the larger breeds of dog where, at 4–5 months of age the ulna may be one and a half times as wide as the radius, while in adult life the latter bone will be considerably wider than the ulna (Figs. 6.8 and 6.9).

(b) The major amount of bone growth occurs at the distal epiphyses of these bones (approximately 70 per cent. in the case of the radius and 85 per cent. in the case of the ulna). To permit this large amount of new bone formation the lower epiphyses become enlarged. This effect is again most marked in the larger breeds where the spreading of the lower end of the metaphysis can be mistaken for evidence of rickets.

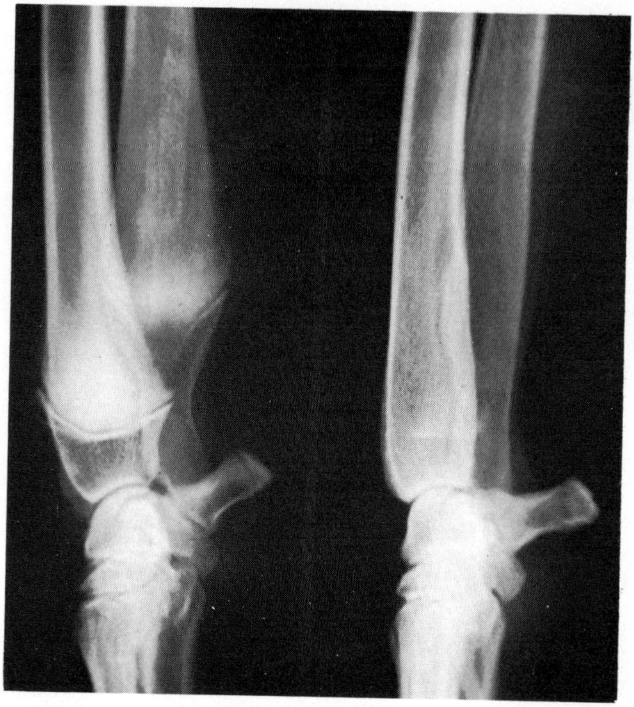

FIG. 6.8.

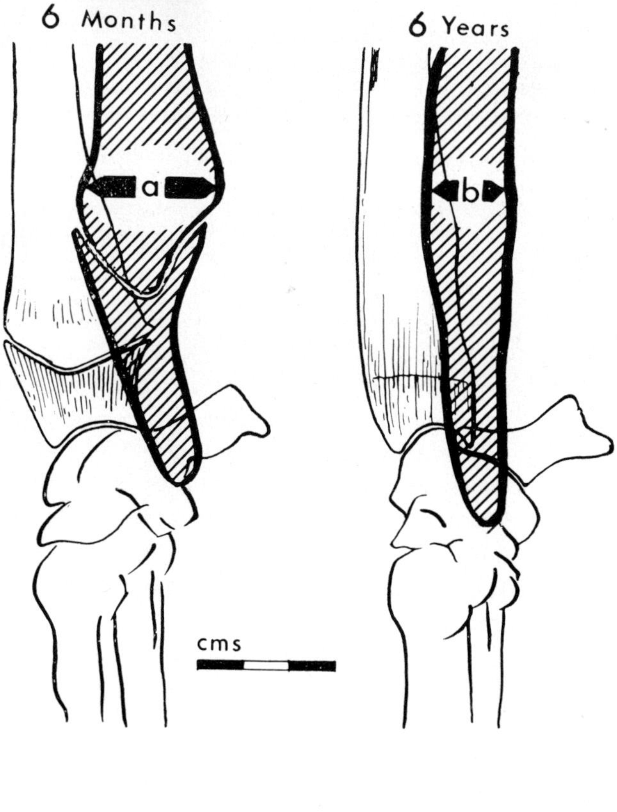

FIG. 6.9.

(c) Since both bones articulate with, and are attached to, the humerus and the carpus they cannot grow independently. Should an injury or other cause, interfere with new bone growth at the lower end of the ulna, this will cause relative shortening of the bone and bowing of the radius.

It has been suggested that it is failure of bone growth at this point which results in the typical bowing of the radius seen in the chondrodystrophoid breeds of dog.

Riser and Shirer (1965) report that similar, but less severe, distortion can occur in larger dogs, due to the presence of a core of cartilage cells within the ulna metaphysis, which fails to undergo normal ossification.

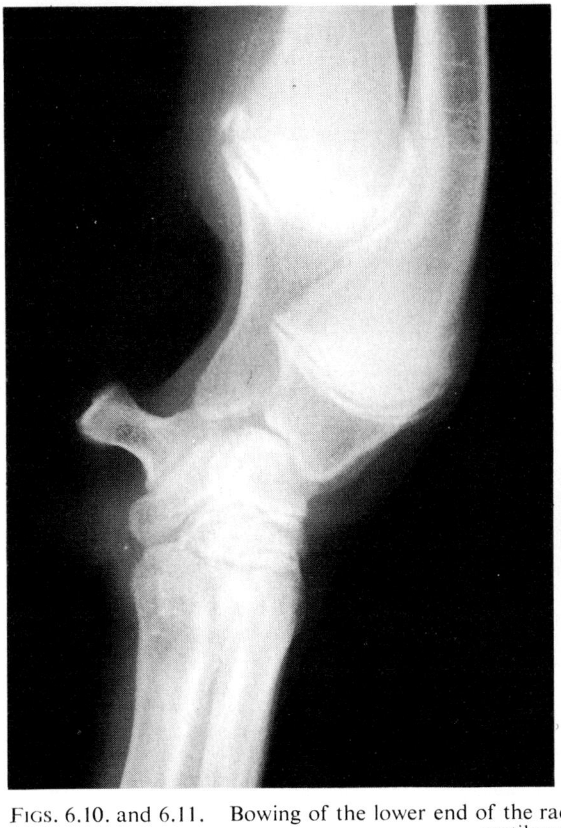

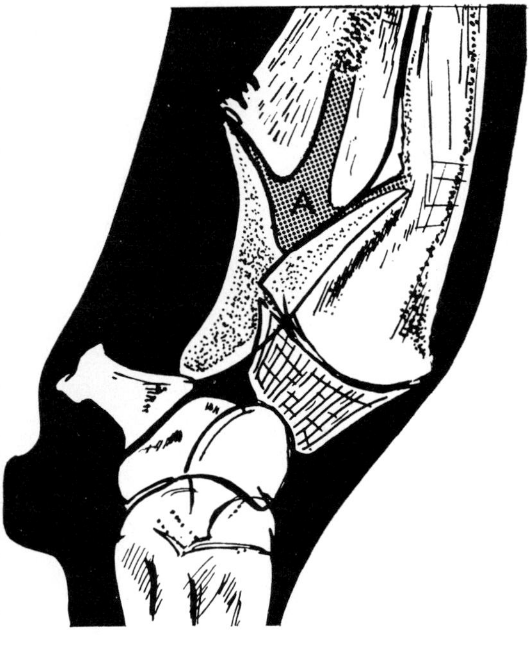

FIGS. 6.10. and 6.11. Bowing of the lower end of the radius and ulna associated with persistance of a core of cartilage (A).

Should an injury to the lower epiphyses of the radius result in cessation of growth, bowing of the bones is unlikely to occur but it is probable that the upper end of the radius will become separated from the humerus.

In chondrodystrophoid dogs, in addition to the bowing of the radius referred to above, radiographs of these bones will show a number of bony projections at the point of attachment of ligaments and tendons.

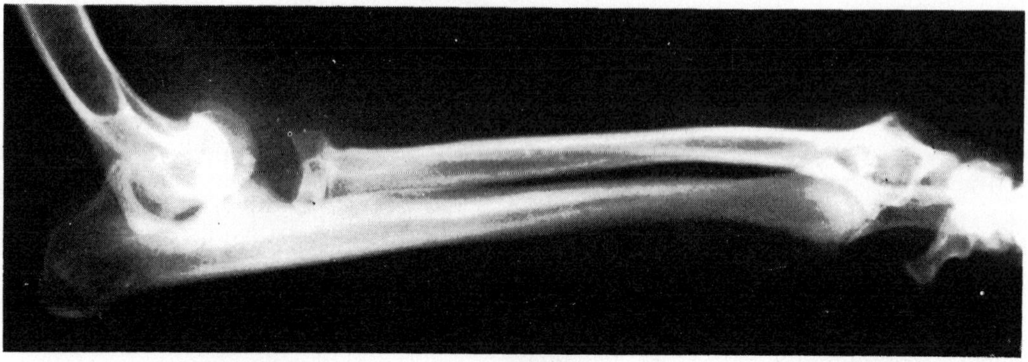

FIG. 6.12. Shortening of the radius, (an injury resulted in premature closing of the lower epiphysis).

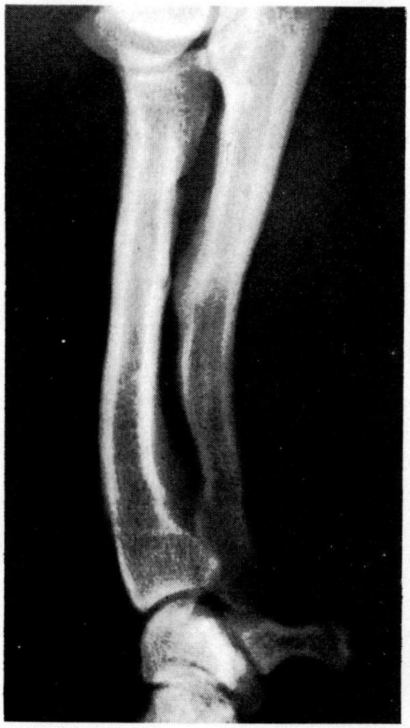

FIG. 6.13. Radius and ulna of a Dachshund.

Carpus

The individual bones of the carpus cannot be demonstrated radiologically at birth as they are still cartilagenous. Centres of ossification begin to appear during the second week of life, but complete demonstration of each bone will not be possible until 2–3 months (there is variation between different dogs). While standard lateral and antero-posterior projections will demonstrate the area satisfactorily, oblique views can be advantageous in showing certain carpal bones.

The common reason for radiographing this joint is the investigation of acute or chronic injuries sustained by the racing greyhound. The bone usually involved is the accessory carpal (pisiform). In acute injuries fractures of this bone may be demonstrated, while with more chronic lesions subsequent radiography is likely to show small ossified spurs as the result of pulling of ligamentous insertions into the bone.

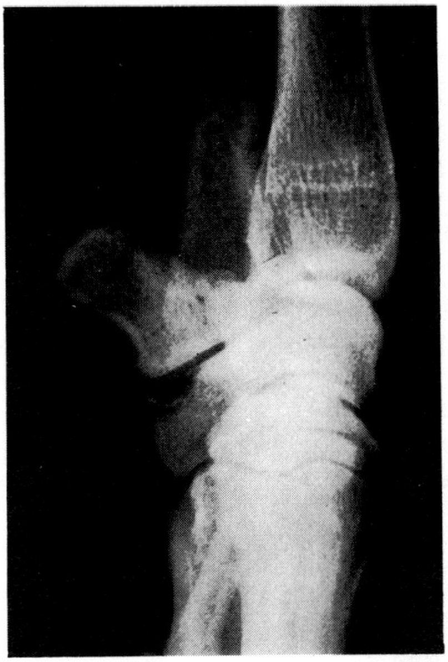

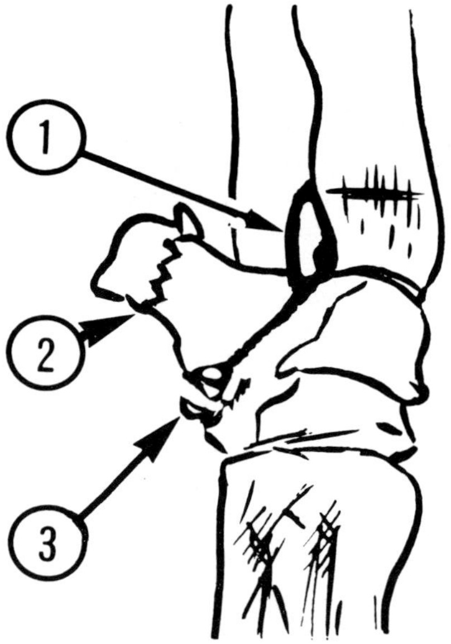

FIGS. 6.14 and 6.15. Multiple fractures involving, (1) the radius, and (2 and 3) the accessory carpal bone.

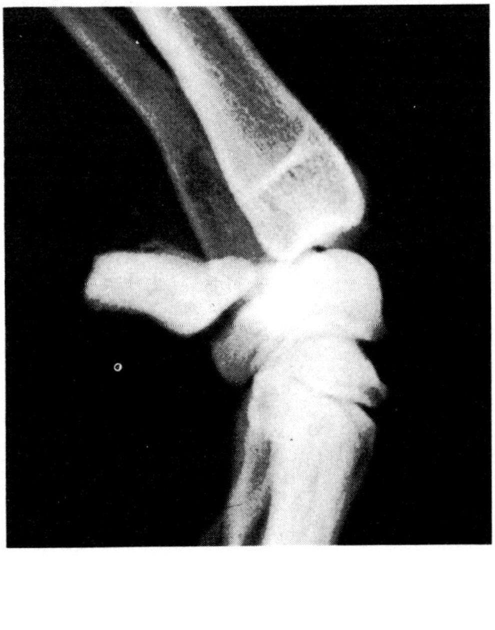

FIG. 6.16. Separation of a fragment of bone and roughening of the dorsal aspect of the accessory carpal bone, due to pulling of a tendinous insertion at this site.

Metacarpus

Since the individual bones are closely applied a fracture of a single bone may not be obvious if little displacement occurs. The normal presence of volar sesamoids (and occasionally of dorsal sesamoids) at the lower end of these bones is not always recognised.

Digits

The digits are the site of traumatic injuries which may need to be investigated radiologically. Fractures and dislocations occur and should be obvious, but the evidence of more chronic injuries may not be so apparent. In anteroposterior projections it is important to extend and flatten the region as far as possible in order to avoid foreshortening of the bones or apparent narrowing of joint spaces. In lateral views the digit under investigation should be drawn forward to separate it from adjacent bones.

Subluxation of a digital joint as the result of tearing of the collateral ligaments may show as definite malalignment of the two bones involved, but in many cases the sole evidence will be enlargement of the joint space—and this may not be obvious unless it can be contrasted with a normal joint.

In old standing joint lesions ("knocked up toe") radiography is likely to demonstrate chronic arthritic changes, with comparatively minute roughening and spurring around the joint and increased density of adjacent bone.

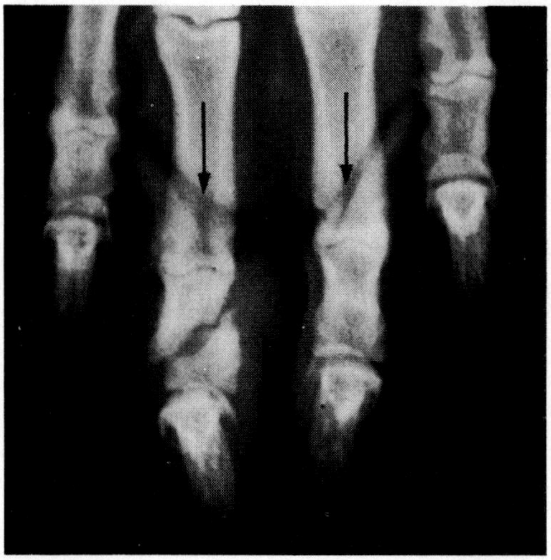

FIG. 6.17. Fracture of a second digit (note the outline of the pad of the foot creating a false effect of a fracture of the first digits).

Pelvis

The pelvis is a relatively complex bone and is best considered in relation to the two standard projections, since there is considerable difference between these, both in relation to their appearance and to their diagnostic value.

Ventro-dorsal projection This is the most informative and, in many instances, may be the only view required. However, if it is to be of diagnostic value, it is essential that the patient should be carefully positioned to ensure that the long axis of the pelvic symphysis is parallel with the film and that there is no lateral tilting of the bone. Significant deviation in either of these planes can seriously affect the X-ray image and the radiologist should examine the films for evidence of this. Lateral rotation would be shown by the fact that the two halves of the bone (particularly the outline of the obturator foramina) do not correspond exactly. Such a film, as well as preventing comparison between a suspected lesion and the corresponding "normal" half of the bone, would interfere with accurate visualisation of the sacro-iliac joints or precise reproduction of the important hip joints.

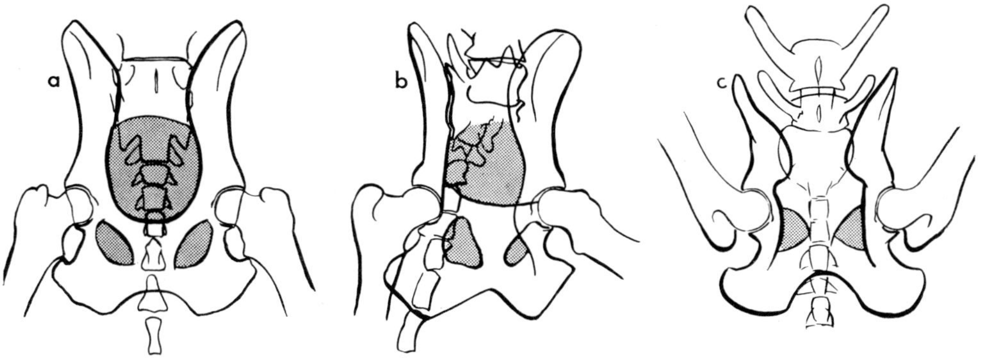

FIG. 6.18. The effect of positioning of the pelvis. (a) Correctly positioned. (b) Lateral rotation (c) Tilted.

Tilting in the other plane can be recognised because it produces a foreshortened appearance of the pubis and ischeum. Such distortion also interferes with accurate demonstration of the hip joint by creating a false effect of added depth to the acetabulum.

In the young growing animal radiographic reproduction of this bone is complicated by the fact that each half of the pelvis is formed from three separate bones and that each of these develops from more than one centre of ossification. The intervening non-ossified areas can, in some circumstances, be mistaken for fracture lines; or small centres of ossification for separated fragments of bone.

The development and radiological appearance of the canine pelvis has been studied and reported in considerable detail by Smith (1964). This author stresses that while there is a general progressive pattern of ossification and fusion of the various parts of the pelvis, there is considerable variation between individual dogs with regard to the precise age at which different stages of this occur. The most important radiological features are:

(a) Only a portion of the pubis, ischium and ilium are ossified at birth, and they are seen as separate bones. These bones are almost completely ossified and united with each other at an age which varies from 4 to 7 months.

(b) A separate centre of ossification (the os acetabuli) develops within the acetabulum at from 6 weeks to 4 months of age. Fusion of this with the surrounding 3 bones permits radiographic visualisation of the acetabulum.

(c) Other centres of ossification appear at the iliac crest (4–8 months), the ischial tuberosity (4–7 months), the ischial arch (5–10½ months) (this may in fact be made up of several centres which fuse), and at the posterior end of the pelvic symphysis.

The age at which these centres appear and at which they subsequently fuse with adjacent bone varies considerably and is spread over the first 4 to 12 months of age. In particular instances the centre of ossification situated at the iliac crest may not merge with adjacent bone until 2 years of age or even older.

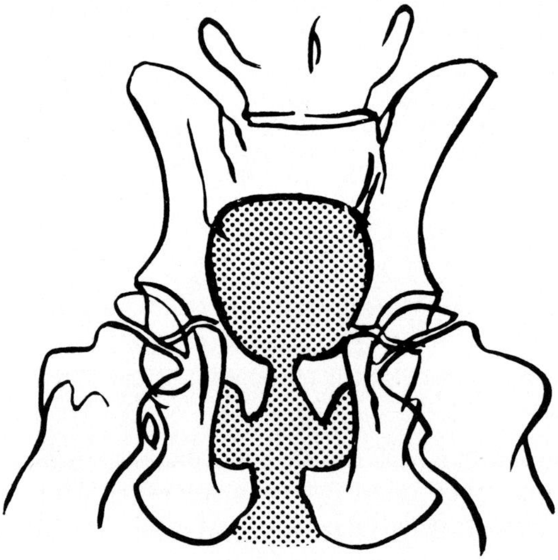

FIG. 6.19. Incomplete ossification of the pelvis at 61 days of age.

(d) Ossification of the pelvic symphysis occurs first at the posterior end and extends slowly anteriorly. Complete bony fusion has not been noted before 2 years of age and it is reported that it may not occur until 5 to 6 years.

In addition to the above progressive changes in the radiographic image of the bone it must be remembered that while there is not normally a bony union between the sacrum and the ilium, this may occur with age.

Clinical Radiology

The chief indication for radiography of this bone is the demonstration of traumatic injuries, which are seldom confined to a single fracture. The majority of such lesions will be obvious, provided that in the young dog, the significance of the non-ossified areas described above, is recognised. However, it will also be found that fractures at the symphysis or of the comparatively thin pubic and ischial bones can be partly obscured by the superimposition of faeces, the scrotum or the os penis.

Pelvic injuries can be complicated by separation of the bone from the sacrum and the radiologist should always check on this junction. In the absence of injury the outline of the inner edge of the shaft of the ilium will be seen to continue smoothly

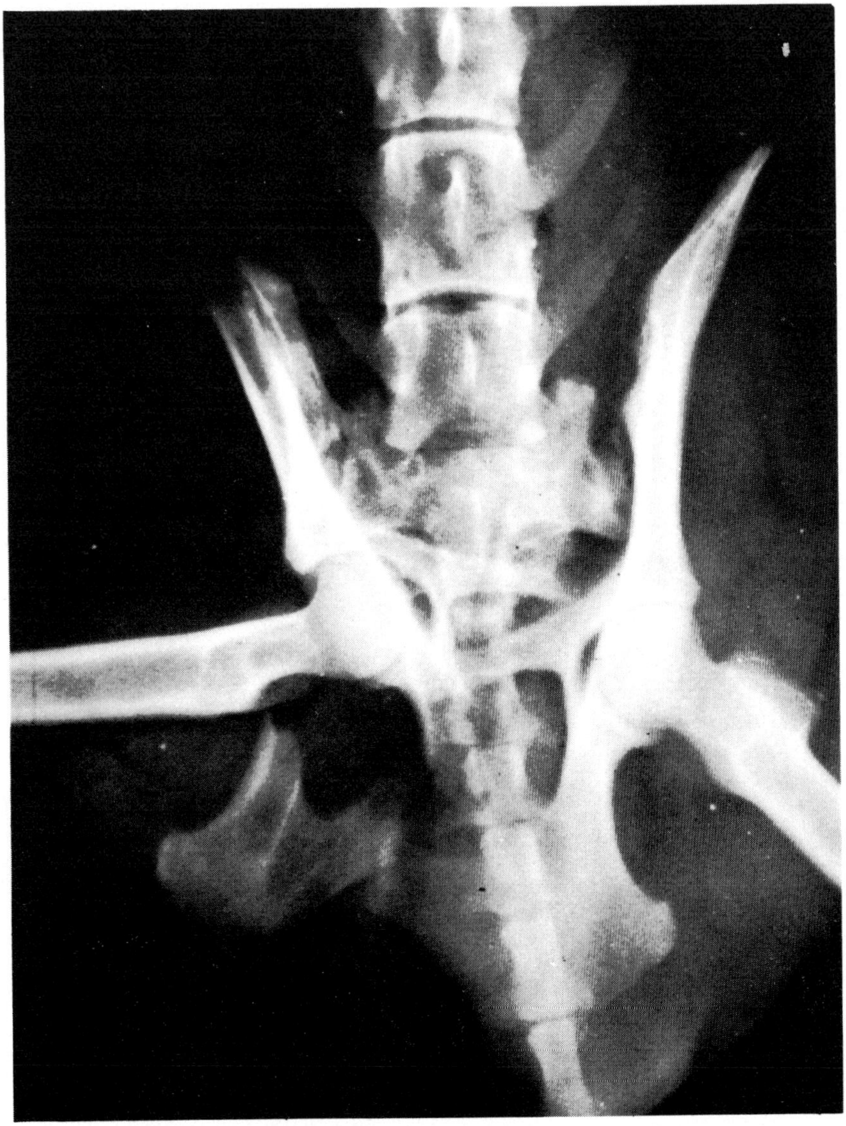

FIG. 6.20. Multiple fractures of the pelvis with separation of the ilia from the sacrum.

into the posterior border of the sacrum, but if sacro-iliac separation has occurred a "step" will be noted at the point of their junction.

While this bone is not a common site of neoplasia, it does occasionally occur.

Lateral Projections

The main purpose of this view is to give further information concerning any pelvic lesion already demonstrated in the other plane, and to show the extent and position of any dislocation of the femur on the pelvis.

Hip

The importance of precise positioning of the pelvis in relation to accurate radiography of the acetabulum has been stressed in the section above. Rotation of the femur on the pelvis can produce marked differences in the radiographic appearance of the other component of the joint, the femoral head, and precise positioning is again essential.

Owing to superimposition, lateral views are of very limited value in demonstrating this joint and ventro-dorsal projections are employed, with the dog placed in one of two positions:

(a) With the hind legs extended fully and uniformly backwards. The limbs should be slightly rotated towards the mid-line so that each patella is centred precisely over the femurs. This is the standard projection of maximum value.
(b) With the hind limbs fully flexed and abducted. It is again important to ensure that the positioning of each limb corresponds precisely. This projection is used when pain prevents full extension of the hip joint, or to alter the position of the femoral head within the acetabulum and to supplement the information obtained by the projection described above.

Anatomy

On account of its particular significance in relation to hip dysplasia, the radiological anatomy of this joint has been studied in considerable detail and the radiologist should be familiar with the following features:

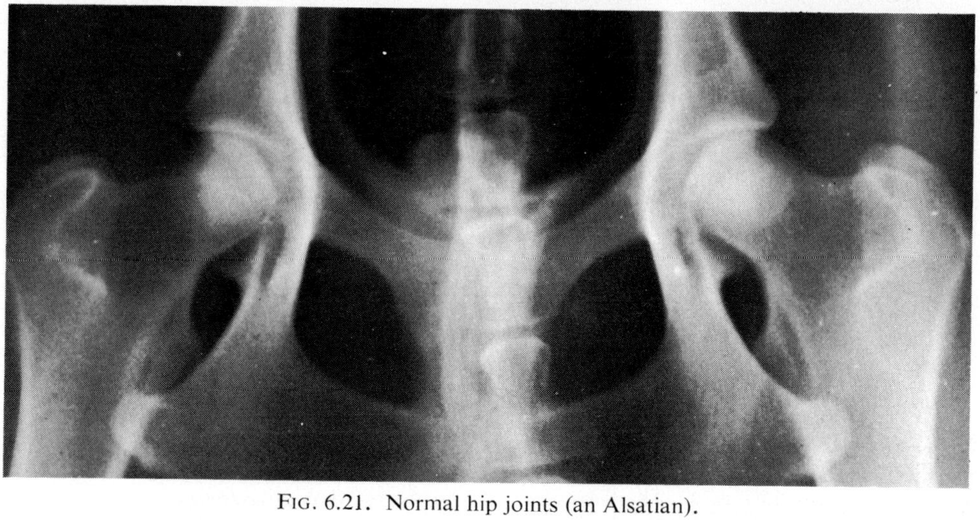

FIG. 6.21. Normal hip joints (an Alsatian).

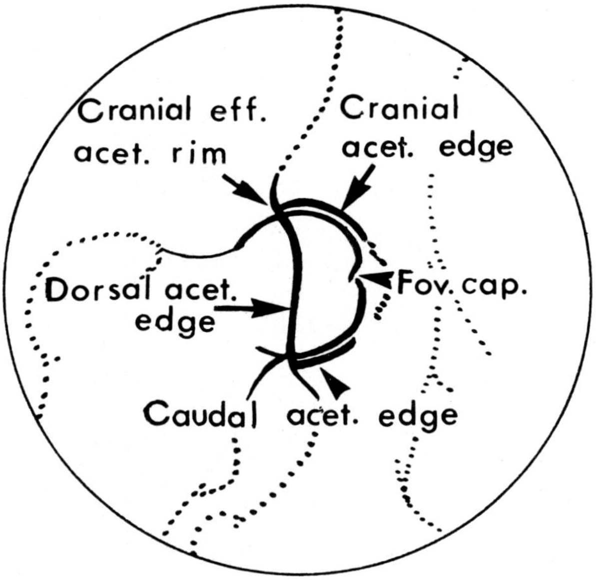

FIG. 6.22.

The Acetabulum

The Dorsal Acetabular Edge is seen as a slightly curved line visualised through the femoral head.

The ventral edge is concave and provides an indication of the depth of the acetabulum. The line of this edge is divided by the Acetabular Fossa into two portions, **The Cranial Acetabular Edge** and **The Caudal Acetabular Edge.** The junction of the dorsal acetabular edge with the cranial acetabular edge forms **The Cranial Effective Acetabular Rim,** a point of considerable importance in the evaluation of hip dysplasia. In the correctly positioned pelvic radiograph this point represents the most lateral portion of the bony acetabulum.

The Femoral Head

The head of the femur is seen as a smooth rounded outline forming roughly two thirds of a circle. When radiographed in the extended position this outline will show a small defect at the site of the **Fovea Capitis** but this will not be apparent in films taken with the limbs in the flexed position.

The Joint Space

This space will be visualised as a regular narrow band between the edge of the femoral head and the ventral acetabular edge. This band will appear distorted at the level of the acetabular fossa and the fovea capitis.

It will not be possible to recognise all of this detail in the young puppy. The acetabulum is formed by the fusion of the ilium, the pubis, the ischium and the small triangular shaped acetabular bone. Complete fusion and ossification of these bones may not be complete until about 6 months of age. The femoral head develops from one single centre of ossification and fuses with the shaft at an age of 6 months and upwards (up to 18 months has been reported).

However the general shape of the acetabulum and its relation to the femoral head can usually be recognised from about 2 months of age.

Pathology

The accurate diagnosis and differential diagnosis of abnormalities of the hip joint is very largely dependent on radiography and the following conditions have to be considered:

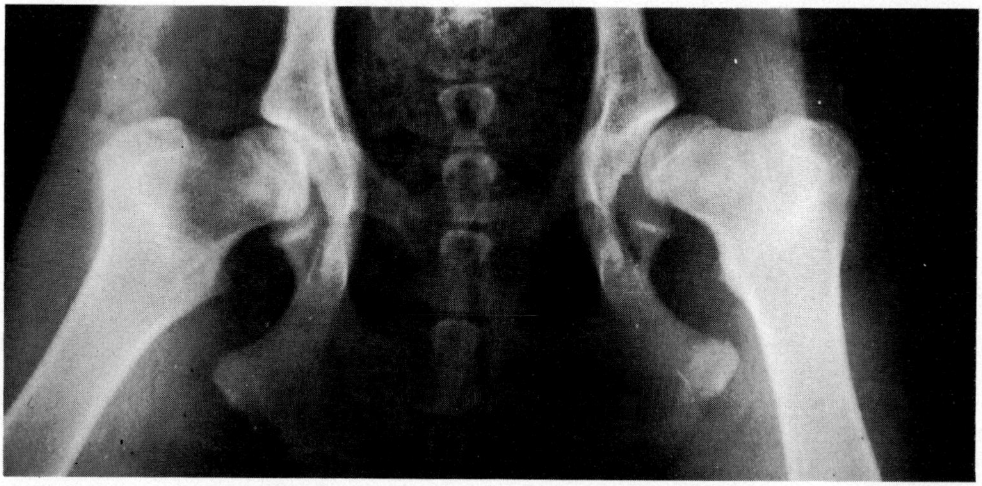

FIG. 6.23. Mild degree of hip dysplasia in a young Alsatian.

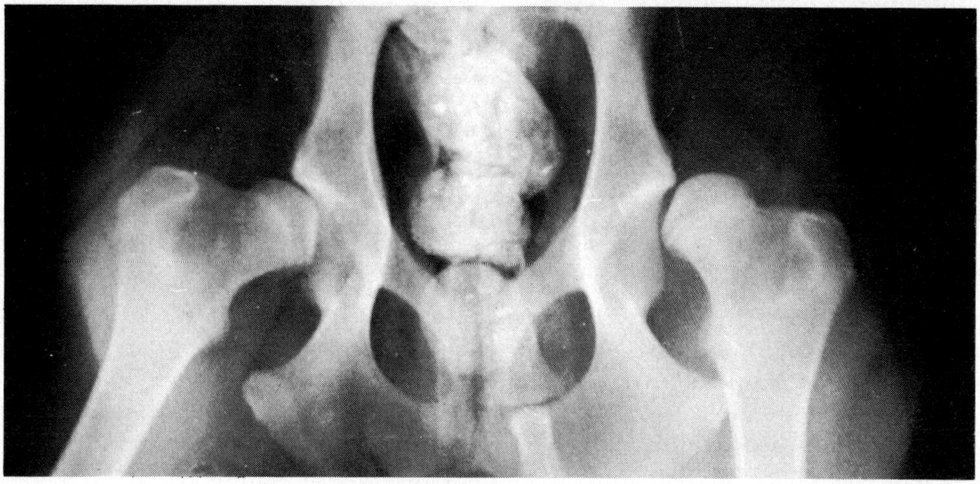

FIG. 6.24. Severe dysplasia of the hips of a 9 month old Alsatian dog.

Hip Dysplasia

The essential radiological features of hip dysplasia depend on:

(a) An irregular fit of the head of the femur within the acetabulum—due to shallowness of the acetabulum or to looseness and subluxation of the femur.

(b) The secondary changes which occur with time around and within the hip as a result of the irregular wear on the joint.

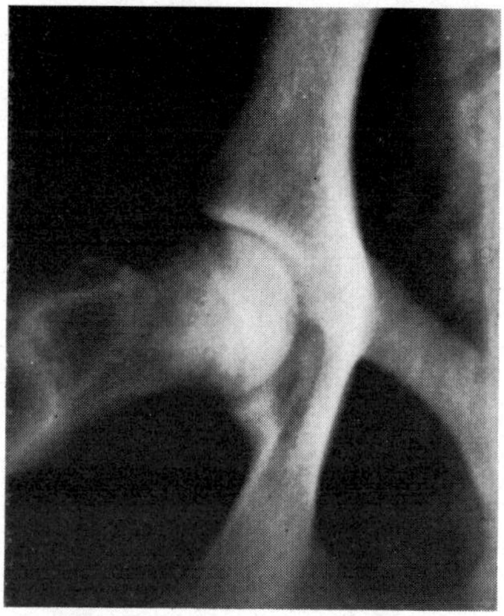

FIG. 6.25.

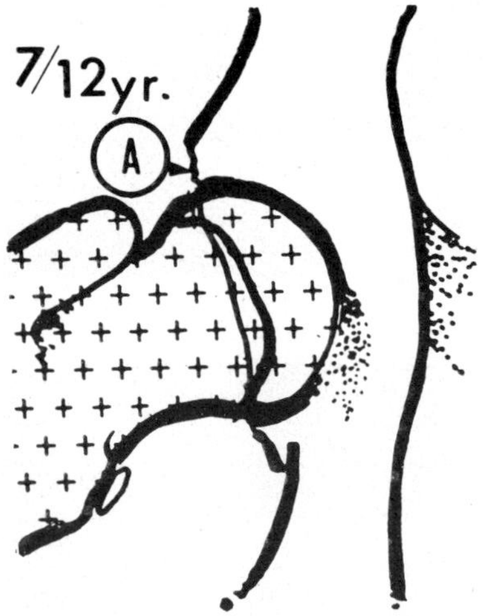

FIG. 6.26.

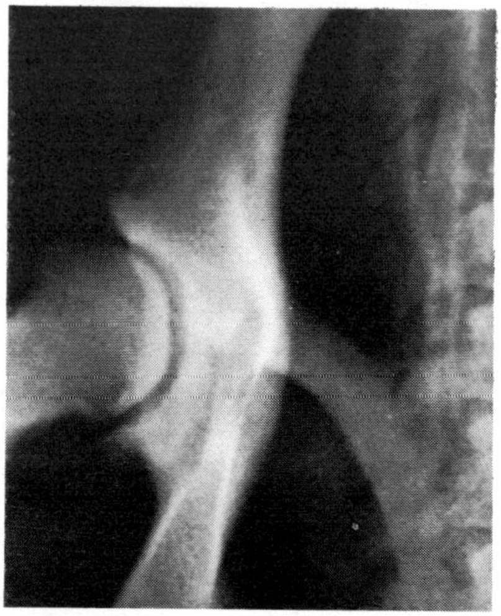

FIG. 6.27.

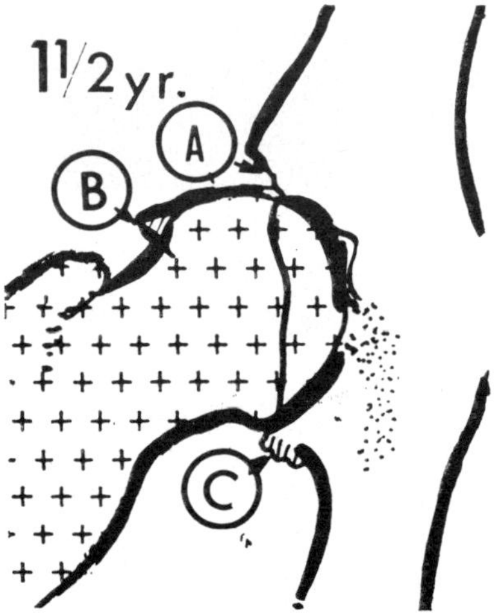

FIG. 6.28.

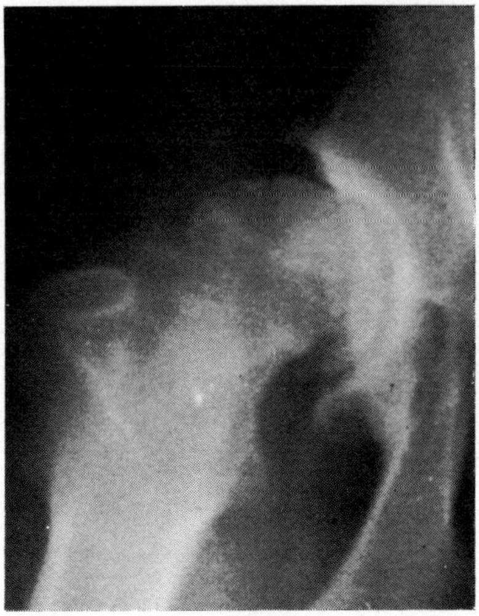

FIG. 6.29.

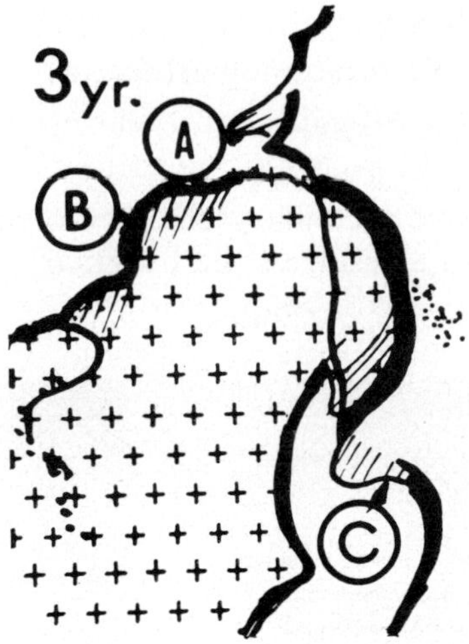

FIG. 6.30.

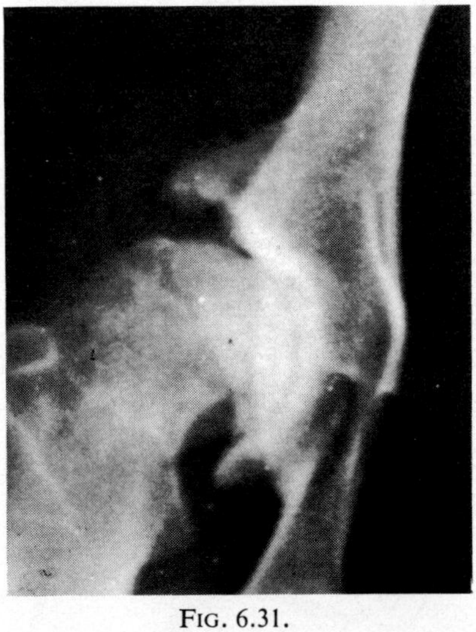

FIG. 6.31.

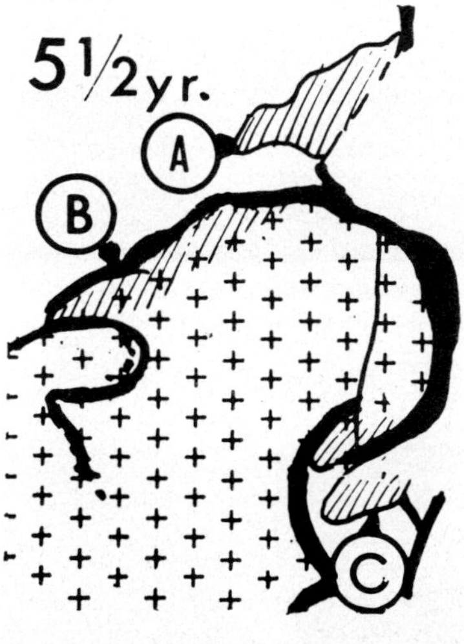

FIG. 6.32.

FIGS. 6.25 to 6.32. Progressive secondary changes of hip dysplasia affecting a Labrador dog over a period of 5 years (A) Bilabiation and new bone formation occurring in the region of the cranial effective acetabular rim. (B) Exostoses around the femoral neck. (C) New bone formation at the posterior limit of the caudal acetabular edge.

Radiologically the displacement of the head of the femur in relation to the acetabulum will be obvious in the more severely affected animals. But in mild and early cases this feature may be less apparent, and is best recognised by the fact that the lines of the cranial and caudal acetabular edges and of the femoral head are no longer parallel, but tend to diverge as they pass backwards.

A more precise and rigid method of estimating shallowness of the acetabulum or displacement of the femoral head is by means of Norberg's method. (See below).

There are three main manifestations of the secondary changes, all of which may, or may not, occur at the same time. The first of these represents an attempt to form a new articular facet to accommodate the altered position of the femoral head. This feature, which is termed "bilabiation" occurs primarily in the region of the cranial acetabular edge, where it produces a divergence of the curve of this edge and a smoothing off of the acute angle at the cranial effective acetabular rim.

The second feature is the development of bony exostoses around the joint which involve the acetabulum and the neck of the femur. The new bone formation involving the acetabulum occurs primarily at the cranial effective acetabular rim where it contributes to the bilabiation effect, but it may also occur on the dorsal acetabular edge and the caudal acetabular edge. The exostoses occurring on the femur produce a thickened, somewhat disorganised appearance of the femoral neck.

The third change takes place in the femoral head which undergoes a certain amount of remodelling and flattening. This, together with the new bone formation around the neck produces a shortened and thickened appearance of the femoral head and neck.

The main radiological characteristics of hip dysplasia have been described above, but it must be stressed that the early recognition of normal or of affected joints for the purposes of hip dysplasia eradication schemes, is a matter requiring precise positioning of the patient, careful radiography, and painstaking examination and interpretation of films.

It would also appear that allowances have to be made for breed variation and that in some of the chondrodystrophoid and brachycephalic breeds (e.g., Pekingese, Bulldogs, Pugs, etc.) radiography may reveal evidence of "loose hips" without this being associated with clinical symptoms or subsequent osteoarthritic changes. The whole subject is of considerable interest and importance to the veterinary radiologist and for further information, attention is drawn to some of a long list of articles on this subject (Olsson 1961, Report of the Panel on Canine Hip Dysplasia 1961, Lawson 1963, 1968).

The Norberg Method of Assessing Hip Dysplasia

This consists of the use of a means of measuring the angle formed by:

(a) A line joining the centres of the two femoral heads.

(b) A line joining the centre of the femoral head on the side being examined to the effective acetabular rim on the same side.

Any measurements of less than 105° are considered to indicate that the femoral head is displaced in relation to the acetabulum and that dysplasia is present.

In order to carry out such measurements it is necessary to prepare a suitable scale on a thick sheet of perspex or similar transparent material as follows:

Draw a series of closely applied concentric circles and make a small hole at the exact centre.

Draw a base line passing through the hole, and from the hole draw two other lines at an angle of 105° to the base line.

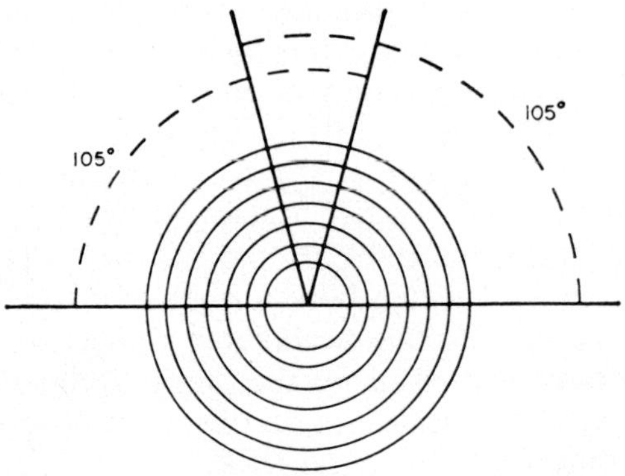

FIG. 6.33. Norberg scale.

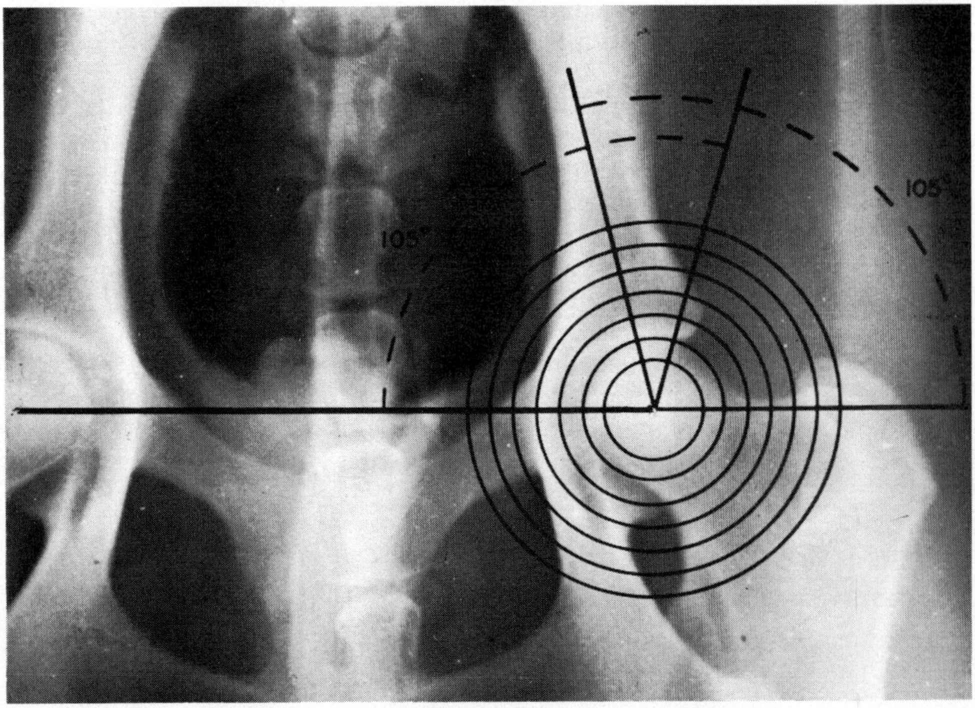

FIG. 6.34. The Norberg scale in use.

In use the scale is placed over each femoral head on the radiograph in such a way that the circles correspond with the femoral outline and a pin or pencil can be passed through the hole, to mark the exact centre. These points are then joined by a line and the scale is replaced on the radiograph so that its base line corresponds with the line just drawn and the hole in the scale coincides with the centre of the femoral head of the joint being examined. It should then be apparent if the angle of the position of the effective acetabular rim is more or less than the specified amount.

While this can be an accurate method of demonstrating displacement of the femoral head, it requires a carefully prepared scale and exact positioning of this on a high quality radiograph, if the method is to be of any value.

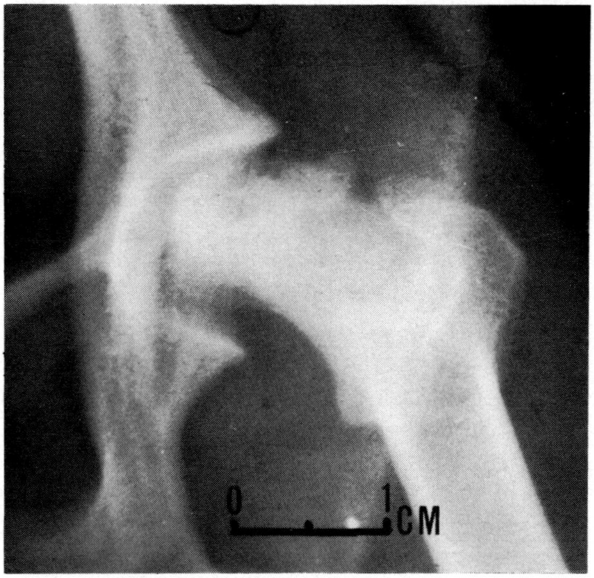

FIG. 6.35. Osteochondritis of the hip of an 18 month old miniature Poodle (illustration slightly enlarged).

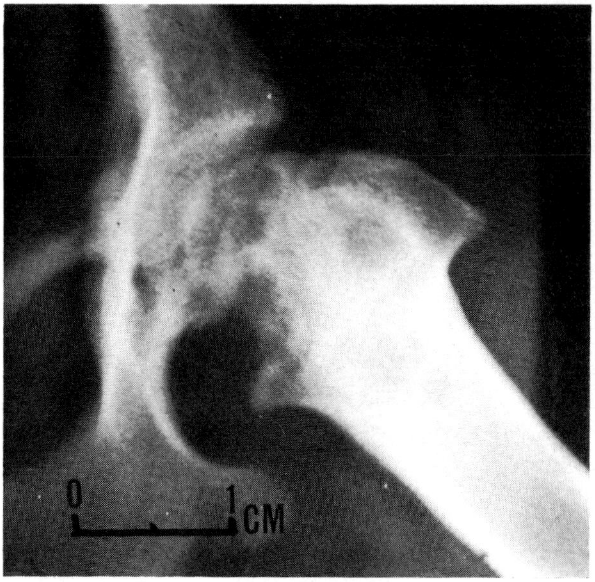

FIG. 6.36. Particularly severe lesion of osteochondritis affecting the hip of a 10 month old Pekingese (illustration slightly enlarged).

Osteochondritis (Osteochondritis Juvenilis, Spontaneous Aseptic Necrosis of the Head of the Femur, Legg-Perthes' Disease)

The essential changes which occur in this condition seen in the smaller breeds of dog are an aseptic necrosis and subsequent collapse of the femoral head, followed by secondary changes in the acetabulum and the femoral neck.

Because of its comparatively insidious onset radiography is not usually undertaken until the lesion is comparatively advanced. In the early stages radiological changes are confined to the femoral head which is ill-defined, irregular in outline and shows areas of increased and decreased bone density (Figs. 6.35 and 6.36).

In the later stages some remodelling of the whole region occurs—the femoral head is flattened and irregular but more distinctly outlined, the femoral neck is thickened and denser and a compensatory flattening of the acetabulum occurs.

Slipped Upper Femoral Epiphysis

Symptoms may again be insidious in onset and secondary changes have often occurred by the time that radiography is undertaken. In an early case the radiological changes are typical but not very obvious, and comprise a widening of the epiphyseal line and the development of a "step" in the contour of the femoral head at the end of the epiphyseal line. In old standing cases an irregular distortion of the femoral head and thickening of the femoral neck will occur and can closely resemble that seen in advanced osteochondritis.

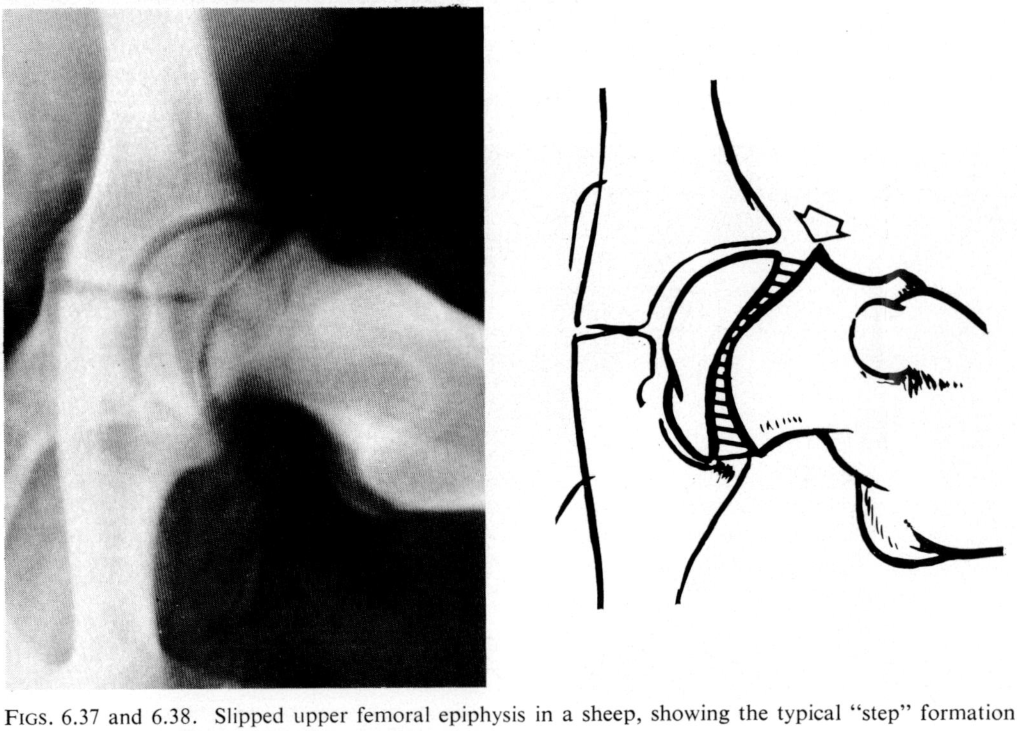

FIGS. 6.37 and 6.38. Slipped upper femoral epiphysis in a sheep, showing the typical "step" formation.

Distinguishing features are that this condition shows less collapse and flattening of the femoral head and more definite angulation of the head in relation to the neck.

Complete Separation of the Femoral Head

This condition is usually of sudden onset and therefore likely to be examined before secondary changes occur. The fracture and separation along the epiphyseal line should be obvious in a radiograph. However, it is possible in a dorso-ventral radiograph for the femoral neck to appear to be still attached to the head, unless a lateral projection is obtained to show the separation.

If the lesion is radiographed at a considerably later date, some atrophy and an absorption of the femoral head, and rounding and thickening of the femoral neck will be evident.

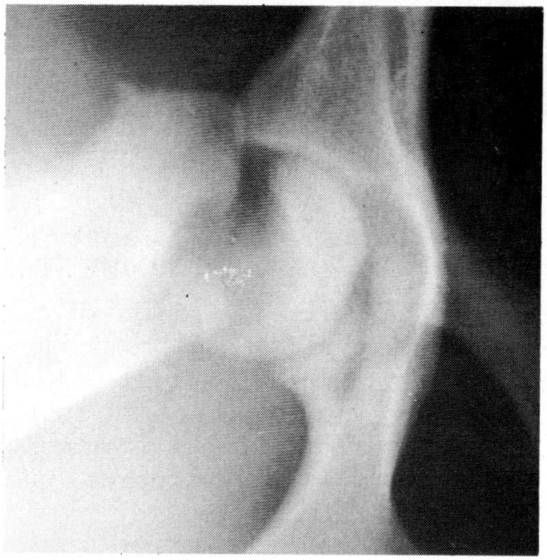

FIG. 6.39. Complete separation of the femoral head.

Fracture of Femoral Neck (see below)

Dislocation

There is normally no difficulty in recognising dislocation of the hip joint in a radiograph. Occasionally the head of the femur may be superimposed on the acetabulum in ventro-dorsal projections and the dislocation may not be obvious unless lateral views are consulted. Such views are also important in providing information concerning the direction of the displacement of the femur.

Dislocation of this joint can be complicated by fracture of the acetabulum or of a portion of the femoral head, and the radiograph should always be checked for this, as it can interfere with correction of the injury and also have an important bearing on the prognosis.

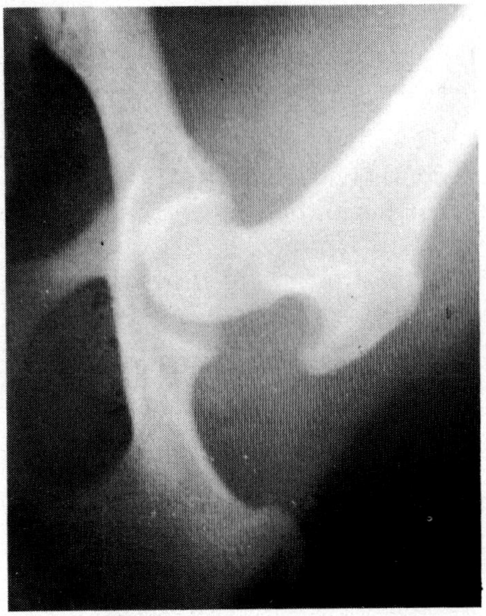

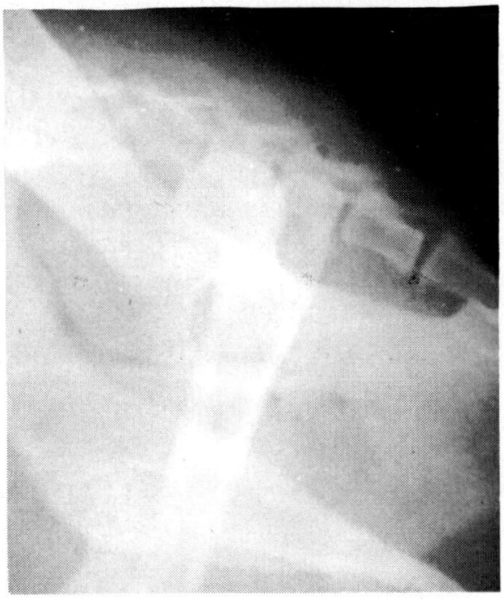

FIGS. 6.40 and 6.41. Two projections of the same hip joint showing that the dislocation could have been overlooked in the ventro-dorsal view.

Femur

As with the humerus, there is a marked difference in the amount of muscle and soft tissues surrounding the two ends of the femur. Therefore, care must be taken to ensure that the long axis of the bone is parallel with the film if a reasonably accurate reproduction is to be obtained (important when measuring the length of the bone before cutting an intermedullary pin). For the same reason, exposure factors will need to be adjusted for optimum demonstration of either end of the bone.

Pathology

This bone is a common site of fractures and of neoplasia and the radiographic demonstration of the majority of such lesions should be straightforward. However, injuries involving the upper and lower epiphyses can be less obvious and it is worth drawing attention to these:

Fractures of the Femoral Neck require to be distinguished from separation of the femoral head (described above) since they may carry a different prognosis, and the exact level of the fracture has to be carefully checked. Fractures at this level (particularly in cats) can be complicated by additional fractures involving separation of the epiphysis at the great trochanter.

Fractures of the Lower Epiphysis are usually self-evident, but injuries involving a single condyle or a portion of it can be overlooked unless radiographs are taken in both planes.

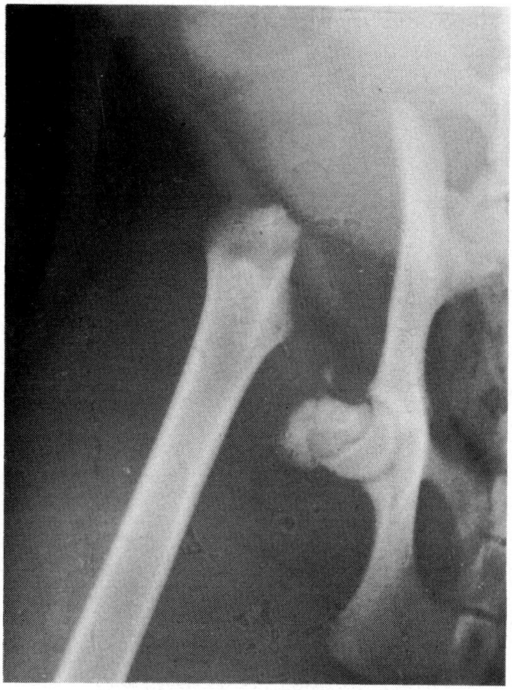

Fig. 6.42. Fracture of the femoral neck of a cat.

Stifle

It is necessary to emphasise that antero-posterior and postero-anterior projections of this joint do not produce comparable radiographs. The latter views are preferable as the film can be placed closer to the bone and a more accurate reproduction can be obtained. Even in this projection, care must be taken to align the X-ray beam correctly, or a false effect of narrowing of the joint will be produced.

Pathology

This is a common site of lameness in the dog and radiography is frequently employed in its investigation. However, even in cases of severe disability, the lesions which can be demonstrated by radiography may be far less than expected.

Some comment on the following conditions of this joint is necessary:

Dislocation of the Patella

In general, radiography has little advantage over clinical examination in demonstrating luxation of the patella. It must also be borne in mind that an oblique view of the joint can create a false impression of displacement of this bone; or that the dislocation can reduce spontaneously while the patient is being positioned.

Once the condition is diagnosed, however, radiography can provide further information which may influence the treatment or prognosis. Thus "skyline" views of the intercondylar groove, can be employed to show if the normal groove of the trochlea is present or if the tendency to luxation is associated with a poorly formed medial ridge. Similarly, radiography may be required to demonstrate early rotation and malformation of the femur and tibia as a result of congenital luxation of the patella in a young puppy.

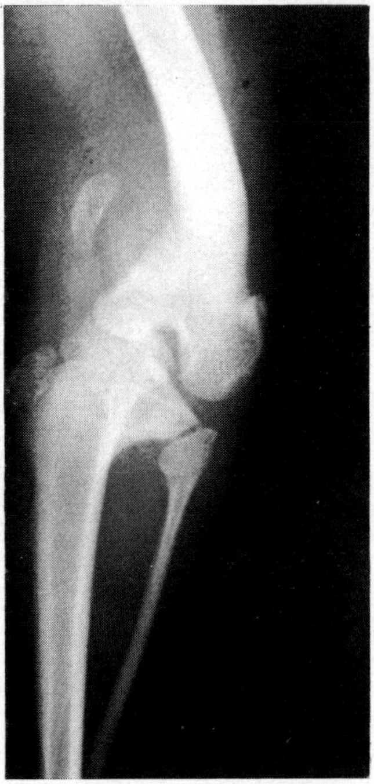

FIG. 6.43. Malformation of the femur and tibia associated with complete dislocation of the patella.

Traumatic Injuries

In recent injuries lateral radiographs might show definite anterior or posterior displacement of the tibia in relation to the femur, thus visualising the anterior or posterior "draw sign" considered to be diagnostic of rupture of the anterior or posterior cruciate ligaments. Similarly, lateral or medial displacement of these bones in an antero-posterior projection would be an indication of rupture of the collateral ligaments. (It must be borne in mind that negative findings in either of these circumstances do not mean that the injury was not present, but merely that there was no displacement at the time of radiography.)

Injuries to the menisci can be difficult or impossible to demonstrate by radiographic means. While the use of air arthrography is sometimes advised in such circumstances, little has been reported concerning the lesions demonstrated by these means.

In more chronic traumatic conditions some evidence of osteoarthritis is likely to be recognised with the development of osteophytes and areas of increased and decreased bone density in adjacent bone.

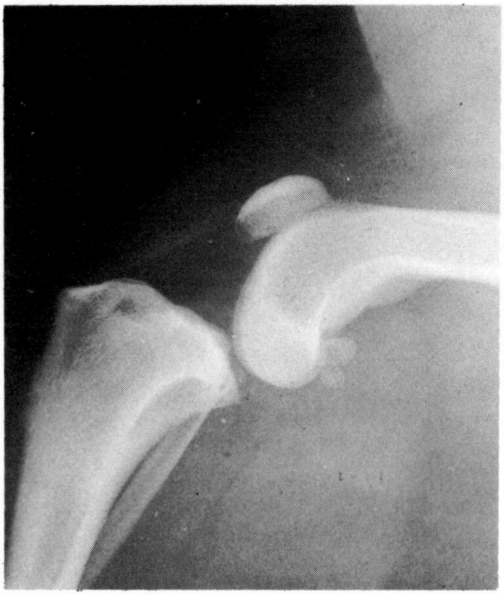

FIG. 6.44. Posterior displacement of the femur on the tibia resulting from rupture of the cruciate ligaments.

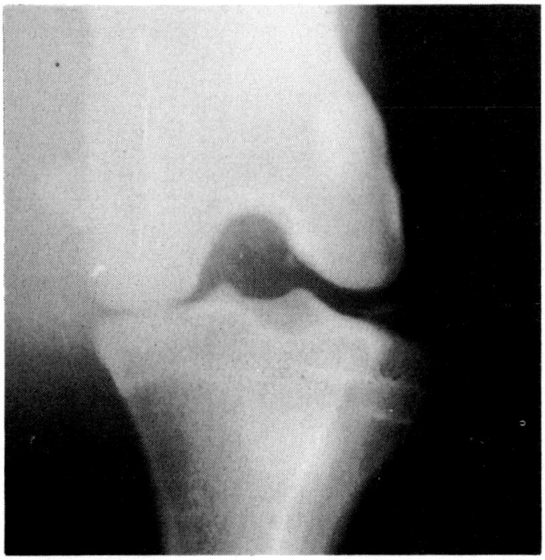

FIG. 6.45. Angulation of the stifle joint due to tearing of the lateral ligament.

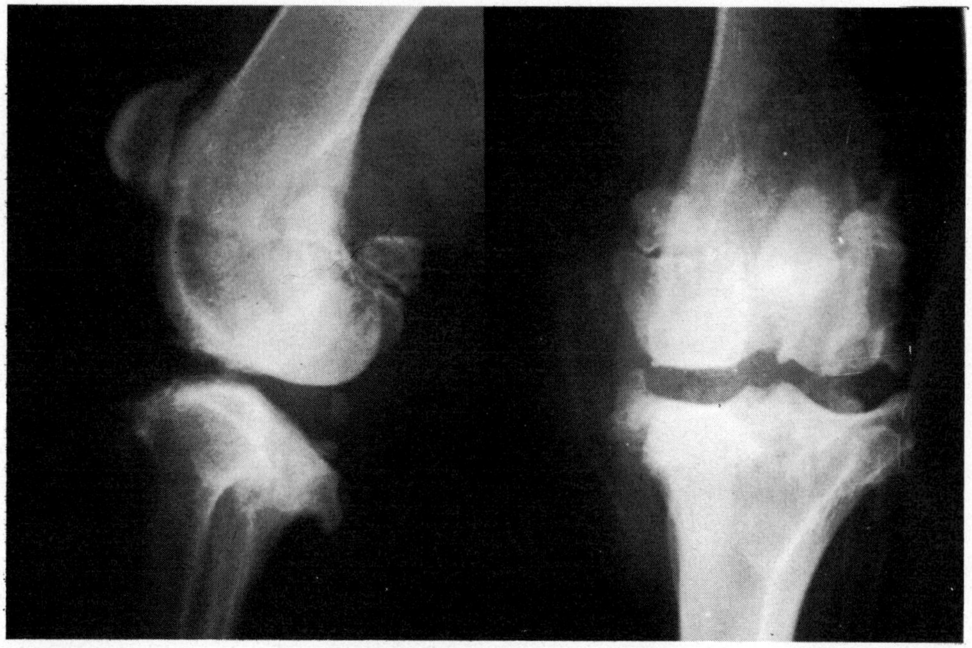

FIG. 6.46. Severe osteoarthritis of the stifle joint.

FIG. 6.47. Radiographic tracings of the tibia and fibula of a Dachshund (a and c) and a Greyhound (b and d).

Tibia and Fibula

There are two points relating to radiological anatomy which should be mentioned:

(a) The marked bending and distortion which is seen in the radius and ulna of chondrodystrophoid breeds of dogs does not occur to the same extent in these bones. However, the relative forshortening of the tibia which occurs in these breeds does give the effect of some curving of the upper end of the bone. Furthermore, in the same breeds, the fibula will show a definite curve—suggesting that it has developed to a greater length than the tibia to which it is attached (cf. radius and ulna, page 97).

(b) The anterior tibial tuberosity develops from a separate centre of ossification and is relatively late in uniting completely with the rest of the bone (Smith and Allcock 1960, report that, in the Greyhound this fusion is not complete until 59 weeks of age). Before this fusion is complete, the comparatively wide non-calcified area can be mistaken for a fracture line, or can make it difficult to recognise an avulsion of this tuberosity when it does occur.

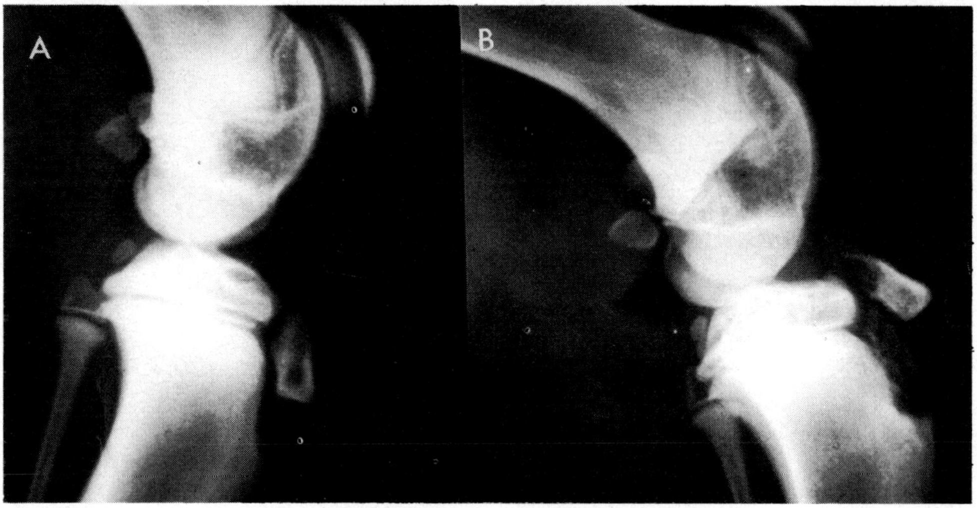

FIG. 6.48. Radiographs of both stifle joints of a 6 month old Greyhound. (A) is normal (B) shows avulsion of the anterior tibial tuberosity.

Tarsus

Anatomy

While the majority of the tarsal bones are cartilagenous at birth and cannot be shown in a radiograph, the tibial tarsal (astragalus) and fibula tarsal (os calcis) bones do normally show small centres of ossification at this age. Ossification of the other bones commences early in life and the outline of all the bones is reasonably complete by about 8 weeks of age.

Pathology

The main reason for radiographing this region is the investigation of traumatic injuries, resulting in dislocations of fracturés of one or more bones, It is not always easy to identify the precise bone or bones involved unless the area is radiographed in both planes and compared with corresponding views of the normal limb.

The commonest injuries are; fractures of the tibial tarsal bone (astragalus) usually with obvious displacement of the upper portion, and fractures of the central tarsal bone (scaphoid) in the racing Greyhound with forward displacement of the fractured portion and some degree of resultant collapse of the whole tarsus. If the latter injury is not investigated until some weeks later, radiographs may show considerable ankylosis and distortion of the whole region making it impossible to identify the precise bone involved.

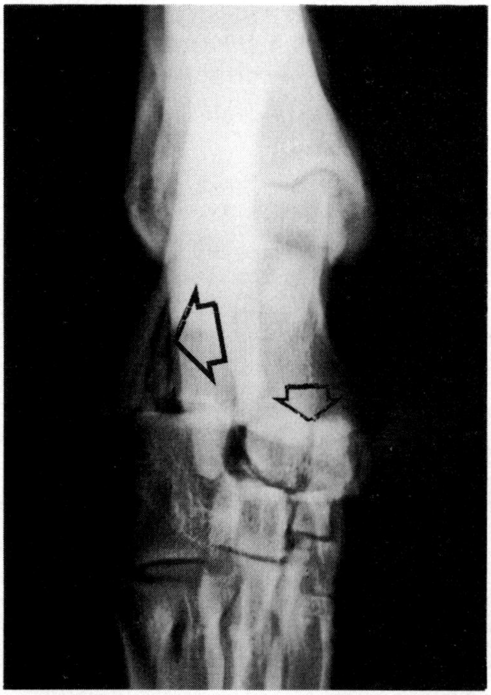

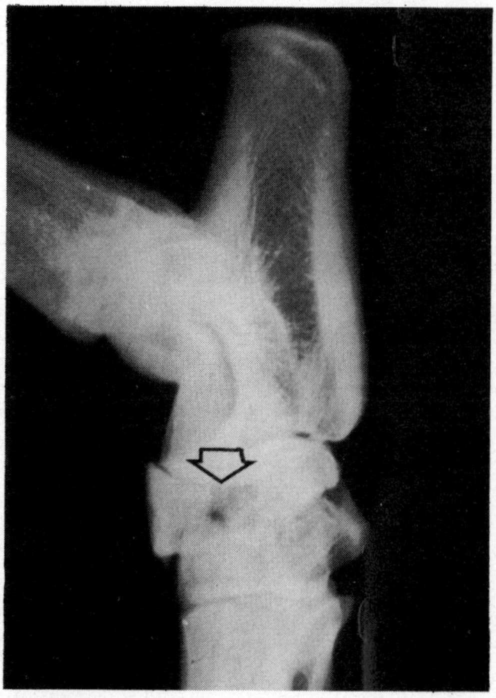

FIGS. 6.49. and 6.50. Two projections of the tarsus showing a small fracture of the tibial tarsal bone and a fracture with displacement of the central tarsal bone.

Metatarsus and Digits

This area corresponds precisely with the fore limb.

REFERENCES

Craig, P. H., and Riser, W. H. (1965), J. Am, vet. Radiol. Soc., **6**, 40.
Evans, P. J. (1968), J. small Anim. Pract., **9**, 55,
Lawson, D. D. (1963), Vet. Rec., **75**, 445.

Lawson, D. D. (1968), Vet. Rec., **83,** 655.
Olsson, S.-E. (1961), Advances in Small Animal Practice. Vol. **3,** page 112. Oxford: Pergamon Press.
Report of Panel on Canine Hip Dysplasia (1961), J. Am. vet. med. Ass., **139,** 791.
Riser, W. H., and Shirer, J. F. (1965), J. Am. vet. Radiol. Soc., **6,** 50.
Smith, R. N. (1964), Vet. Rec. 76, 975.
Smith, R. N., and Allcock, J. (1960), Vet. Rec., **72,** 75.

CHAPTER 7

LARGE ANIMAL RADIOLOGY

A number of factors (e.g., the size of the patient and the low power of most veterinary apparatus, problems of moving and restraining the patient and economic considerations) have all combined to restrict the use which has been made of radiography for the examination of large animals in veterinary practice. Such use has been very largely confined to the investigation of the lower limbs of horses and (to a very limited extent) of cattle, and it is only in this region that any detailed knowledge of veterinary radiological interpretation has been built up. Such radiography as has been undertaken, even within this restricted field, has been principally directed to the investigation of the clinical case and, with a few exceptions, no systematic studies have been directed to normal radiological anatomy and its variation with species, breed and age.

In other body areas and in other large animal species knowledge of the precise radiological anatomy and of the pathological conditions which can be demonstrated by radiography is inevitably limited, although this is beginning to be investigated by those individuals and centres which possess the necessary facilities. In these circumstances the veterinary radiologist should be cautious in making a diagnosis and must depend on his own general experience of radiology and on his knowledge of the anatomy and likely pathology of the part, in interpreting films.

From the above comments it will be obvious that at the present time the chief value of the radiographic examination of large animals is in the investigation and diagnosis of acute and chronic conditions of the skeletal system.

Most gross fractures of large animals can be recognised on clinical examination and as transportation of the patient is difficult and treatment is not often practicable radiography is seldom required for precise demonstration of the extent of the injury. It is, however, of importance in the demonstration of less obvious fractures of the smaller bones (the carpus and tarsus, the phalanges, the sesamoids, etc.) which may be suitable for treatment.

The other common indication for the use of radiography in these species is in the investigation of chronic inflammatory lesions, particularly in the horse. Such lesions may show any of the radiological manifestations of bone disease described in Chapter 3, but in the horse they usually take either or both of two main forms:

(a) Periostial Reaction (Periostitis)

This inflammatory condition of the periosteum usually results from traumatic injury (pulling or tearing of adjacent muscular and tendinous insertions) but could be due to infection. The first radiological evidence of this process would be indefinite and would be seen as soft tissue swelling in the affected area. The more typical bony changes will take time (a matter of weeks or months) to develop and will be recognised as osteophytic outgrowths from the surface of the bone. Such new bone formation may be small and localised, and if this is to be demonstrated satisfactorily care must be taken to avoid over-penetration of the part and to direct the X-ray beam at an appropriate angle (oblique projections may be necessary in addition to the standard views).

In many instances radiography, as well as showing the site and extent of such lesions, can provide some indication as to whether they are likely to be stationary or progressive. Thus an active extending process will show an ill-defined edge with the bone-forming process extending into the surrounding tissues, while a particularly distinct outline would suggest that the inflammatory process had subsided. In doubtful cases such impressions would, of course, be confirmed by repeating the radiographic examination of the part some weeks or months later.

(b) Osteoarthritis

This is characterised by two pathological processes which can be demonstrated radiologically to a varying degree.

The first of these, erosion of the cartilagenous joint surface, will not initially be recognisable in a radiograph. If the process extends, however, it will be visualised by distortion or collapse of the joint space or by osteoporosis of underlying bone (e.g., in navicular disease). Radiography may also show compensatory sclerosis of the area of bone adjacent to the eroded part.

The second process—the development of hypertrophic changes around the edge of the joint is usually accompanied by new bone formation and this will be demonstrable in a film. The amount of such bone can vary from small osteophytes at the margin of the joint, to large formations of new bone which may result in ankylosis.

THE HORSE

The Shoulder, Humerus, Elbow, Radius and Ulna

While in some circumstances the general outline of these bones and joints can be demonstrated by radiography in the standing animal, the films produced will be of poor quality and will not show fine detail. Furthermore, in most clinical conditions affecting this region, the patient will not tolerate the extension of the limb necessary for radiography. Casting and anaesthetisation of the animal, together with the use of a good quality grid and relatively high exposure factors, are necessary to permit accurate demonstration of the area.

Radiography of the lower half of the radius is straight forward but visualisation of the ulna in this region can be very variable. Morgan (1965) has studied differences in the radiological appearance of the distal ulna in a number of normal horses. This author reports that in some instances the lower end of the ulna is not ossified and perceptible in a film, but where ossification has occurred, it may appear narrow or wide and may occasionally show lack of continuity suggesting a "fracture". It is also noted that variation between opposite limbs may occur on the same animal.

The Carpus

This joint can be radiographed without difficulty but some overlap and superimposition of individual bones will occur in all projections.

Fractures The ease with which fractures of individual carpal bones can be recognised will depend on the amount of displacement that occurs, and in doubtful cases films will require careful comparison with similar projections of the opposite limb.

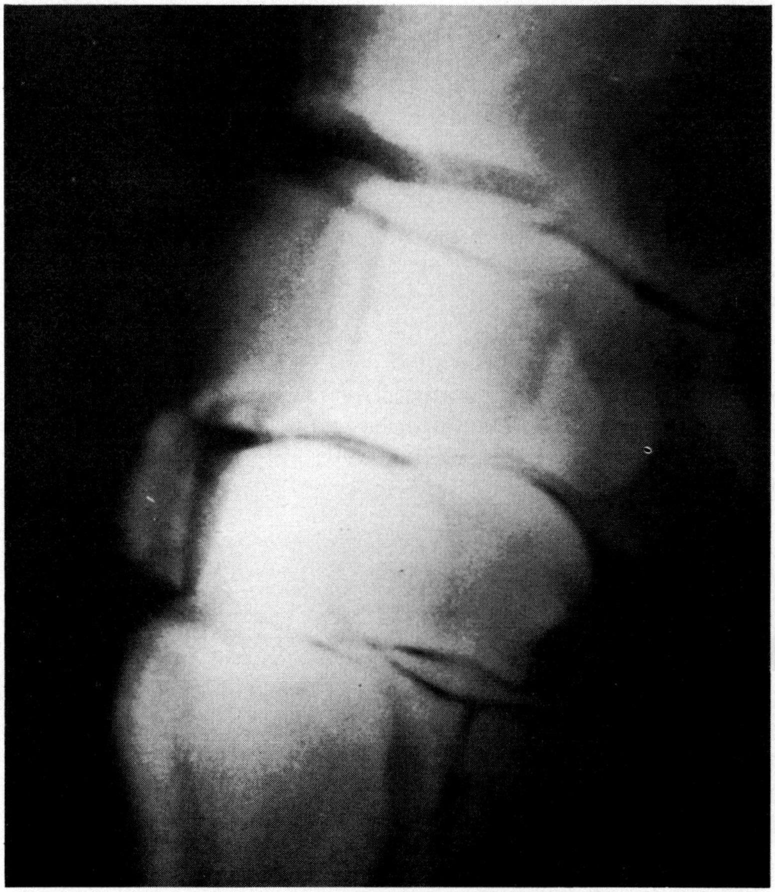

FIG. 7.1. Fracture of a small portion of the radial carpal bone.

A fairly common carpal fracture which can be lost in the standard antero-posterior and lateral views is separation of a fragment of bone from the antero-medial aspect of the radial carpal as a result of pulling of a ligamentous insertion.

Carpitis This term is used for chronic inflammatory conditions of this joint with characteristic osteoarthritic changes. Such changes usually commence on the anterior surface of the joint and will be recognised first in lateral projections. As the process extends new bone formation may occur on the lateral and medial aspects of the joint and within the intercarpal joint space (best demonstrated by lateral projections of the flexed joint).

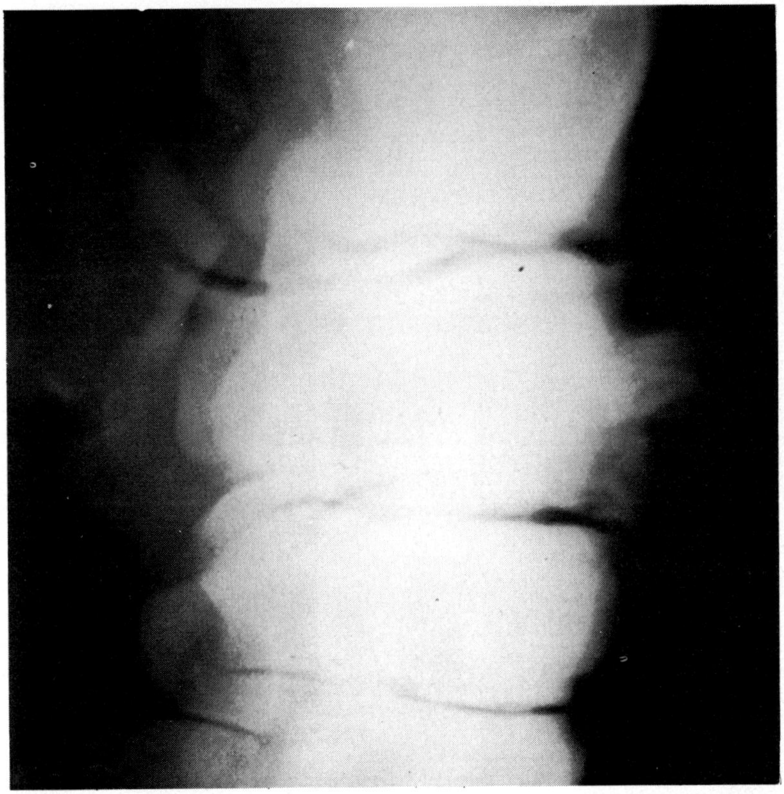

FIG. 7.2. Carpitis, with considerable new bone formation on the anterior surface of the upper row of carpal bones.

The Metacarpus

The large (third) metacarpal bone is easily radiographed and may be examined to show the full extent of fractures or of lesions of periostitis.

At birth this bone shows a distinct distal epiphysis but no proximal epiphysis.

The small (second and fourth) metacarpal bones do not show any evidence of a separate epiphysis at birth. These bones are frequently radiographed to show evidence of periostitis—the condition commonly termed "splints". The condition is characterised by new bone formation which distorts the outline of the bone and tends to result in fusion of the affected bone with the adjacent large metacarpal bone.

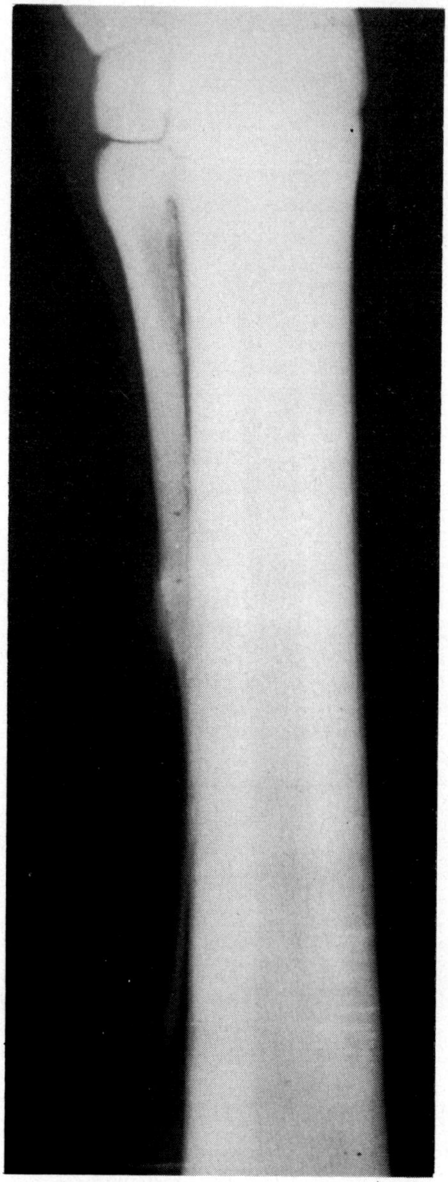

FIG. 7.3. Early splint formation.

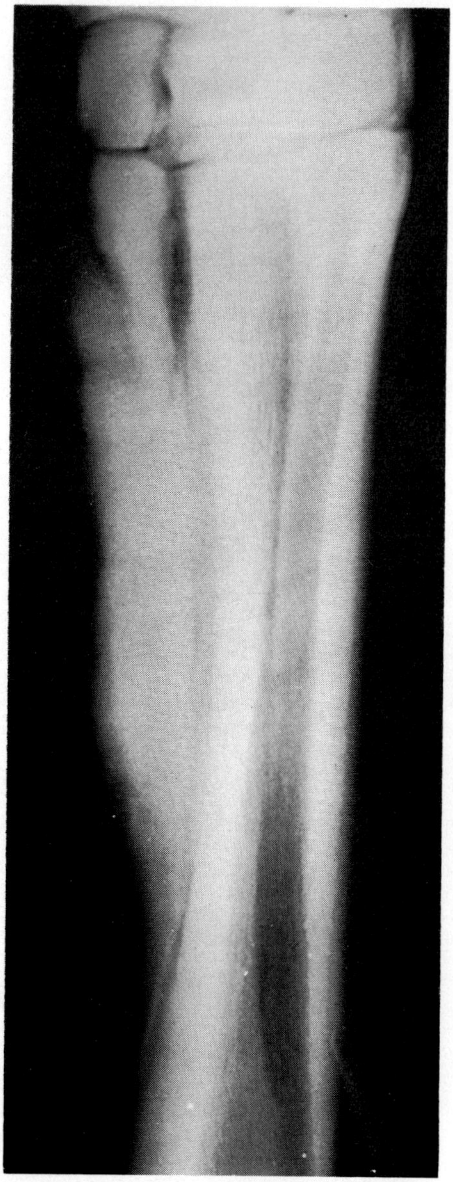

FIG. 7.4. Gross periosteal new bone formation around the small metacarpal bone.

Where such changes are slight they will only be visualised in oblique projections of the region but larger lesions will project beyond the large metacarpal bone and will be visible in the usual lateral and antero-posterior projections.

Similarly, fractures of these small bones can be overlooked unless oblique views are employed.

The Sesamoids

These small bones can be the site of significant radiological lesions which may require careful radiographic technique for their demonstration. Although they are situated completely behind the large metacarpal bone they can be demonstrated in the antero-posterior plane, provided that the exposure factors are adjusted to permit adequate penetration of the larger bone. Obviously lateral views will lead to superimposition and in some circumstances oblique projections may be necessary.

Fractures of these bones tend to occur in the horizontal plane and may, or may not, be associated with displacement of the fragments and in the latter circumstances will not be easily perceived.

Evidence of periosteal damage as the result of pulling of tendinous insertions may be recognised by separation of small fragments of bone or by other evidence of periostitis (areas of osteoporosis and of new bone formation).

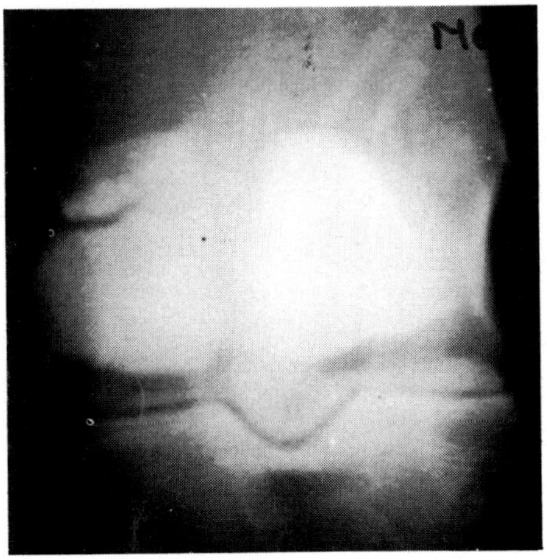

FIG. 7.5

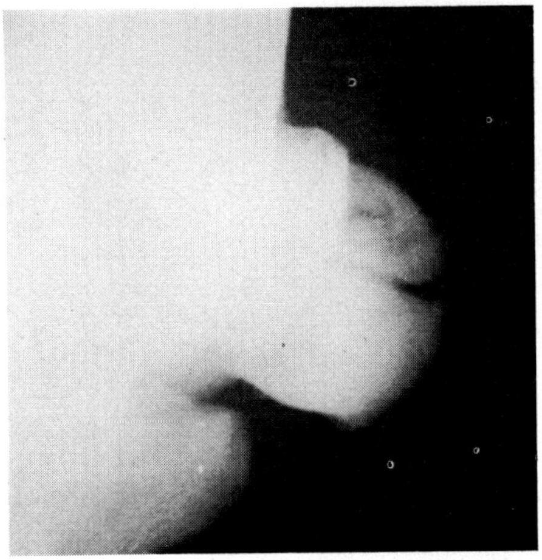

FIG. 7.6

FIGS. 7.5 and 7.6. Antero-posterior and oblique projections of a fracture of a sesamoid.

Metacarpal-Phalangeal (Fetlock) Joint

This joint is subject to osteoarthritis but demonstration and recognition of this poses no particular problems.

The First Phalanx

At birth this bone shows a proximal, but no distal, epiphysis.

This bone can be a site of fissure fractures which do not extend right through the bone and are not accompanied by separation of the fragments. Such injuries can be missed if radiography is confined to one plane.

Lesions of periositis may be demonstrated but are of less frequent occurrence than in the other two phalanges.

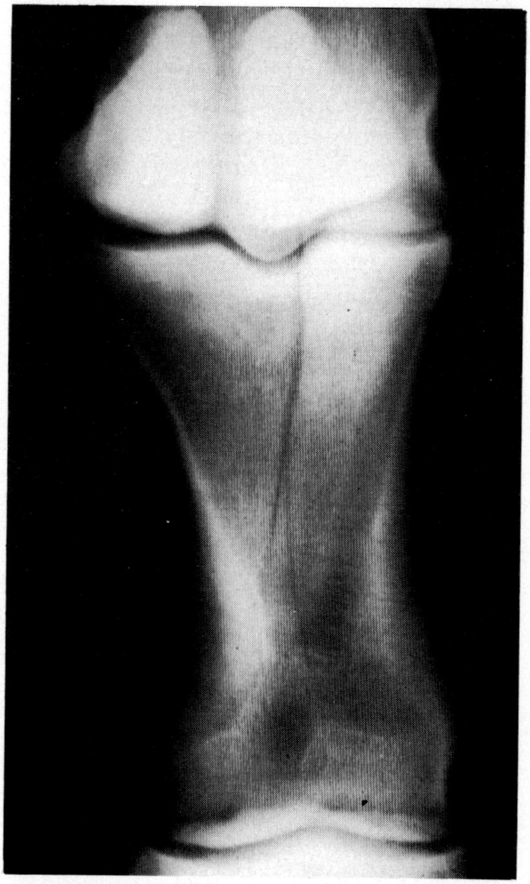

FIG. 7.7. Incomplete longitudinal fracture of the first phalanx (this would not have been visible in a lateral projection).

The First Interphalangeal (Pastern) Joint

This joint is a comparatively common situation for chronic osteoarthritic changes.

The term "ringbone" is used generally for osteoarthritic lesions of the first and second interphalangeal joints and for lesions of periostitis involving the second and third phalanx. This term is qualified in many ways ("true" and "false", "low" and "high", etc.) but such qualifications are not used consistently and will not be employed here. Radiography is extensively employed for the demonstration of the presence and extent of such lesions and, in particular, whether they are likely to interfere with joint function.

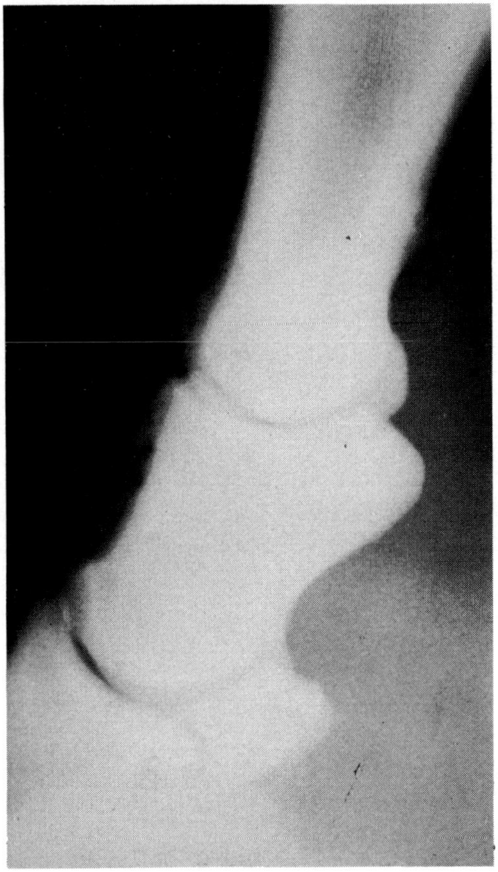

FIG. 7.8. Periosteal new bone formation on the anterior surfaces of the first and second phalanges.

The Second Phalanx

This bone also shows a proximal, but no distal, epiphysis at birth.

Owing to its situation this bone is subjected to considerable pressure and in any fracture the fragments are likely to be considerably displaced and thus very obvious in a radiograph.

As mentioned above, periostitis involving this bone is one of the manifestations of "ringbone".

The Second Interphalangeal (Coffin) Joint

This joint is also a situation in which chronic osteoarthritic changes are seen.

The Third Phalanx (Pedal Bone)

There are at least three accepted positions in which this bone can be placed for radiography in the antero-posterior plane. While each of these methods is capable of producing diagnostic radiographs they will not be exactly comparable and allowance must be made for this when comparing radiographs produced by different techniques.

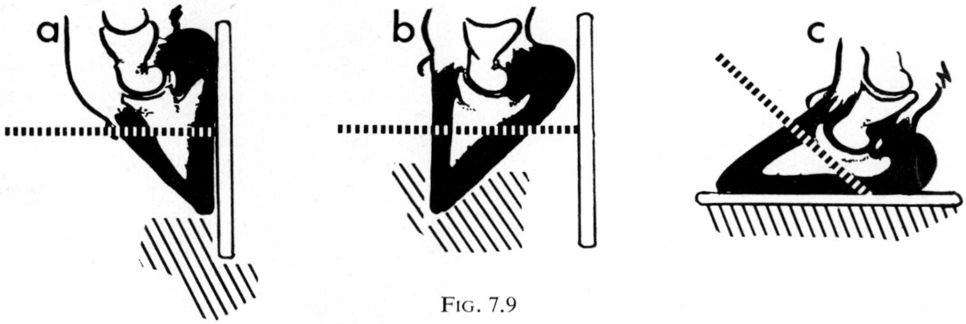

FIG. 7.9

Variations in the thickness of the bone have to be borne in mind when selecting factors for exposures in the antero-posterior plane—those suitable for the denser centre may over-penetrate the periphery.

Lesions can be missed or artefacts mistaken for pathological abnormalities unless the foot is carefully prepared for radiography. It is necessary to remove the shoe, trim back excessive horn, and scrub off dirt and stones.

Radiology

Fractures of this bone are unlikely to be accompanied by much displacement. Bear in mind that superimposition of the lines of the clefts of the foot can simulate fracture lines.

Osteomyelitis The situation of the third phalanx renders it particularly liable to osteomyelitis as a result of penetrating foreign bodies or of misdirected nails. This is likely to be associated with loss of normal bony structure and detail, with osteoporosis and occasionally with the formation of bony sequestra.

Periostitis A further manifestation of "ringbone" occurs—usually characterised by new bone formation in the region of the pyramidal process (best visualised in lateral projections).

Ossification of the Lateral Cartilages (Sidebones) Development of this condition is first shown by new bone formation at the posterior angles of the bone just lateral

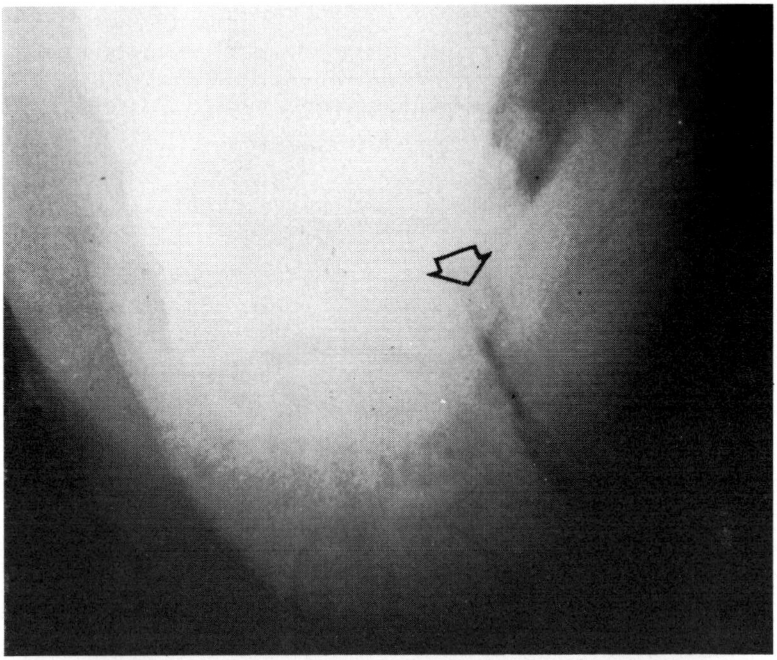

FIG. 7.10. Fracture of the third phalanx (this bone has been positioned slightly obliquely).

FIG. 7.11. Fracture of the pyramidal process of the first phalanx (this is an old-standing injury and considerable new bone formation has occurred around the separated fragment).

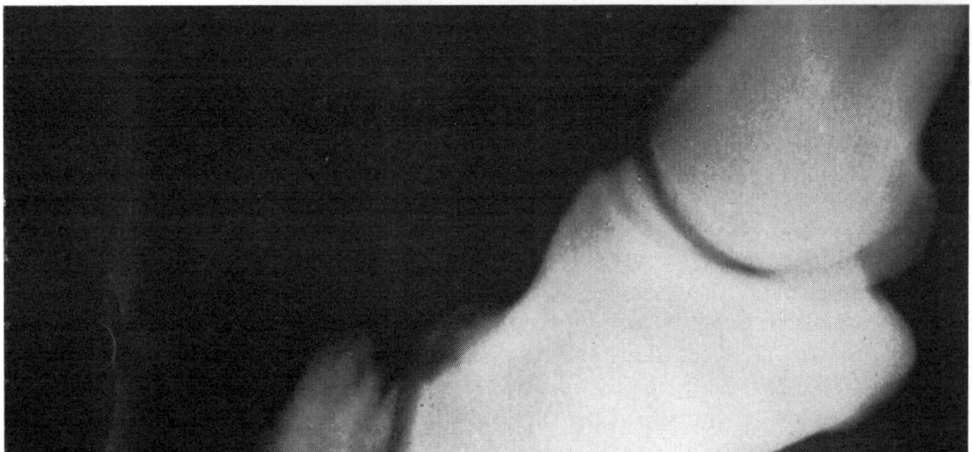

to the navicular. The process of ossification spreads backwards and may involve part of, or the entire, lateral cartilages. Such changes are not necessarily associated with lameness but they are more likely to be of clinical significance if the bony process can be shown to be extending inwards and thus compressing the soft tissues. Accurate visualisation of such changes will require films taken in the antero-posterior as well as the lateral projections.

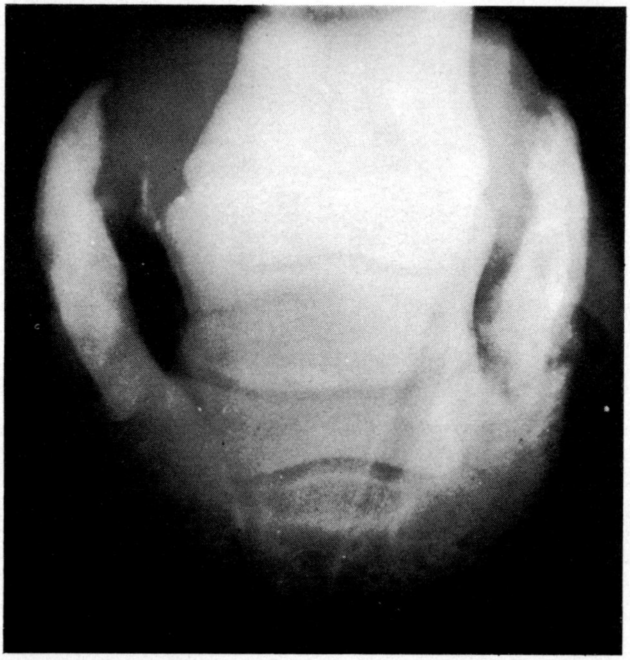

FIG. 7.12. Particularly extensive ossification of the lateral cartilages.

Chronic Laminitis Angulation or rotation of the third phalanx as a result of persistent laminitis can be demonstrated in lateral projections. The significant feature is a downward rotation of the bone with the result that the anterior surface of the bone is no longer parallel with the anterior wall of the hoof, and the point of the bone approaches the sole of the foot and may show evidence of penetrating it.

Pedal ostitis The main change which can be visualised in association with this condition is a roughening of the outline of the pedal bone. This occurs chiefly in the region of the heels and is best seen in antero-posterior and oblique projections. Some loss of detail and blurring of the bone and the development of spicules of bone around its margin, can also be appreciated.

Keratoma Tumours of the hoof are rare and may result in distortion or malformation of the third phalanx which can be demonstrated radiologically.

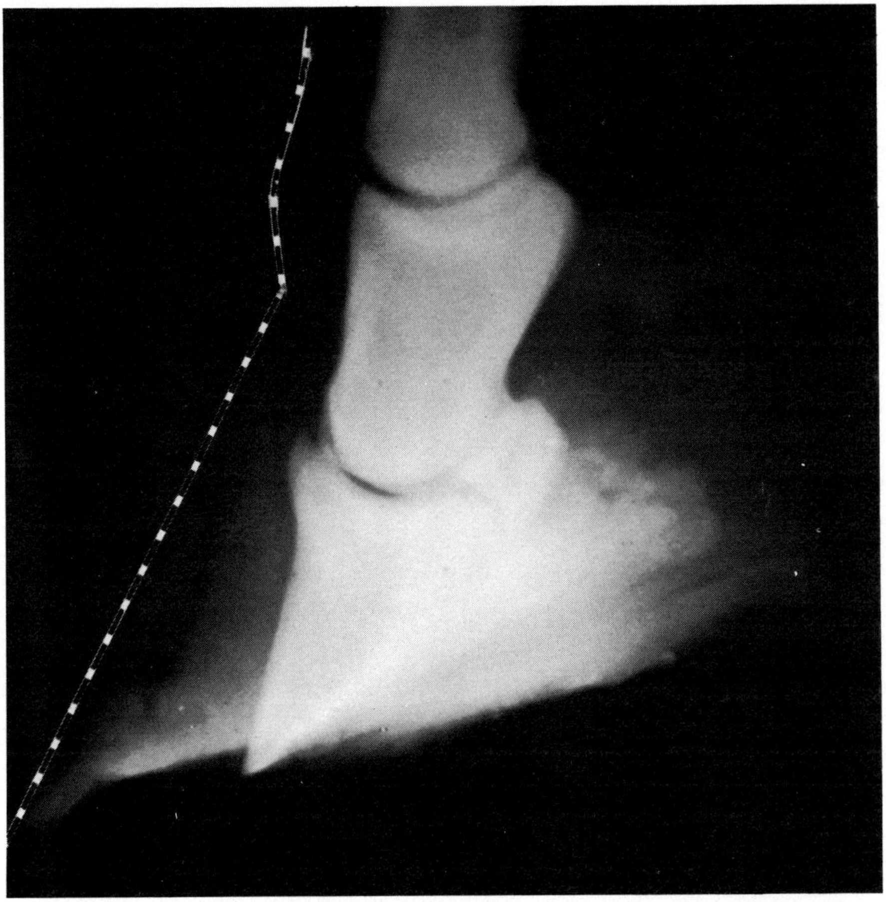

FIG. 7.13

FIGS. 7.13 and 7.14. Angulation of the third phalanx due to chronic laminitis.

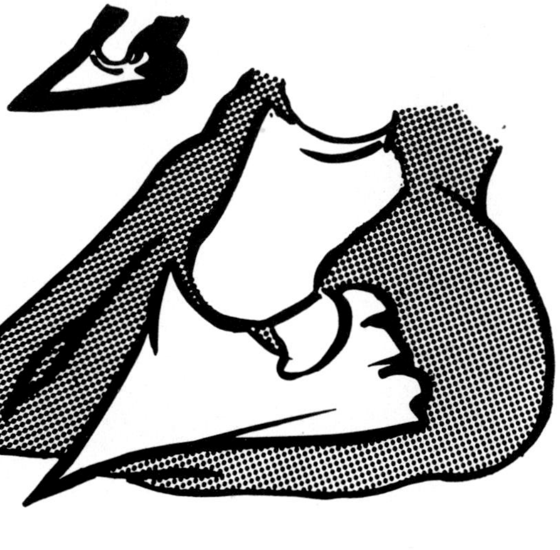

FIG. 7.14

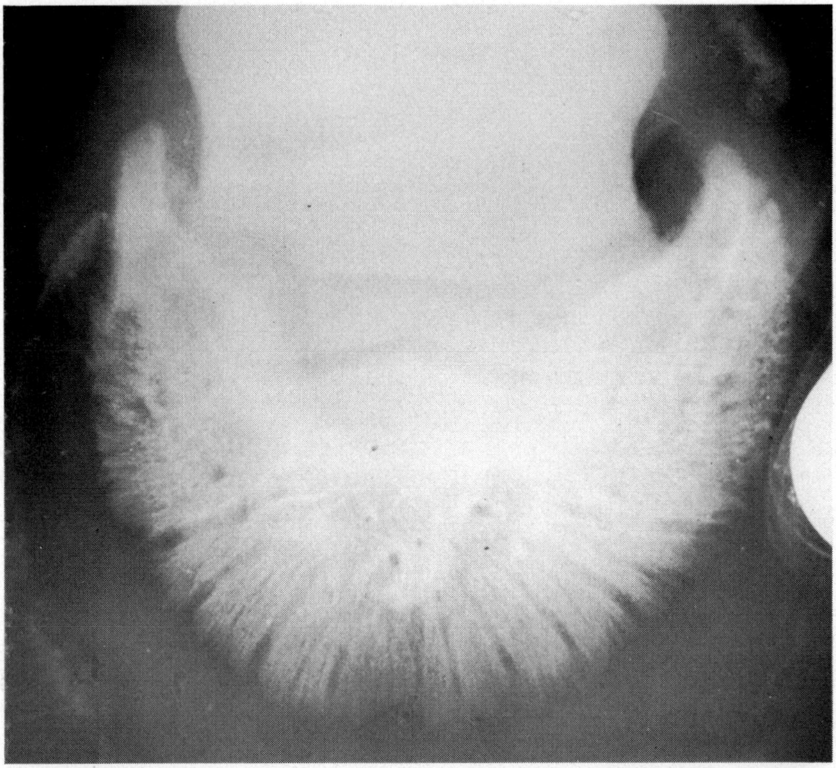

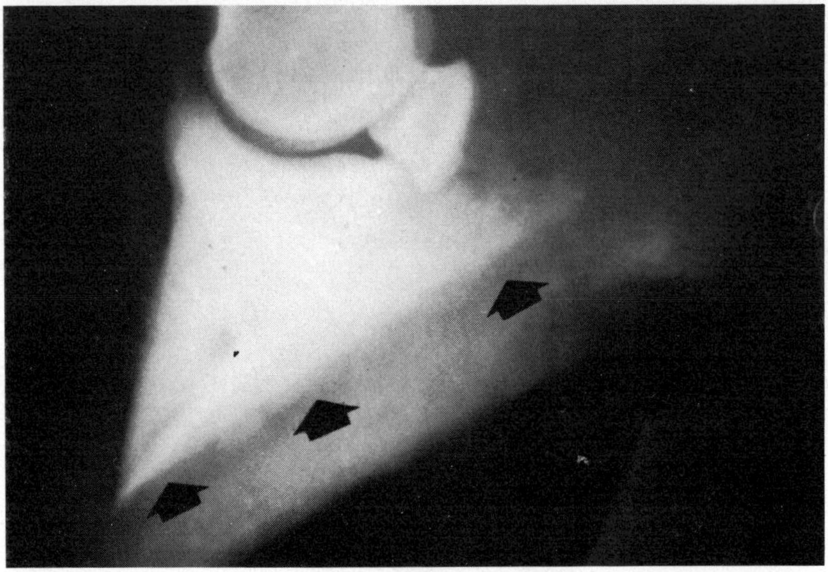

FIGS. 7.15 and 7.16. Roughening of the edge of the pedal bone associated with pedal ostitis.

FIG. 7.17

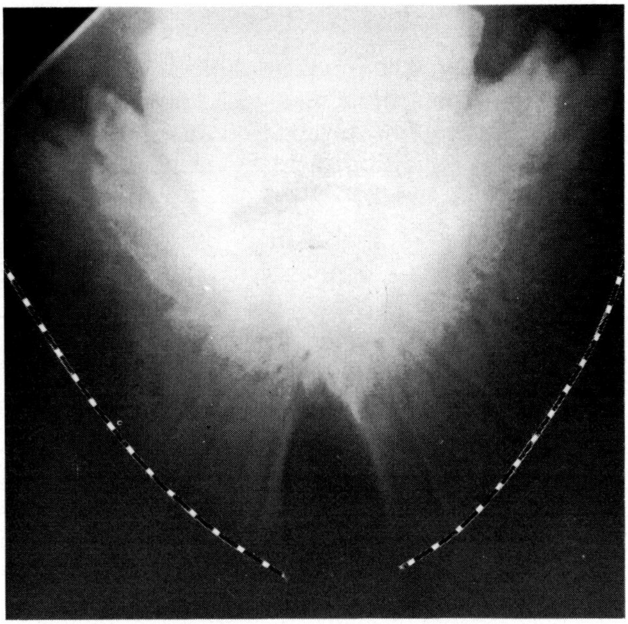

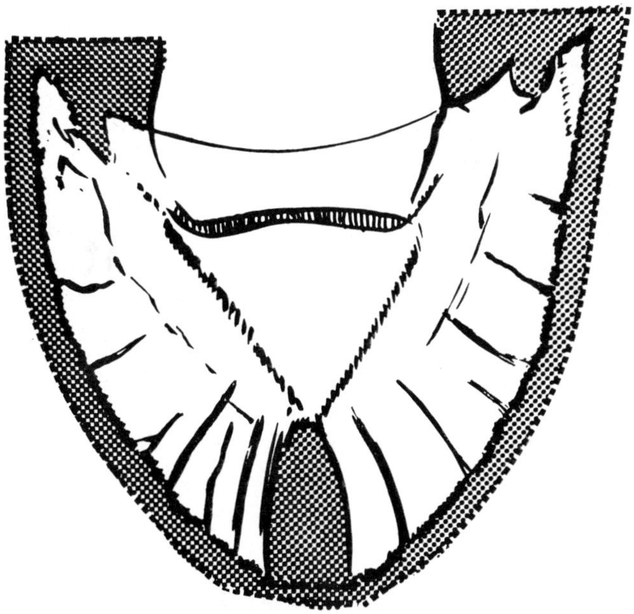

FIG. 7.18

FIGS. 7.17 and 7.18. Malformation of the third phalanx due to the presence of a keratoma.

The Navicular Bone

Radiography The practical difficulties involved in the radiographic demonstration of the navicular bone are well known, but they are reiterated here to help the radiographer in the production of films of maximum quality and to remind the radiologist of limiting factors which must be allowed for when interpreting films. They include:

(a) Similar preparation of the foot to that described for the third phalanx is necessary in order to avoid confusing shadows cast by dirt or other material.

(b) Antero-posterior projections of the bone can only be visualised through the comparatively dense second phalanx. Because of this, the earliest changes associated with navicular disease cannot be appreciated and the more advanced lesions will only be apparent if all radiographic aids to contrast and definition are employed (the use of a grid is essential).

(c) The lower border of the navicular bone can easily be superimposed on and masked by, the line of the second interphalangeal joint and repositioning may be necessary.

(d) Superimposition of areas of decreased density in the foot (in particular, the cleft of the frog) on the image of the navicular bone can produce a false effect of osteoporosis or fracture in a radiograph. Attempts have been made to avoid this artefact by filling the clefts with "horn paste", but most radiogists prefer to recognise the actual areas of the clefts and to allow for this in their interpretation of the films.

(e) It is essential that antero-posterior projections of this region are accurately positioned and that the natural tendency of the foot to rotate outwards is avoided.

(f) Lateral projections of the navicular bone avoid superimposition by other bones, but are of little diagnostic value.

Radiology It should be noted that there are a series of nutrient foramina situated along the lower border of the navicular bone. These are barely perceptible in the young animal but they can become enlarged with age and give an irregular appearance to the lower border of the bone.

Fractures These are not common injuries and care must be exercised in their diagnosis. The actual injury is not very obvious as there is little displacement and it is viewed through the denser second phalanx. In addition, superimposition of one of the clefts of the foot can suggest a fracture—however, if the film is carefully examined this artefact will be seen to extend beyond the limits of the bone and can thus be distinguished from a fracture.

Navicular Disease Radiography is extensively employed for the investigation of suspected navicular disease but radiographs must be interpreted with caution. The following radiological features are usually considered to be characteristic of navicular disease. Clinical cases of the condition may show, any of these features, a combination of them, or no recognisable radiological evidence of the disease.

(a) Osteophytic outgrowths which produce an effect of spur development at one or both ends of the navicular bone.

(b) Irregularities along the upper or lower border of the bone. In the lower border such changes are due to enlargement of the nutrient foramina and while they are indicative of the disease when seen in the young horse they are not necessarily of clinical significance in the older animal. This feature is the least characteristic of the three and care must be taken in making a definite diagnosis when this is the only radiological finding. Irregularities along the upper border can be difficult to visualise and are usually caused by new bone formation rather than by osteoporosis.

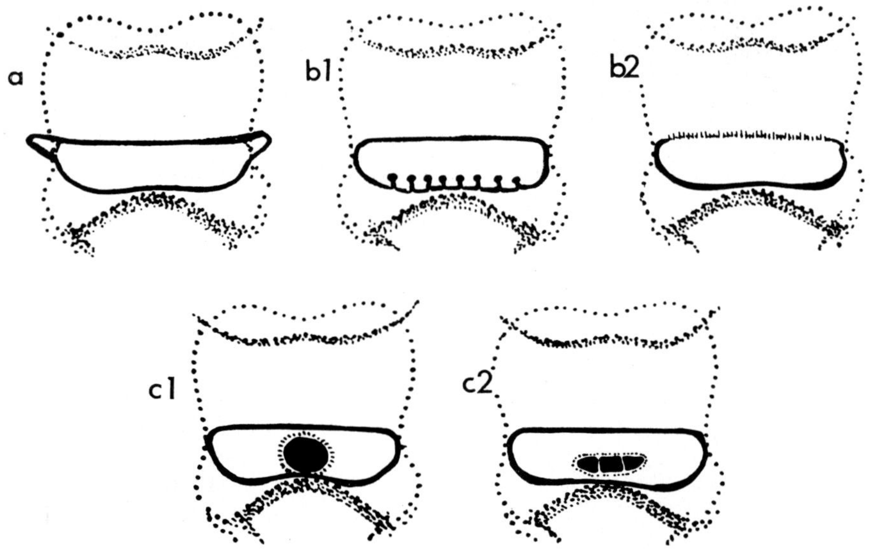

FIG. 7.19. Diagrammatic representation of the features of navicular disease.

(c) Distinct areas of osteoporosis in the central area of the bone. Care must be taken to eliminate artefacts due to superimposition of the clefts of the foot. In doubtful cases radiography should be repeated after altering the angle of the beam so that the apparent position of the navicular bone in relation to the second phalanx is moved. If the osteoporotic area moves with the navicular, it can be judged to represent an area of cavitation within the bone and not an artefact.

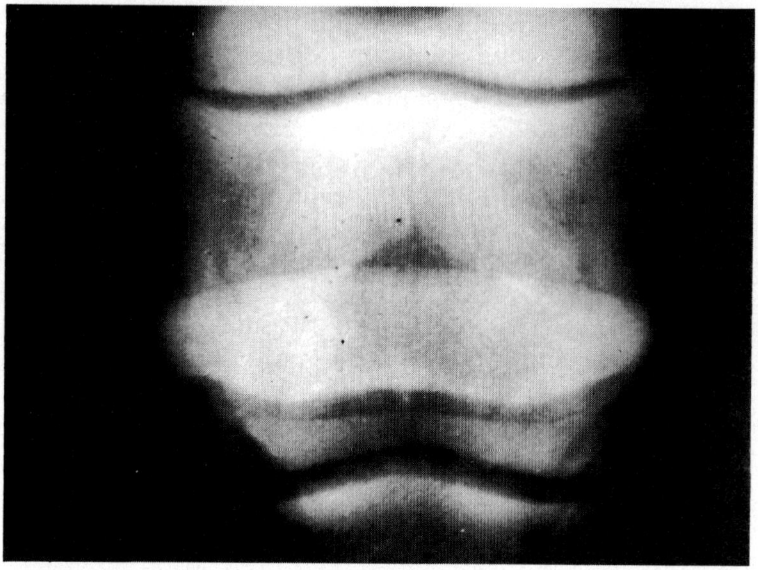

FIG. 7.20. Normal navicular bone.

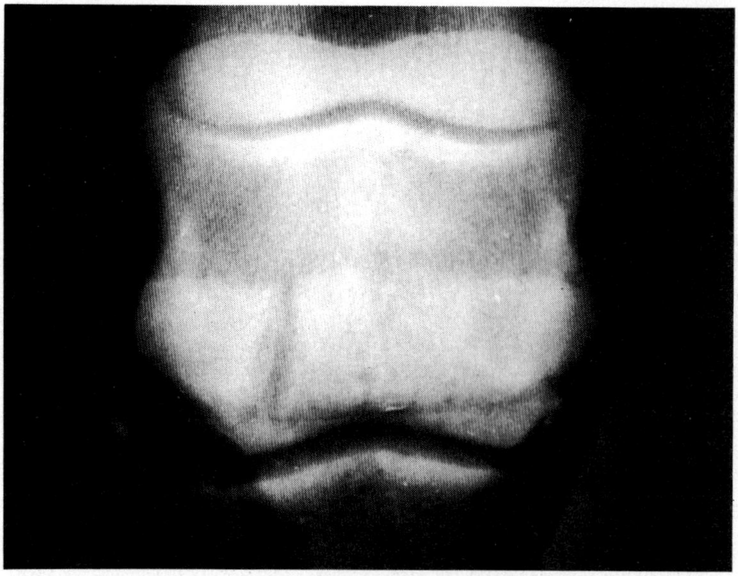

FIG. 7.21. Fracture of the navicular bone.

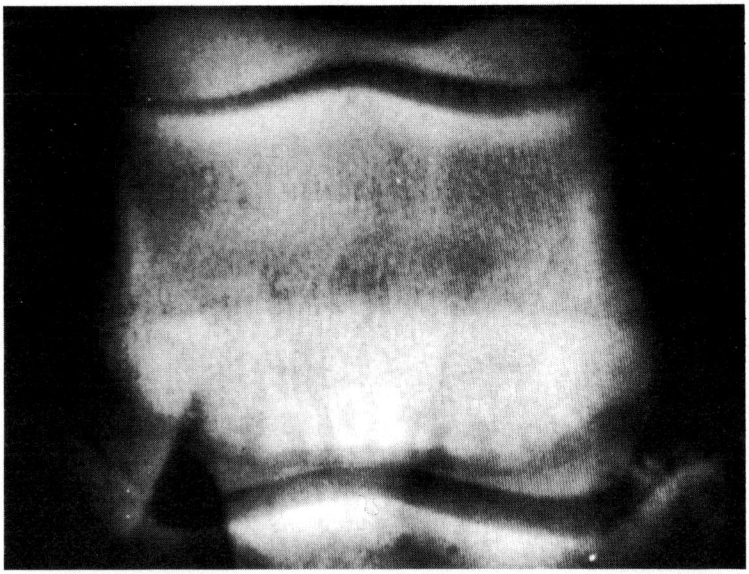

FIG. 7.22. Navicular disease—irregularities of the lower border.

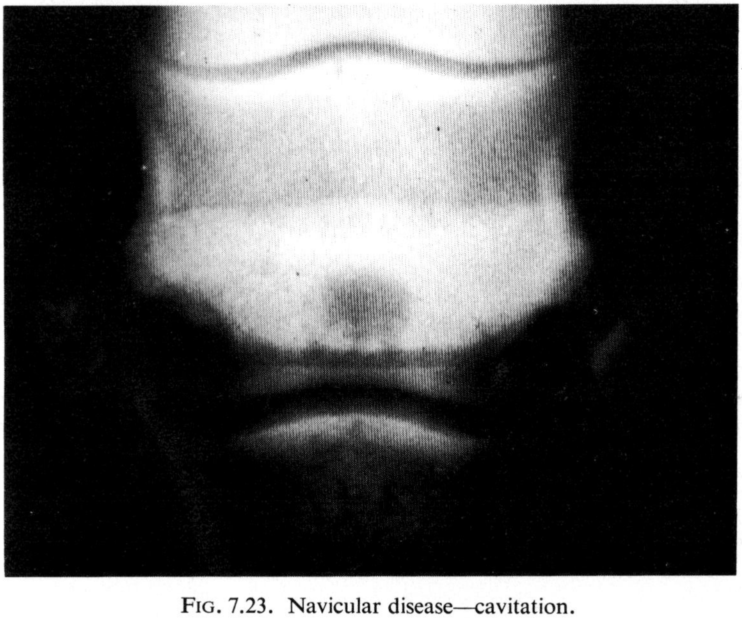

FIG. 7.23. Navicular disease—cavitation.

The Pelvis, Hip Joint and Femur

This region can only be radiographed if the patient can be cast and anaesthetised and the legs fully flexed, and if apparatus of at least medium output (60—100mA and 80—90 kV) is available.

The Stifle Joint

In many instances the upper portion of this joint (i.e., the femoral condyles) cannot be adequately demonstrated in the standing animal.

The Tibia and Fibula

Demonstration of these bones is reasonably straightforward in both lateral and postero-anterior projections.

The Tarsus

The two standard projections permit adequate demonstration of the joint and of its bone for most purposes.

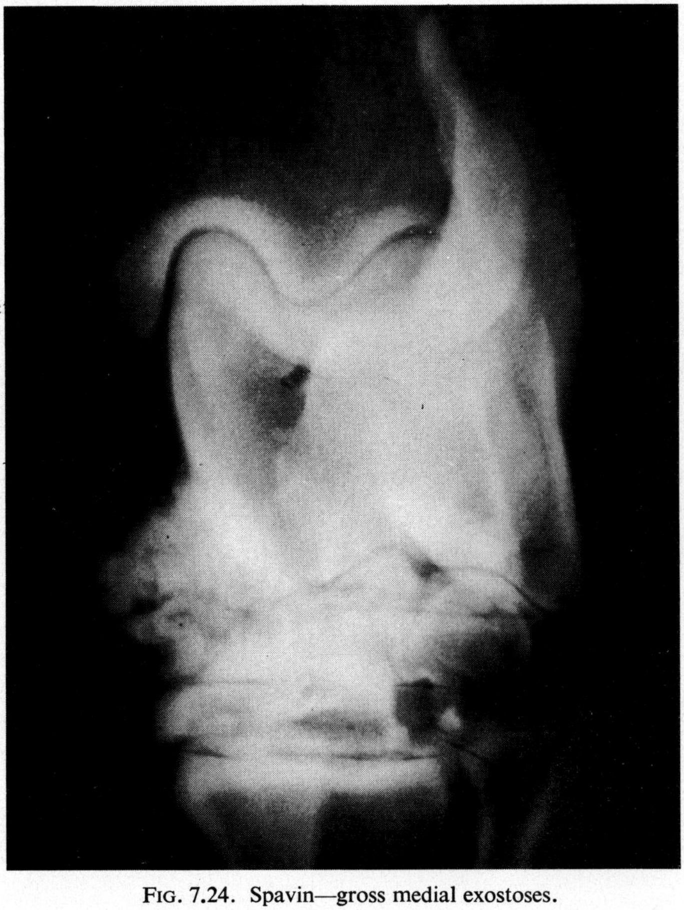

FIG. 7.24. Spavin—gross medial exostoses.

Fractures Such injuries are rare and most likely to involve the fibula tarsal bone.

Spavin This condition is characterised by the development of osteophytic outgrowths on the medial and anterior aspects of the lower row of tarsal bones and the upper end of the large metatarsal bone. In advanced cases fusion of the new bone is likely to result in ankylosis of some or all of the bones involved. The condition is most obvious on the medial aspect of the joint and therefore best visualised in antero-posterior projections but lateral and when necessary oblique, views should also be employed to visualise the full extent of the changes.

For obvious practical reasons very little use has been made of radiography for the examination of the remainder of the equine skeletal system. Under particular circumstances it might be of value in the following regions.

The Cervical Vertebrae

Provided the animal is quiet or can be immobilised reasonable lateral projections of the cervical vertebrae can be obtained in all but the largest horses with apparatus of medium output. Not more than two or three vertebrae can be included even in the largest films and a series of radiographs will be necessary to examine the whole neck. Difficulty will be experienced in adequately visualising the seventh vertebra.

Radiography of this region has been employed for the investigation of suspected fractures and for the demonstration of ankylosis of the vertebrae in association with tuberculosis.

The Skull

Casting, and usually also anaesthetisation, of the patient is essential before this region can be investigated. This is a large and complex area and at present only limited experience of the radiography and radiology of the region is available. The authors have discussed some of the problems and techniques of radiography in Principles of Veterinary Radiography. In our experience radiology may be of some assistance in the investigation of the following clinical problems.

Conditions of the Teeth Owing to superimposition and the size and density of the mandibles and the molar teeth very little detail can be visualised in lateral and dorso-ventral projections. Conditions of individual teeth (fractures, malpositioning and evidence of infection) may be demonstrated by the use of intra-oral films or by oblique projections. A connection between a sinus about the head and a particular tooth can sometimes be demonstrated by the introduction of a probe or of contrast agent into the sinus.

Fractures While gross fractures are usually clinically obvious, radiography may be of assistance in showing those cases in which little or no displacement has occurred. Such injuries may be best demonstrated by "sky-line" projections showing the outer contour of the bone.

Conditions of the Nasal Chambers and of the Frontal and Maxillary Sinuses These regions of the skull are normally distinctively outlined in a radiograph by the air which they contain. For this reason radiography can be employed to show the

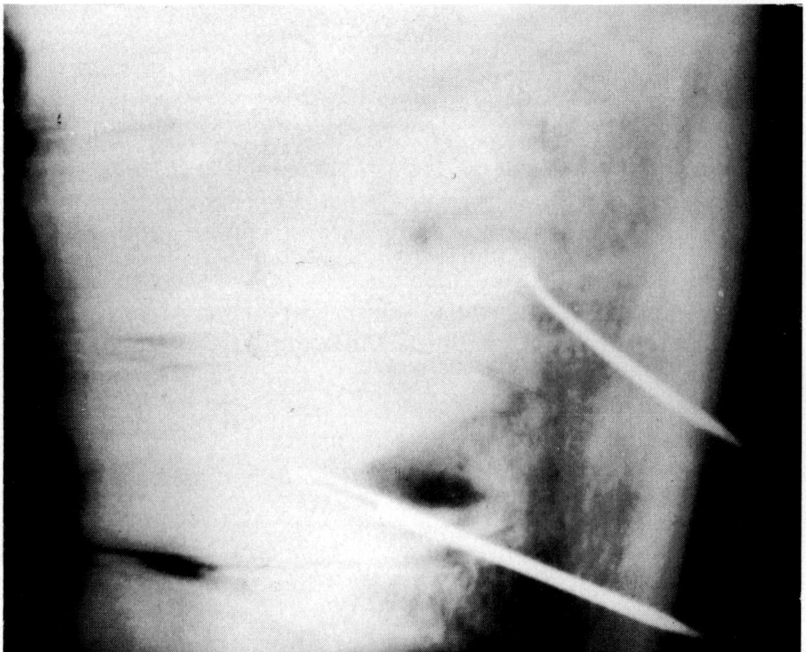

FIG. 7.25. Localised osteoporosis due to infection around the roots of the molar teeth (the associated sinuses are demonstrated by metallic probes).

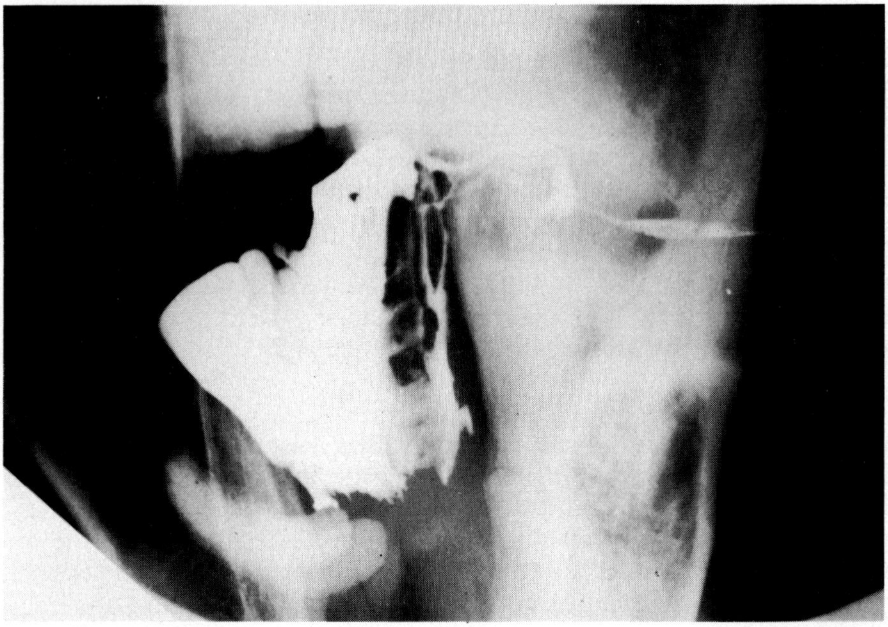

FIG. 7.26. Communication of an external sinus with the interior of the mouth demonstrated by the injection of a contrast agent (a considerable quantity of the agent has accumulated within the mouth).

accumulation of pus or other material within these cavities. If the skull can be so positioned that the X-ray beam can be directed horizontally, it may be possible to show fluid levels within the sinuses.

THE OX

It is practicable to radiograph most of these regions of the ox which correspond with those areas described above for the horse. For economic reasons and because there appear to be few clinical indications, the use of radiography is very largely confined to examination of the foot. There are two main clinical indications for this (obviously the foot must be cleaned and prepared as carefully as that of the horse).

Fractures Such injuries of the pedal bone may be more common than is generally recognised. They are associated with little displacement and require careful radiography in both the usual planes for their demonstration.

Osteomyelitis This term is used here rather generally to indicate any suppurative process involving the bones of the foot. Radiography can be of considerable value

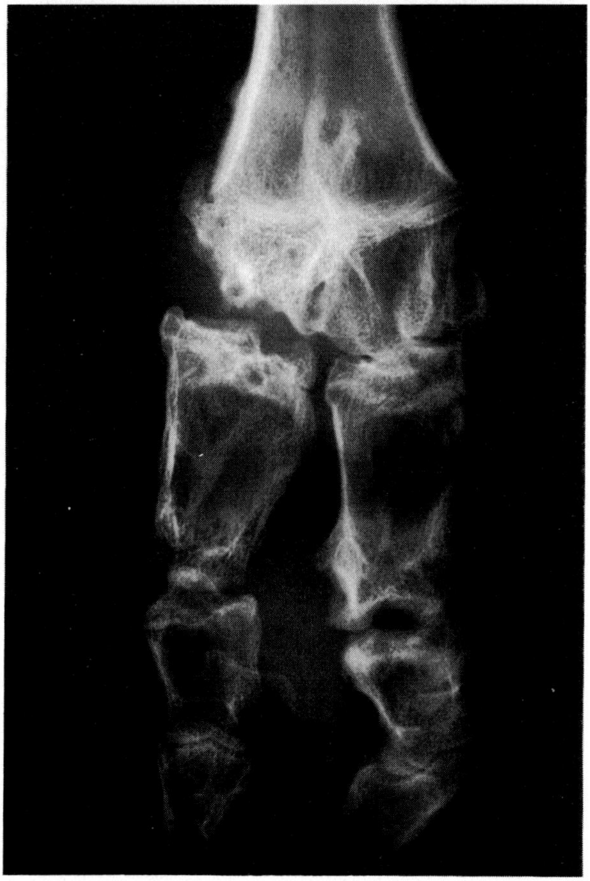

FIG. 7.27. Healed septic arthritis of the foot of a calf (there is obvious loss of bone but the structure and outline of the bones are re-established and clearly demarcated).

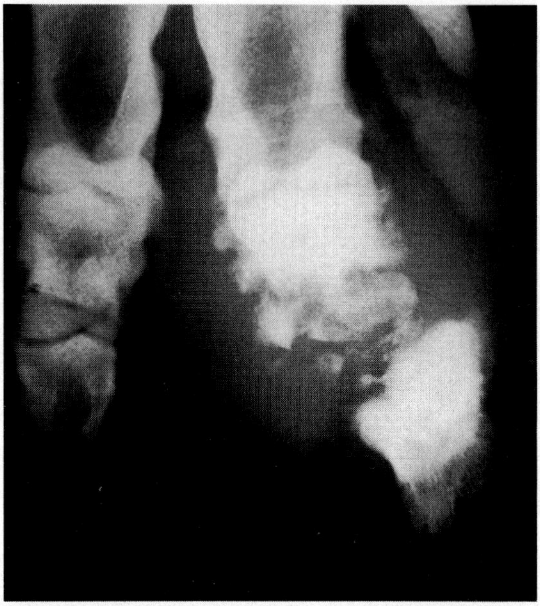

FIG. 7.28. Active septic arthritis of the foot of a pig (there is disorganisation of bone with considerable lysis and sclerosis, and the edge of the bones is vague and poorly defined).

in demonstrating the extent and progress of bony involvement and the practibility of surgical excision. If seen in the early stages the infective process is likely to commence in the third phalanx as a result of a penetrating wound, or in the second interphalangeal joint by spread from "foul in the foot". Films may show any of the usual evidence of bone infection—loss of detailed bone structure, areas of osteoporosis, the development of sequestra, new bone formation, etc.

THE PIG AND THE SHEEP

The smaller size of these species means that, provided the animal can be immobilised, most portions of the skeletal system can be investigated radiographically (some areas of the adult pig can be difficult to penetrate). While this has been used in the examination of fractures and other injuries of the more valuable animals, little is known concerning other clinical conditions which could be demonstrated radiologically in these species.

REFERENCES

Morgan, J. P. (1965), J. Am. vet. Radiol. Soc. **6,** 78.

The following work is again recommended as a reference book for normal radiological anatomy.

Schebitz, H., and Wilkens, H. (1968), Atlas of Radiographic Anatomy of Dog and Horse, Berlin, Paul Parey.

PART THREE

SOFT TISSUES

CHAPTER 8

THE RESPIRATORY SYSTEM

General Radiographic Considerations

As most of the respiratory system is contained within the chest, it is advisable to consider the general problems relating to the radiography and radiology of this region, before studying the individual parts of the system in detail.

In man, radiography is one of the most important means of investigating pathology of the chest and its routine use has permitted the recognition of disease before it could be appreciated or diagnosed by other means. The potential value of radiography as an aid to the diagnosis of lesions of the respiratory system in animals is also great and, similarly, it may reveal pathological changes before they result in clinical symptoms (e.g. the first stages of secondary neoplasia). It must be realised, however, that the use of this procedure is accompanied by certain inherent limitations, particularly:

(1) Some blurring of radiological detail due to respiratory movement is likely to occur unless respiration can be controlled by general anaesthesia (possibly employing a relaxant), or unless a sufficiently short exposure time (0·02—0·05 sec.) can be used.

(2) The great depth of an animal's chest (particularly noticeable when compared with man) renders precise positioning for dorso-ventral radiography difficult, results in geometric distortion, and also complicates the subsequent radiological interpretation of the radiographs produced.

Radiography of the chest in the dorso-ventral plane rather than ventro-dorsally is advisable as positioning an animal on its back will result in displacement of the heart. Radiographs taken in this plane will need to be supplemented by lateral views, but these exposures will show superimposition of the lungs and will be less informative. However, if dorso-ventral exposures are to provide readable films, it is essential that great care should be taken to ensure accurate positioning of the patient and correct alignment of the X-ray beam.

Another problem encountered in radiographing the chest in this plane is associated with the additional amount of muscle which occurs in the region of the scapulae. This will produce an effect of increased density in the anterior half of the chest (particularly noticeable in Boxers and other thick-set dogs), unless the use of more powerful apparatus permits this to be "evened out" by employing higher kilovoltage and lower milliamperage factors. (This technique requires the use of a grid).

Further apparent variations in the density of the lung parenchyma are due to the stage of respiration at which the exposure is made, and a radiograph taken at expiration will suggest that the lungs are denser than one taken at full inspiration. It is usual to endeavour to expose chest films at inspiration, so that the contrast effect of the increased amount of air contained in the lungs will improve the detail which can be appreciated. The use of general anaesthesia and a relaxant eliminates respiratory movement and permits slight over-aeration of lung tissue. This results in the production of maximum detail, but obviously films taken under these conditions are slightly exaggerated and not directly comparable with those obtained from the conscious animal.

RADIOLOGY

As mentioned in the Preface, subtle but important features which can be appreciated in clinical radiographs are often lost in the process of reproduction, and where this appears likely to happen to a marked degree, diagrams traced from appropriate films are shown instead of the original radiographs. Obviously the use of such diagrams over-emphasises the definition and density which can be visualised in a film.

It is unfortunate but inevitable, that such substitution of diagrams will become more necessary in this third section and particularly in this and the subsequent chapter. As far as practicable, diagrams have been employed in the first half of the chapters when individual radiological features are being considered, and radiographs are shown in the latter half to illustrate pathological entities. Since both methods of illustration have their limitations, each should be considered in relation to the other.

The Examination of Chest Radiographs

The way in which radiographic technique can affect radiological interpretation has already been discussed in Chapters 1 and 2, but this is of considerable importance in relation to the respiratory system, where even slight variations in positioning, in exposure factors, or in the stage of respiration can simulate pathological change. It is particularly important, therefore, that the radiologist should check the technical quality of a chest film, before proceeding to consider any pathological changes which may be present. Such a check, which can be carried out comparatively quickly once it becomes a matter of routine, will involve posing and answering the following questions:—

(1) Is the film correctly exposed? (loss of detail in lung parenchyma can be due to emphysema or to pneumothorax, but it can equally well result from over-exposure of the film). The density of the radiographic shadows of the bony structures of the chest is likely to be directly related to the exposure factors used, and examination of this portion of the film will, in the light of experience, provide the most reliable evidence of under or over-exposure.

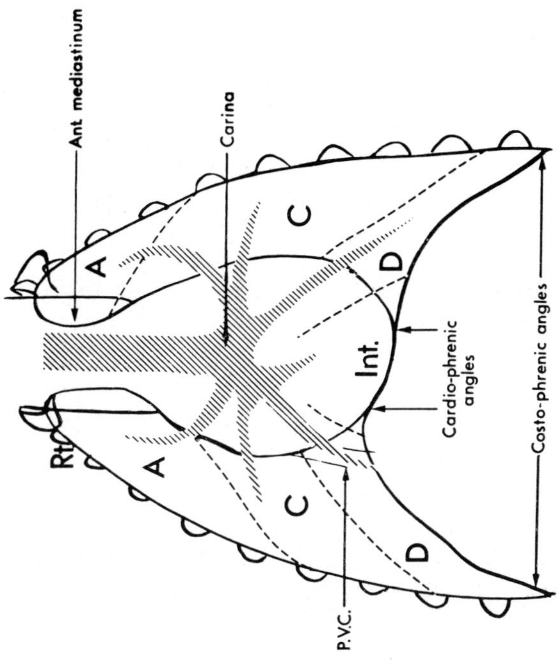
Ant mediastinum
Carina
Rt
A
A
C
C
D
D
Int.
Cardio-phrenic angles
Costo-phrenic angles
P.V.C.

FIG. 8.2.

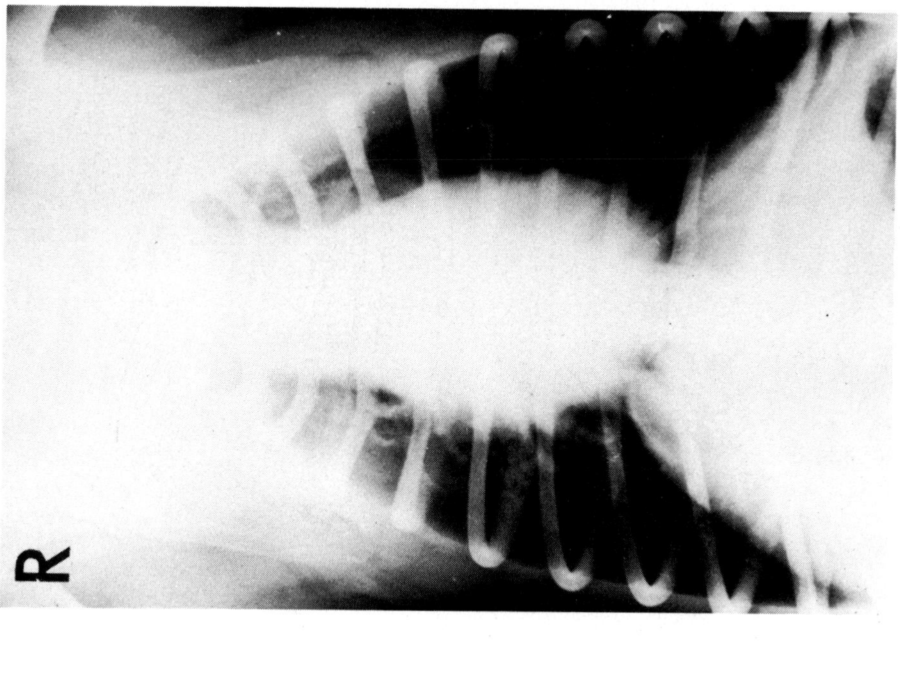
R

FIG. 8.1.

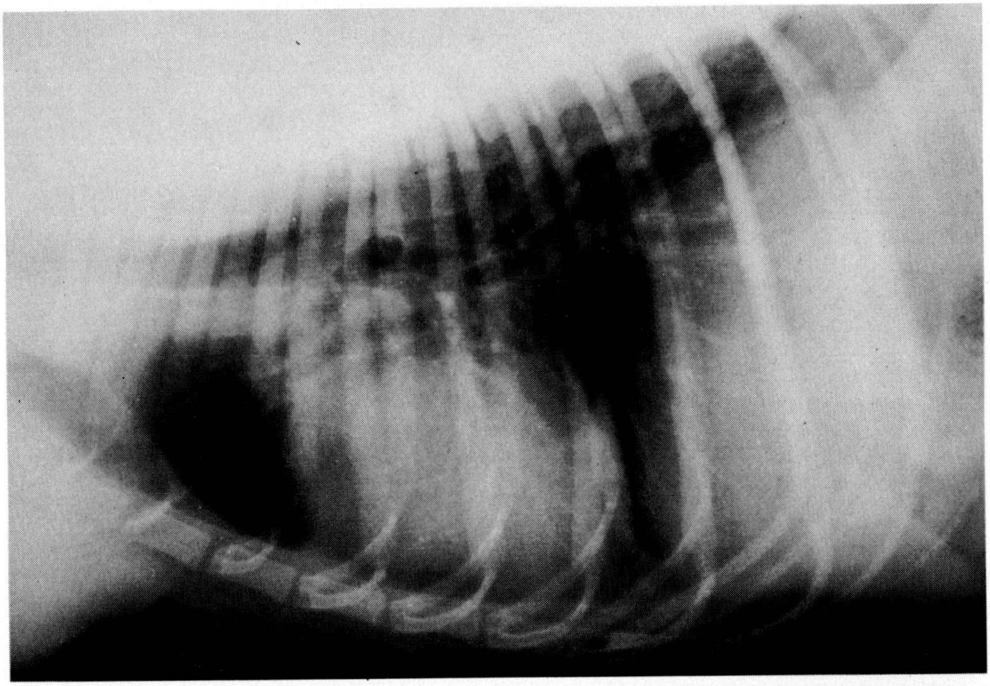

FIG. 8.3.

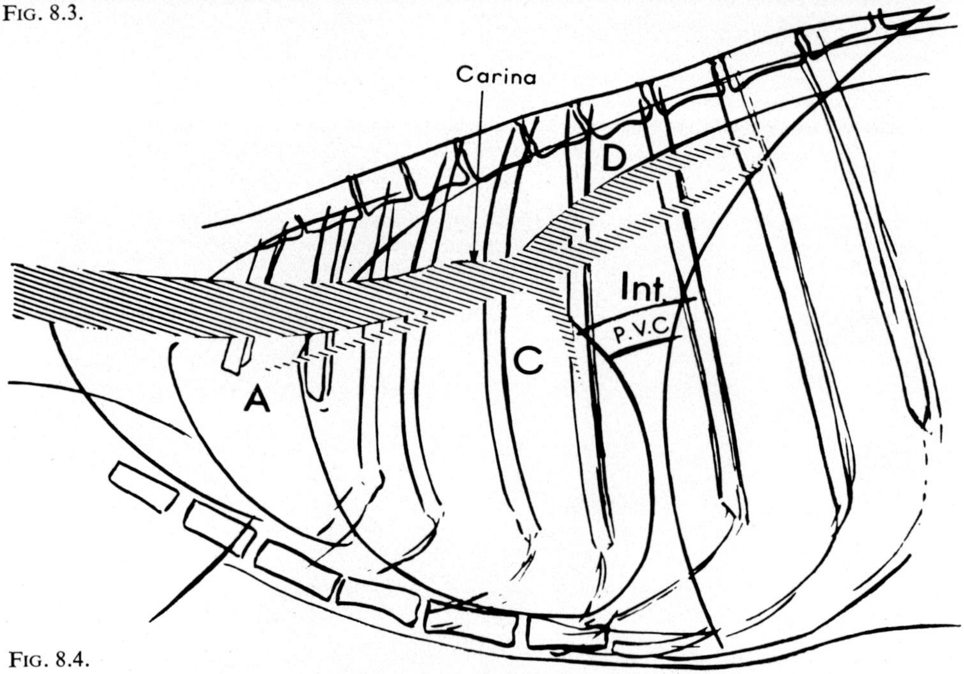

FIG. 8.4.

FIGS. 8.1 to 8.4. Dorso-ventral and lateral projections of the normal canine chest. The approximate areas of the apical (A) cardiac (C) diaphragmatic (D) and intermediate (Int) lobes of the lungs are indicated.

(2) Is the patient and the X-ray beam correctly positioned? In dorso-ventral views correct positioning of the patient will be indicated by the fact that the outline of the sternum is directly superimposed on the thoracic vertebrae and that the two halves of chest are comparable. Centring too far forward or back will result in distortion of the outline of the heart.

Positioning for lateral views is not so critical, but it is important to ensure that the fore limbs are drawn as far forward as possible and that the trunk is not rotated.

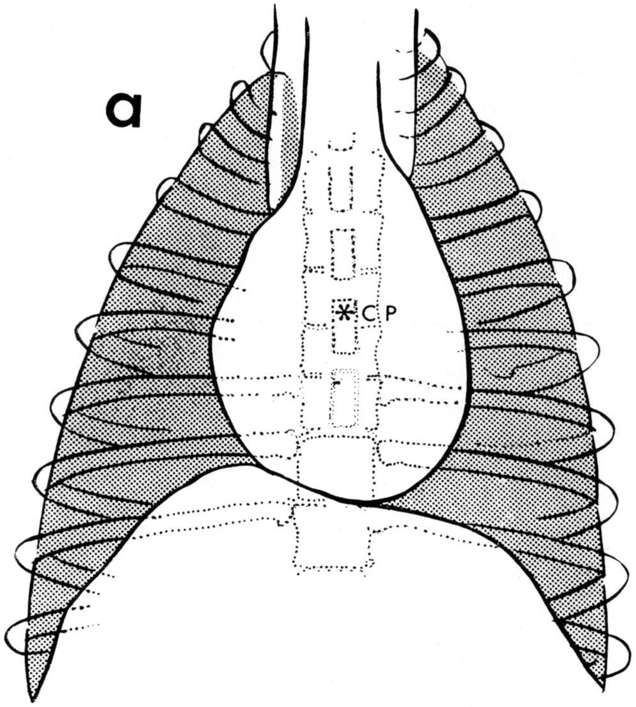

FIG. 8.5.

FIGS. 8.5. to 8.7. The effect of positioning of the patient and the X-ray apparatus on the resultant radiograph.

(a) correct positioning
(b) rotation of the patient
(c) apparatus centred too far posteriorly.
(CP = centring point)

(3) Was the film exposed at inspiration or expiration? The stage of respiration can be judged by noting the position of the diaphragm. This is seen most clearly in lateral views. At expiration the anterior line of the diaphragm extends forward to the level of the fifth or sixth ribs and merges with the posterior border of the heart. When radiographs are taken at inspiration the line of the diaphragm is seen to be more curved, to be distinct from the heart, and to extend only to the region of the seventh or eighth rib. (The effect of inspiration and expiration on the position of the diaphragm is discussed further on page 164).

(4) Are any artefacts present? A common source of confusion in chest radiographs is the presence of longitudinal linear marks which can suggest the presence of

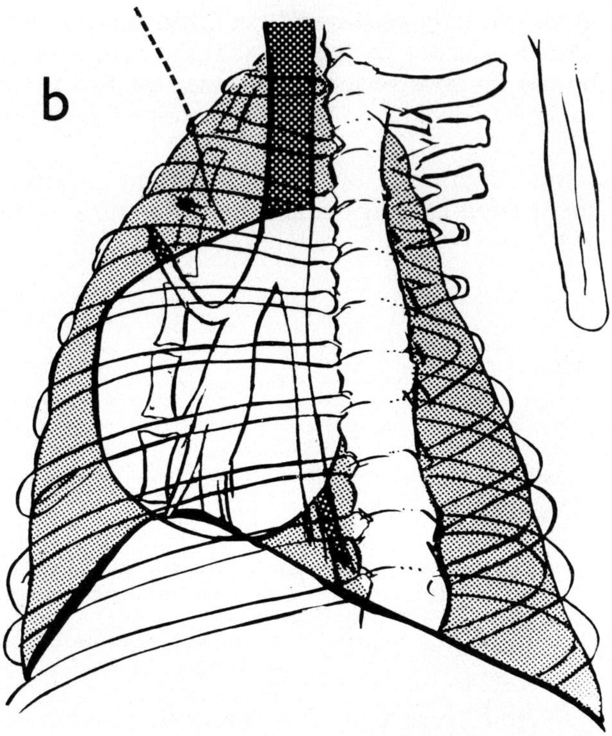

FIG. 8.6.

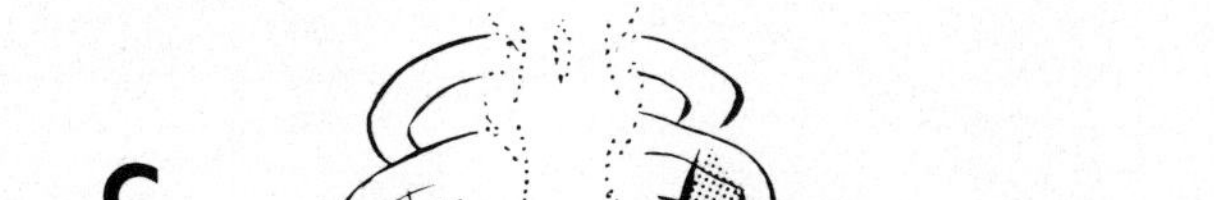

FIG. 8.7.

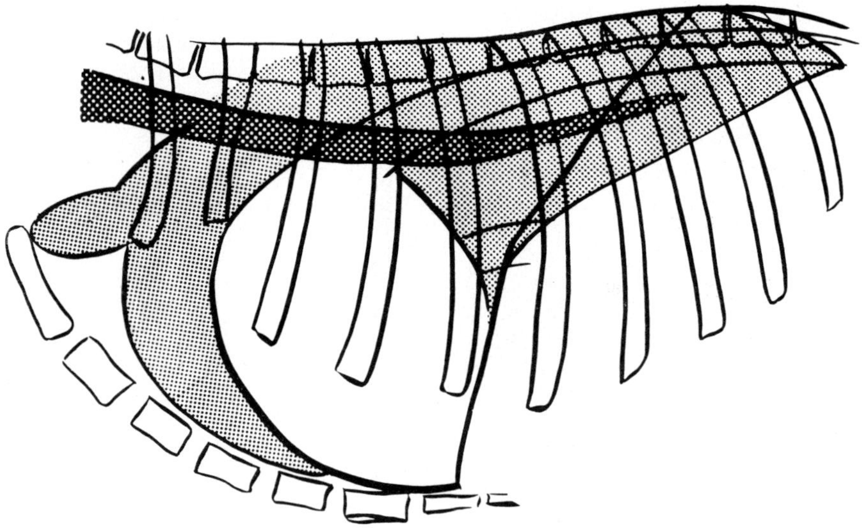

FIG. 8.8. Expiration.

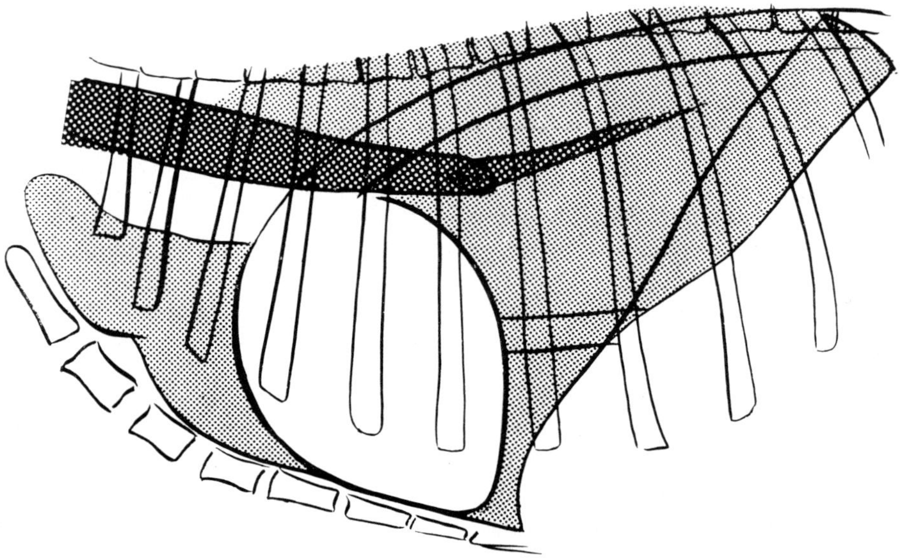

FIG. 8.9. Inspiration.

pneumothorax, but are in fact due to folds of loose skin or other normal anatomical structures. Careful examination will normally show that these lines extend beyond the thoracic cage and that they cannot be part of the lung structures.

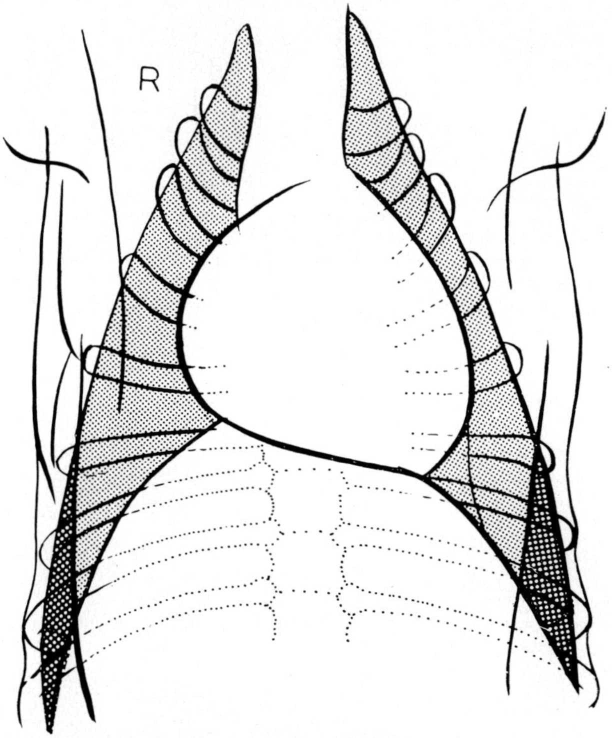

FIG. 8.10. Skin folds.

In Bassett Hounds and possibly some other breeds, there is a peculiar concavity in the contour of the chest which can result in the appearance of pneumo-thorax in dorso-ventral radiographs.

Occasionally superimposition of the anterior mammary glands of the bitch can suggest localised dense areas within the posterior lung fields.

(5) Are any variations present, due to the breed or age of the patient and therefore to be considered as "normal"? It will be appreciated that there is considerable variation in the contour of the canine chest between different breeds (e.g., between the Greyhound and the Pekingese). Since there are so many breeds these differences cannot be listed, but the general shape both of the chest and of the air passages of the particular animal being considered must be borne in mind while examining the radiographs.

Similarly, certain minor radiological changes must be expected to occur with age. While no particular age limit can be quoted, linear markings and small nodular densities within the lung parenchyma, pleural thickenings, and an increased density of tracheal and bronchial walls, have all been reported (Reif and Rhodes, 1966) in chest films of the older dog.

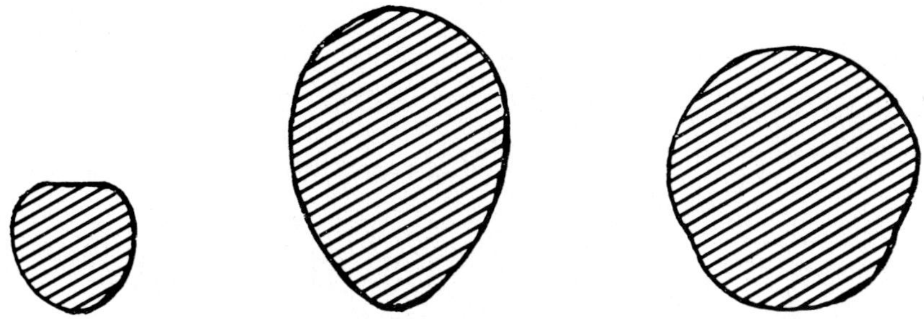

FIG. 8.11. Cross section of the canine thorax in three contrasting breeds.

INDIVIDUAL RESPIRATORY STRUCTURES

Since the respiratory system is a complex structure the normal and abnormal radiology of its component parts will be considered in some detail, before discussing the radiographic findings associated with the common pathological conditions involving the system.

The Nasal Passages

These have been described in Chapter 4.

The Larynx

In a lateral view the air-filled larynx should be easily identified immediately behind and below the angle of the jaw. Some of the component cartilages and also the bones of the hyoid apparatus can be completely lost in over-exposed films. In contrast, the transverse hyoid (basihyoid) will be seen "end on", which gives it a particularly dense appearance and can lead to it being mistaken for a foreign body.

Dorso-ventral projections are seldom of value as the larynx will be obscured by the cervical vertebrae.

Pathological changes in the structure of the larynx itself are rarely recognised, but compression or displacement in either plane can occur in association with adjacent soft tissue masses.

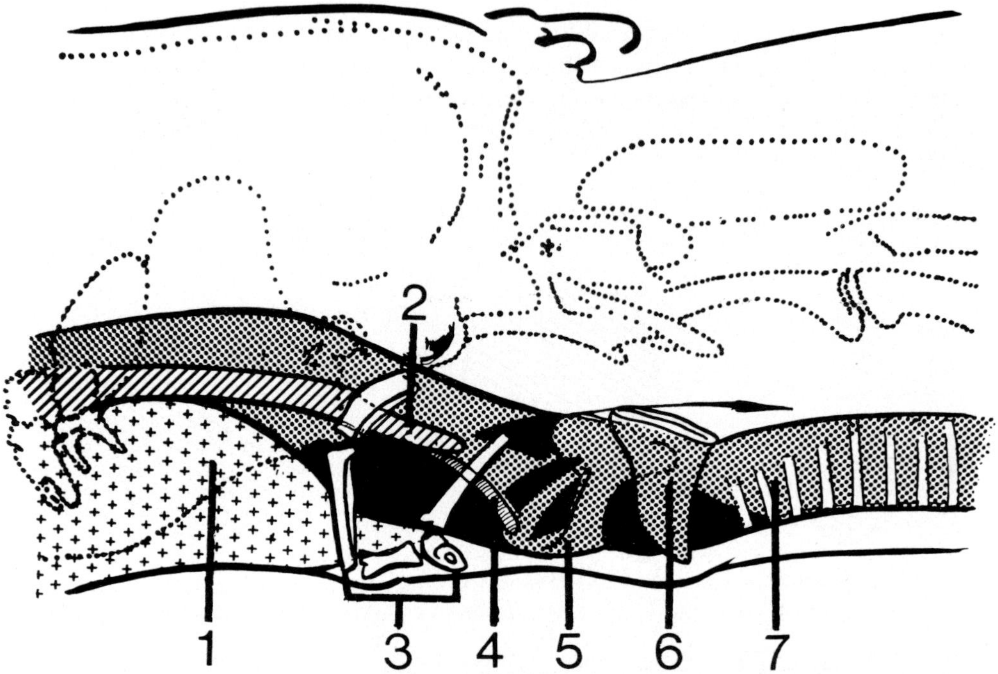

FIG. 8.12.

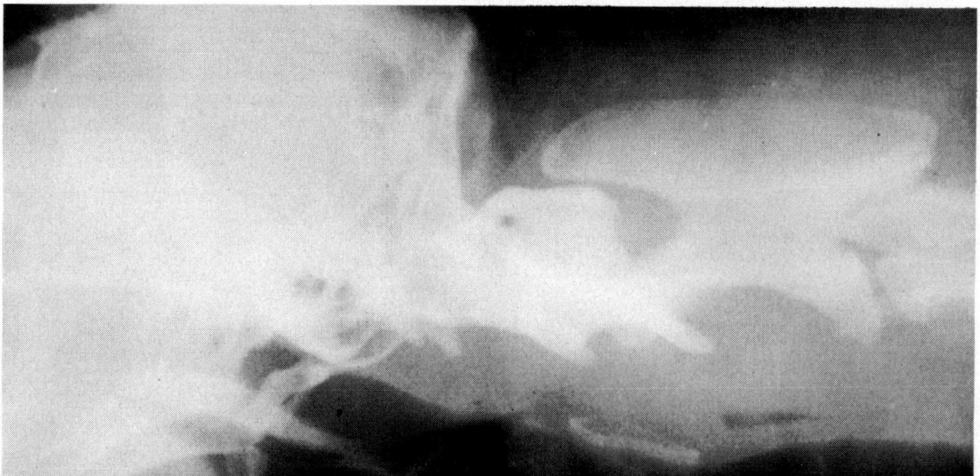

FIG. 8.13.

FIGS. 8.12 and 8.13. Normal lateral radiograph of the pharyngeal area.

(1) tongue (2) soft palate (3) hyoid apparatus (4) epiglottis (5) thyroid cartilage (6) cricoid cartilage (7) tracheal ring.

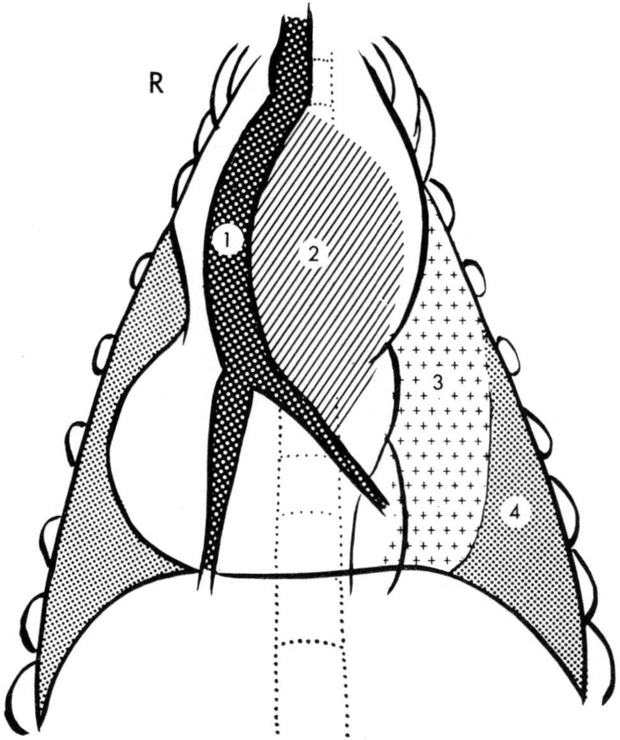

FIG. 8.14.

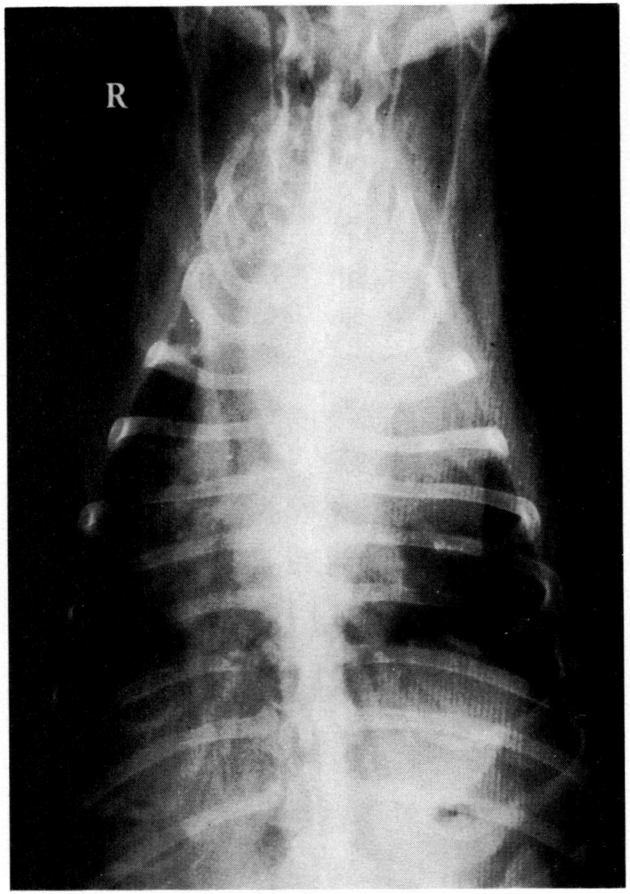

FIG. 8.15.

FIGS. 8.14 and 8.15. Displacement of trachea by mediastinal tumour.

(1) displaced trachea (2) mediastinal mass
(3) consolidation of lung (4) normal lung parenchyma.

The Trachea

The position of the trachea is similarly visualised by the air which it contains, although in the dorso-ventral plane it is partially obscured by the denser shadow of the cervical and thoracic vertebrae.

In a lateral view the trachea roughly parallels the line of the cervical and anterior thoracic vertebrae. It curves downwards towards the heart and finally terminates in the bifurcation (carina) which may be reproduced in some films as a particularly dark, nearly circular shadow (Fig. 8.4).

Displacement of the trachea from its normal position can be an indication of the presence of inflammatory or neoplastic lesions in the neck, or of enlargement of a mediastinal lymph gland (Fig. 8.15).

Tracheal collapse resulting in respiratory obstruction has been reported in dogs (O'Brien, Buchanan and Kelly, 1966) and lateral films of clinical cases will show marked narrowing of the trachea at the thoracic inlet. However, in the authors' experience similar narrowing can sometimes be demonstrated in radiographs of clinically normal dogs if the head and neck are over extended at the time of radiography. Thus caution must be exercised in ascribing symptoms of respiratory obstruction to this finding in a single radiograph.

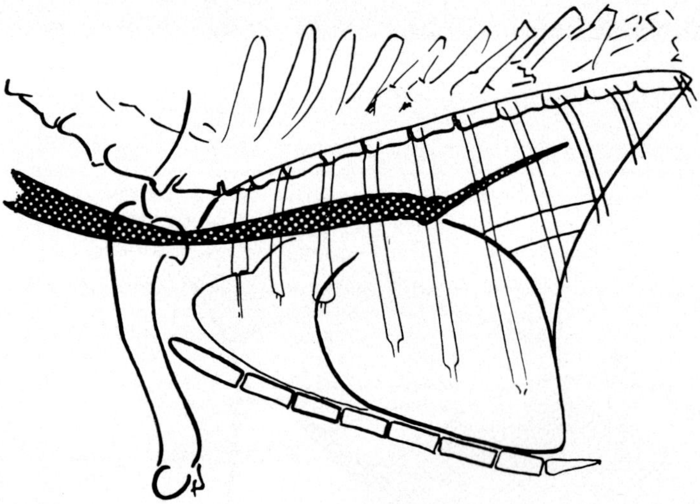

FIG. 8.16. Narrowing of the trachea due to positioning.

The Bronchial Tree

At the carina the trachea divides into the right and left main bronchi, which in turn give rise to the apical, cardiac, diaphragmatic, and (on the right side only) intermediate bronchi. These main bronchi, which are outlined by the air they contain, can usually be identified in radiographs, provided that the radiologist is familiar with the anatomy of the bronchial tree and that radiographs taken in both planes are available for comparison.

Radiological recognition of the smaller bronchi is not normally possible as they become confused with the shadows cast by the pulmonary blood vessels. Both small bronchi and blood vessels radiographed "end on" will cast comparatively dense shadows which can be mistaken for small neoplastic foci.

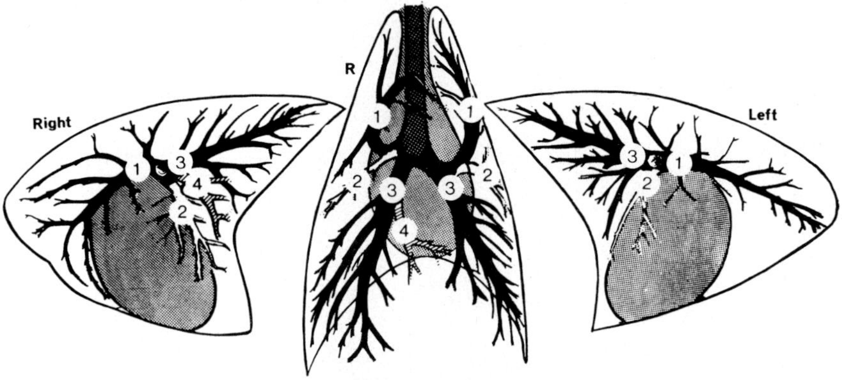

FIG. 8.17. Bronchial tree
(1) apical bronchus. (2) cardiac bronchus. (3) diaphragmatic bronchus. (4) intermediate bronchus.

For detailed demonstration of the bronchial tree bronchography (Douglas and Hall, 1959) is necessary. Since this procedure is usually only carried out on one half of the chest at one time it renders lateral views considerably more informative.

The actual substance of the bronchial wall is not clearly defined in a normal chest radiograph and pathological changes are also difficult to recognise. Bronchitis would result in a slight increase in the radio-density of the bronchial tree but this is seldom sufficiently marked to permit a diagnosis on radiological grounds alone.

The nodules arising from bronchial wall in the region of the carina as a result of infestation with Filaroides osleri have been demonstrated radiologically (Lauder and Lawson, 1959), but their presence can be confirmed more accurately by other methods.

Gross bronchial changes are not common but severe bronchiectasis has been demonstrated (Douglas and Hall, 1959). This condition should be suspected on films showing a dense irregular bronchial outline together with loss of the usual air-filled lumen, but can probably only be diagnosed conclusively after bronchography.

The demonstration of bronchial foreign bodies will depend: (a) on their radio-opacity, (b) on the amount of local reaction they provoke. A localised broncho-pneumonia of the base of the diaphragmatic lobe of lung due to a non radio-opaque foreign body (a head of wheat) has been reported (Burriss, 1961). The authors have encountered similar radiological findings in the same area of lung and due to a similar foreign body. Consideration of the anatomy of the bronchial tree suggests that foreign material passing down the trachea would most naturally pass into the diaphragmatic bronchus and that this is the site to examine for evidence of its presence.

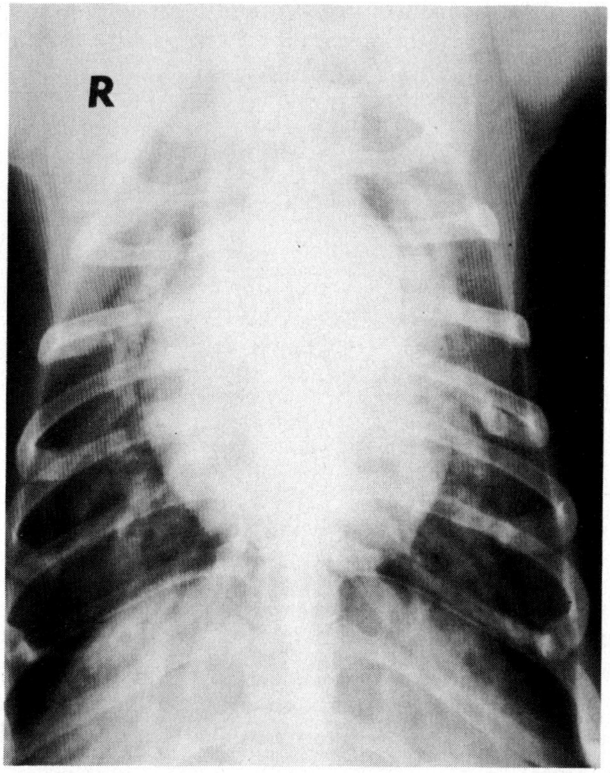

FIG. 8.18.

FIG. 8.19.

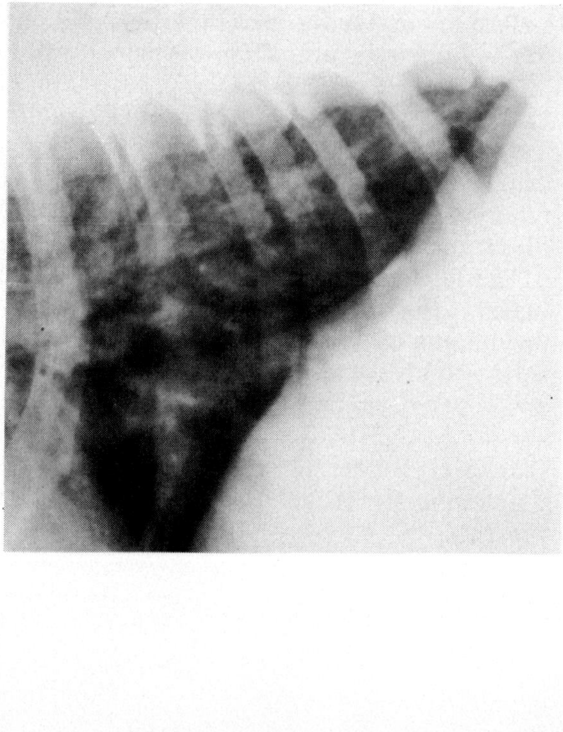

FIGS. 8.18 and 8.19. Peribronchial density associated with severe tracheobronchitis.

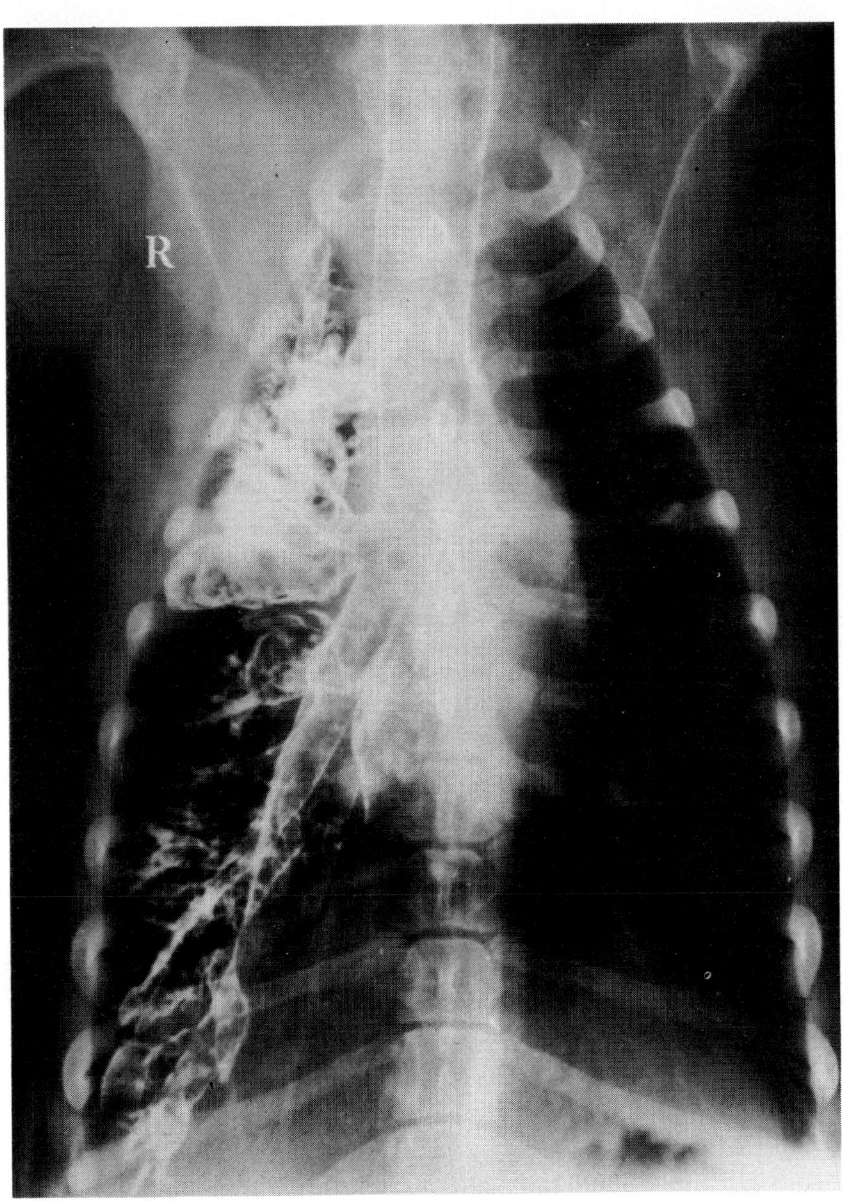

FIG. 8.20. Bronchogram of the right chest of a Corgi dog demonstrating saccular bronchiectasis.

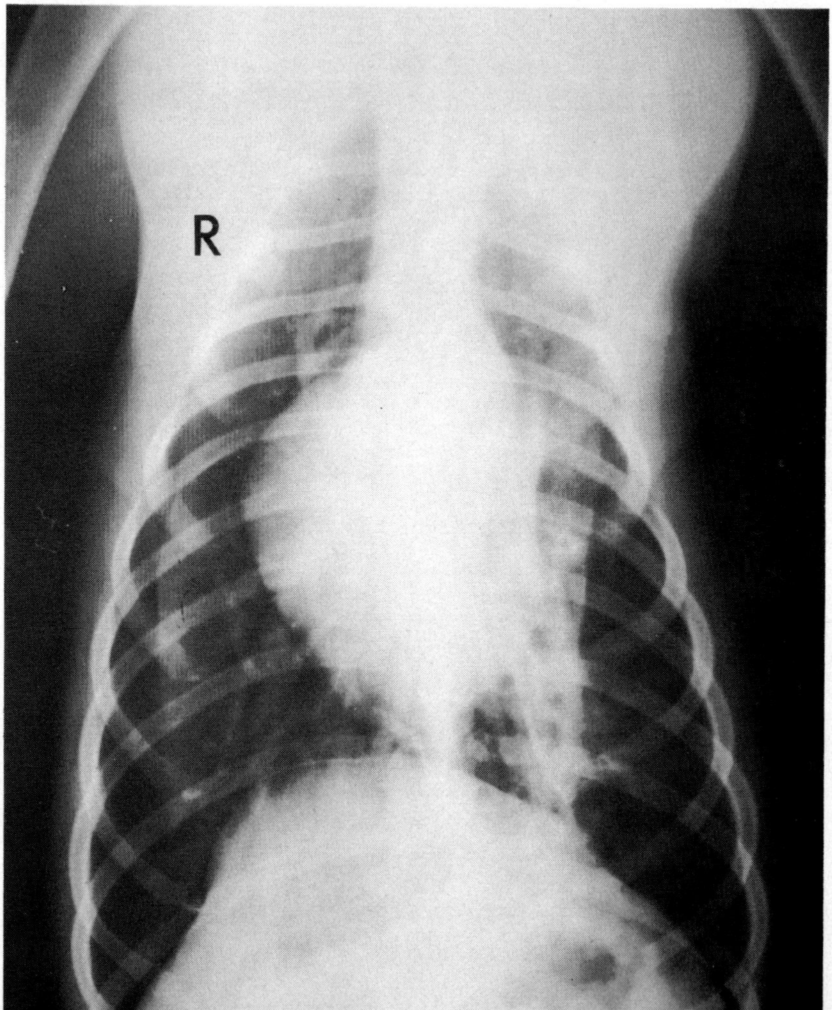

FIG. 8.21. Collapse and consolidation of an area of the left diaphragmatic lobe of lung in a mongrel, due to the presence of a barley head within the bronchus.

The Lungs

It is important to be familiar with the lobular structure of the lungs. The division between individual lobes is not appreciable in a radiograph of normal lungs, but demonstration of these fissures can be the first evidence of the presence of fluid within the pleural cavity.

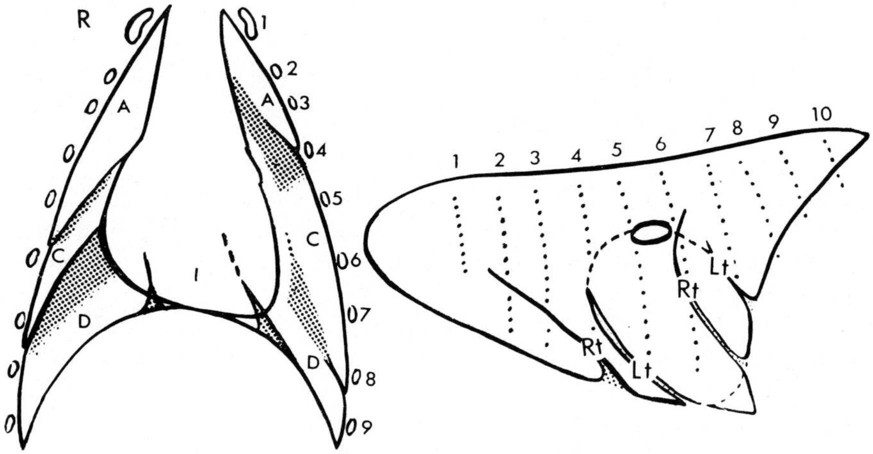

FIG. 8.22. Composite diagram to indicate the approximate divisions between the lobes of the lungs, as visualised radiologically following the accumulation of small amounts of fluid.

The fact that the intermediate lobe of the right lung extends into the left half of the chest is shown by the thin oblique line of demarcation (termed the diaphragmatico-pericardial ligament by Carlson, 1967) seen in most dorso-ventral chest radiographs.

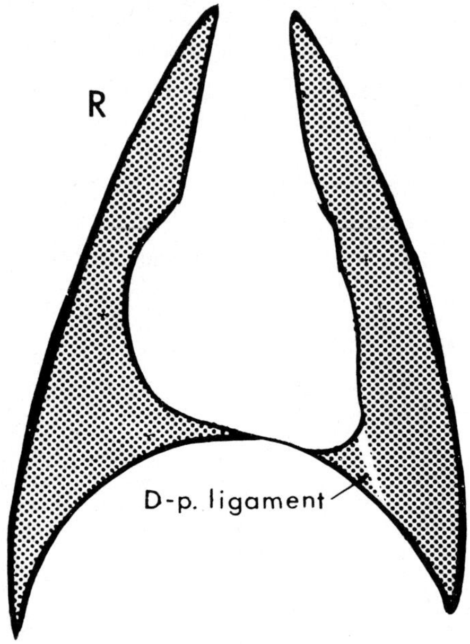

FIG. 8.23.

Normal lung parenchyma is almost imperceptible radiologically and the extent of lung substance is very largely indicated by the bronchi and pulmonary vessels.

These become progressively smaller and indistinct towards the periphery of the lungs but they can usually be identified as extending almost to the bony thoracic cage, thus indicating that the lungs are fully filling the chest cavity. Collapse of the lungs is shown, by an increased density of the affected lung tissue, by recognition of a distinct outline to the collapsed lobe, and by complete absence of vascular or bronchial markings in the zone between lung and chest wall.

Areas of increased density in lung substance may be associated with various forms of pneumonia, with neoplasia, and with haemorrhage into the lung. The chief characteristics of these conditions are discussed later in the chapter but any areas of consolidation must be examined critically if their significance is to be accurately assessed. Comparison of dorso-ventral and lateral projections will enable the extent of the lesions and their relation to other structures to be judged (e.g., is the density confined to one lobe of lung? or, does the condition follow the bronchial pattern and suggest bronchopneumonia?). The demarcation of the area is also of significance —a diffuse edge is typical of infection while, in general, neoplasia is more discretely outlined. Subsequent radiographs will provide information as to the spread or regression of the condition, but if this is to be of value it is essential that exposures are made under identical conditions.

The Pleural Cavity

This potential cavity is bounded by the rib cage and by the diaphragm but it will not be appreciable in a radiograph of a normal animal.

The first evidence of pathological change is likely to be visualisation of the pleural cavity by the presence of air or fluid within it. This is recognised as a zone extending around the collapsed lobes of lung, in which no lung tissue can be identified, and which is dark and radiotranslucent when due to pneumothorax, or light and dense when due to the presence of fluid. These areas usually extend around the lobe or lobes of lung (i.e., on the diaphragmatic and lateral surfaces in dorso-ventral views, and on the diaphragmatic, dorsal, and ventral surfaces in lateral fields) and may be associated with displacement of some of the thoracic organs.

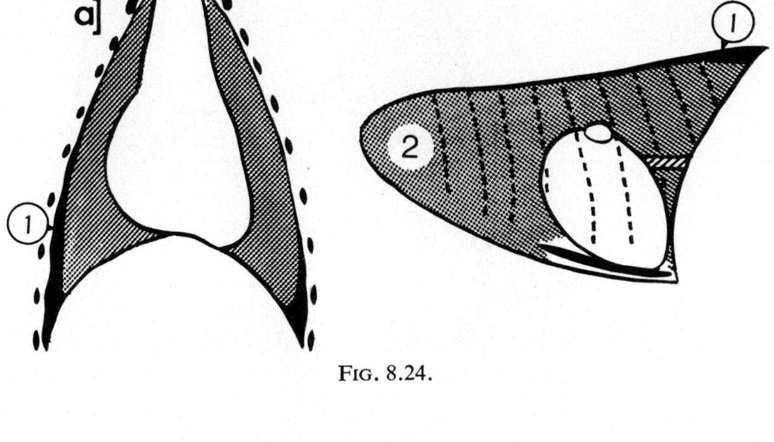

FIG. 8.24.

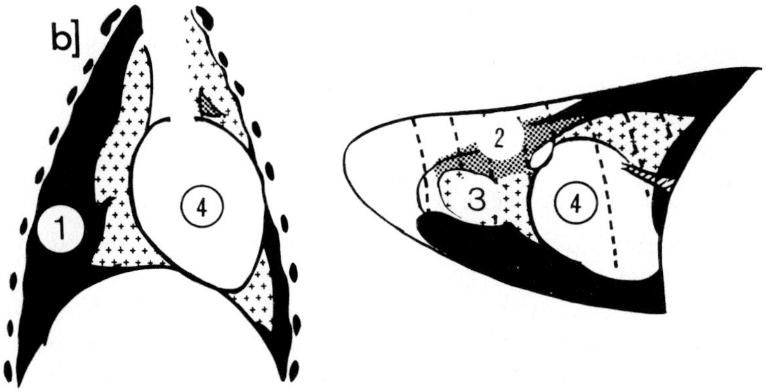

FIG. 8.25.

FIGS. 8.24 and 8.25. Tracings from radiographs of mild (a) and severe (b) cases of pneumothorax.
(1) air in thoracic cavity
(2) normal lung parenchyma
(3) collapsed lung
(4) displaced heart.

The development of fluid within the pleural cavity may be insidious in onset and difficult to diagnose with certainty. A characteristic and helpful feature at this stage can be the presence of arrowed projections of fluid extending into the fissures between the lobes of lung. As more fluid accumulates there will be a diffuse increase in density throughout the chest and all detail will be lost. Lateral radiographs taken with the patient in the standing position will cause the fluid to gravitate and permit demonstration of a "fluid line". While this positioning renders a portion of the lungs visible in the dorsal portion of the chest, they are invariably compressed and an accurate radiological examination of the underlying chest pathology can only be undertaken after aspiration of most of the fluid from the thorax.

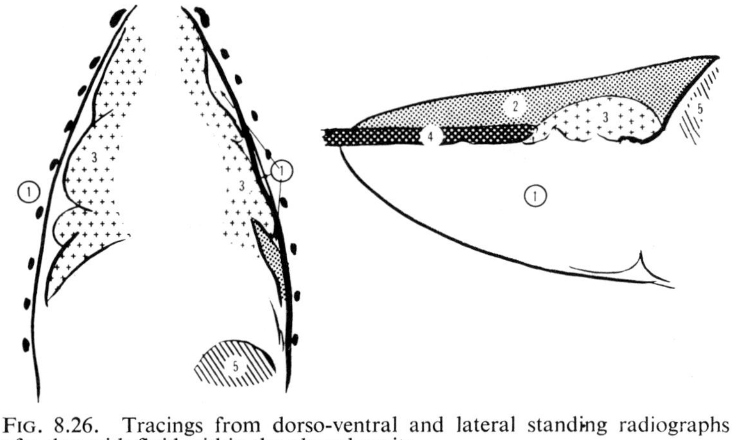

FIG. 8.26. Tracings from dorso-ventral and lateral standing radiographs of a dog with fluid within the pleural cavity.
(1) pleural fluid (2) normal parenchyma
(3) consolidated lung (4) Trachea
(5) stomach gas.

The Rib Cage

This has been described in Chapter 5. Since the ribs are less dense than might be expected, lesions of these bones can be overlooked unless they are very carefully examined.

The Diaphragm

In the normal animal the line of the diaphragm is clearly indicated by the contrast between the air-filled chest anteriorly and the dense liver posteriorly. However, since the diaphragm is a domed structure, it must be appreciated this "line" indicates only the most anterior portion of the diaphragm and that the posterior edges of the diaphragmatic lobes of lung and the peripheral portion of the diaphragm extend further back. This fact is responsible for the appearance of a "double line" in the dorsal region of lateral films, and for the recognition of lung markings situated apparently posterior to the diaphragm in dorso-ventral projections.

The fact that the position and appearance of the line of the diaphragm varies with the stage of respiration has already been mentioned. This is best visualised in lateral radiographs where, at the stage of expiration, it will be seen that the diaphragm has a domed outline. The lower half of this line tends to merge with the posterior edge of the heart, and the upper half is angled backwards reaching the spine at the level of the tenth or eleventh thoracic vertebra. At inspiration this domed effect is lost and the diaphragm is a comparatively straight line quite distinct from the cardiac outline, and, in the upper two-thirds situated at least a full intercostal space behind the expiratory line.

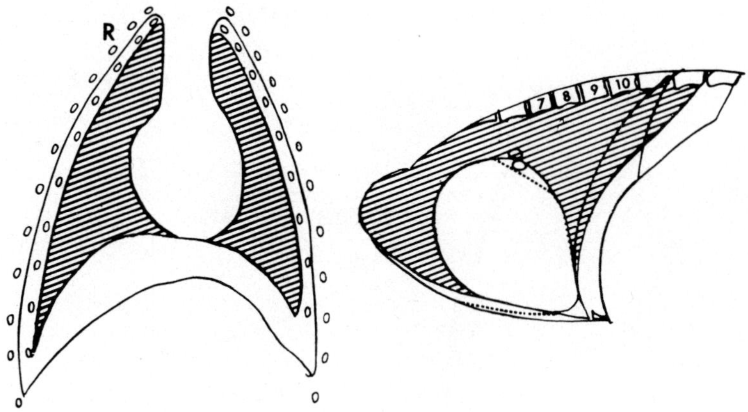

FIG. 8.27. Tracings of superimposed chest radiographs taken at inspiration and expiration.

In dorso-ventral projections the line of the diaphragm is seen to be slightly bilobed in structure and it will be noted that the two halves do not exactly correspond—the right half is set at a sharper angle and extends further forward than the left half.

In expiratory films this line is again situated approximately one intercostal space anterior to the inspiratory line.

In clinical cases localised anterior distortion of the line of the diaphragm is likely to be the result of adhesion to the lungs associated with a previous infection, while marked displacement in either direction will result from thoracic or abdominal pressure due to fluid or neoplastic mass.

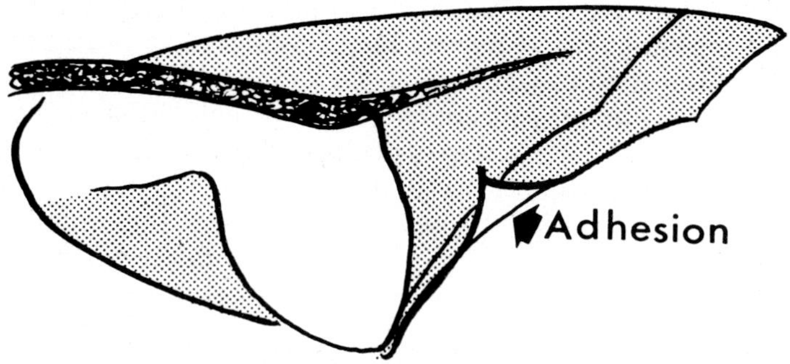

FIG. 8.28.

Failure to identify the diaphragm line may be due to consolidation of the diaphragmatic lobes of the lungs and thus to lack of contrast with the liver, but it is always suspicious of the presence of a rupture of the diaphragm and further evidence to prove or disprove this must be sought.

The Mediastium

Most of this region is not clearly outlined in thoracic radiographs and its extent is best demonstrated by the organs which it contains (the heart, the major vessels, and the trachea). However, in correctly positioned dorsal-ventral projections the anterior mediastinum is recognised in the mid line reaching from the cardiac shadow to the anterior limit of the lungs and extending on each side of the vertebral column. Because of the superimposed shadows of the spine and sternum little detail can be appreciated, but the air-filled trachea is usually just visible.

In clinical cases recognition of mediastinal shift (displacement of the shadow of the mediastinum and its contained structures to one side) indicates either, increased intra-thoracic pressure on one side of the chest or, decreased pressure on the other side. The former might occur in association with the presence of a thoracic neoplasm or herniated abdominal contents, while the latter situation might result from atelectasis (collapse of a portion of lung—usually resulting from obstruction of the bronchus supplying the area).

The Heart and Major Blood Vessels

See Chapter 9.

The Thoracic Oesophagus

See Chapter 11.

COMMON PATHOLOGICAL CONDITIONS AFFECTING THE CHEST

Pneumothorax

The distinctive features of this condition are the demonstration of some degree of collapse of the lungs and the presence of air within the pleural cavity. This is indicated by the typical dark band of air (in which no lung markings can be recognised) surrounding and outlining the collapsed lungs (which have receded from the chest wall and appear denser than usual).

The features seen in lateral projections will vary with the position of the animal at the time of radiography. If the dog is placed in lateral recumbency, the films will show the usual zone of air around the periphery of the lung and, in most instances, a typical upward displacement of the heart. If, however, the examination is carried out with the animal in the standing position, the displacement of the heart is corrected and the air tends to accumulate in the dorsal areas of the chest.

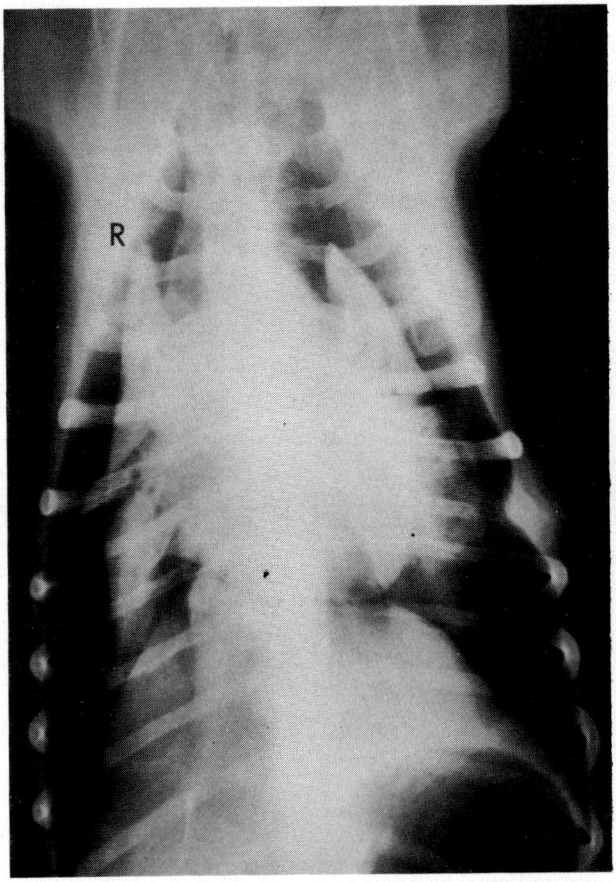

FIG. 8.29.

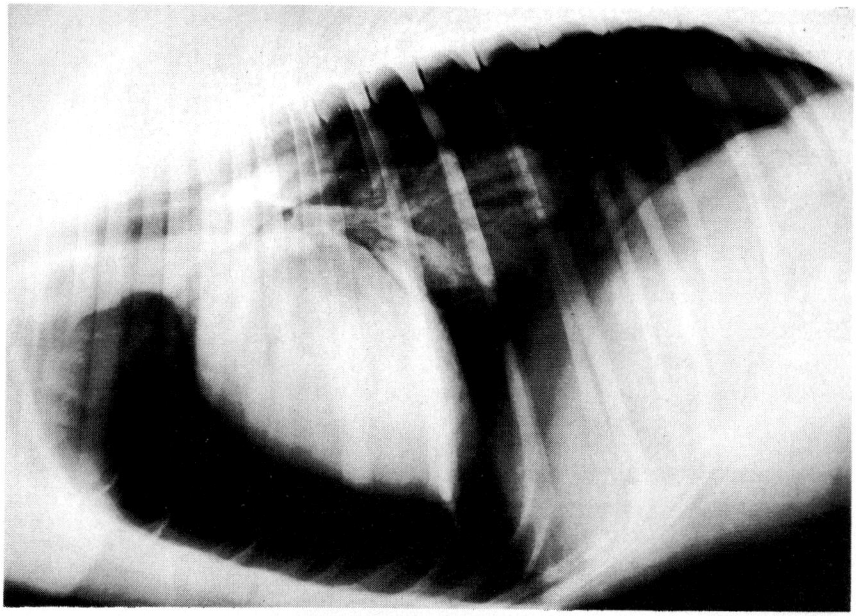

FIG. 8.30.

FIGS. 8.29 and 8.30. Bilateral pneumothorax with collapse of all lobes of lung.

Over-exposure, skin folds, and certain anatomical abnormalities can all give rise to a false impression of pneumothorax.

If the condition is likely to have been traumatic in origin a particularly careful examination of the film should be made for evidence of further injury. Close inspection of the rib cage may reveal a fractured rib or ribs and this can be associated with the presence of air in the overlying soft tissues (emphysema). A marked increase in density of the collapsed lung could be associated with haemorrhage into its substance.

Fluid in the Pleural Cavity

The presence of fluid within the pleural cavity may be associated with a number of thoracic conditions (respiratory infections, the presence of abdominal viscera or thoracic neoplasia, cardiac abnormalities, leakage from the chyle duct, haemorrhage, etc.). In each instance radiography is likely to be of value in confirming the presence of fluid but may be of little assistance in distinguishing its nature or cause. In particular, as the condition advances, the accumulation of large amounts of fluid will prevent the recognition of associated chest pathology and it may be necessary to aspirate this before any further radiological diagnosis can be undertaken.

Intrathoracic Haemorrhage

Haemorrhage into the thorax is encountered as a result of severe trauma, or following the ingestion of Warfarin rat poison. Such haemorrhage may occur into the lung substance, or into the pleural cavity, or into both areas simultaneously.

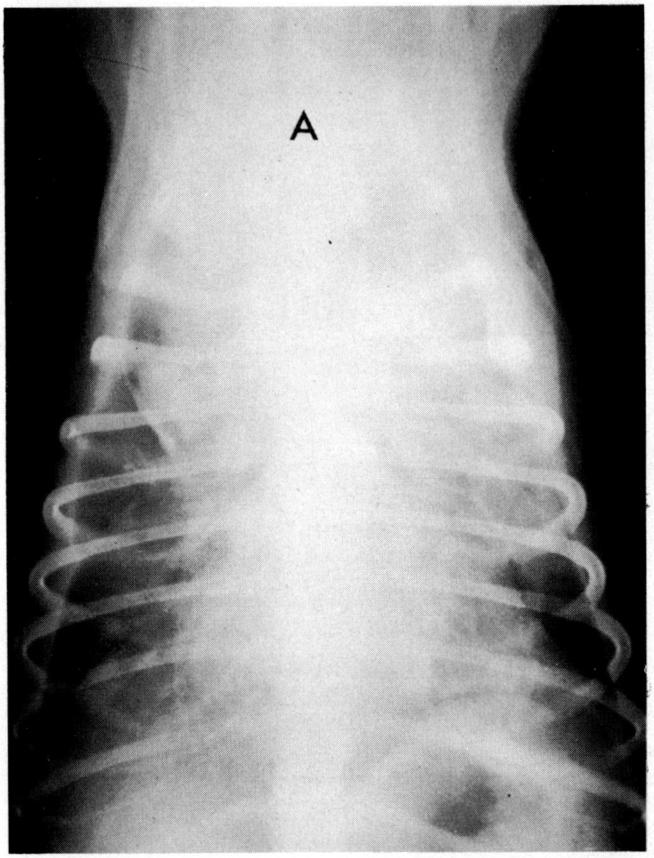

FIG. 8.31.

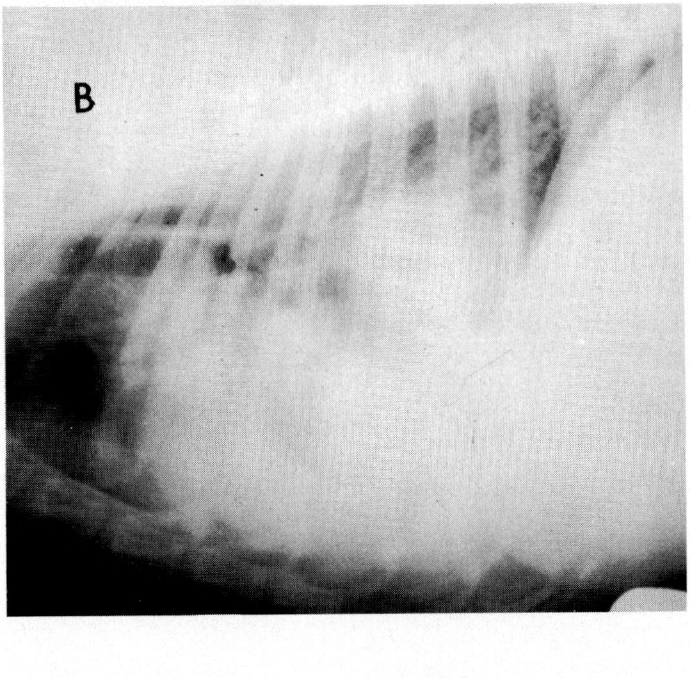

FIG. 8.32.

FIGS. 8.31, 8.32 and 8.33. Fluid within the pleural cavity associated with the presence of secondary neoplasia.

(A) Dorso-ventral film showing visualisation of the fissures by fluid.

(B) Film taken with dog in lateral recumbancy and revealing a diffuse opacity of chest.

(C) Standing lateral film demonstrating a fluid line.

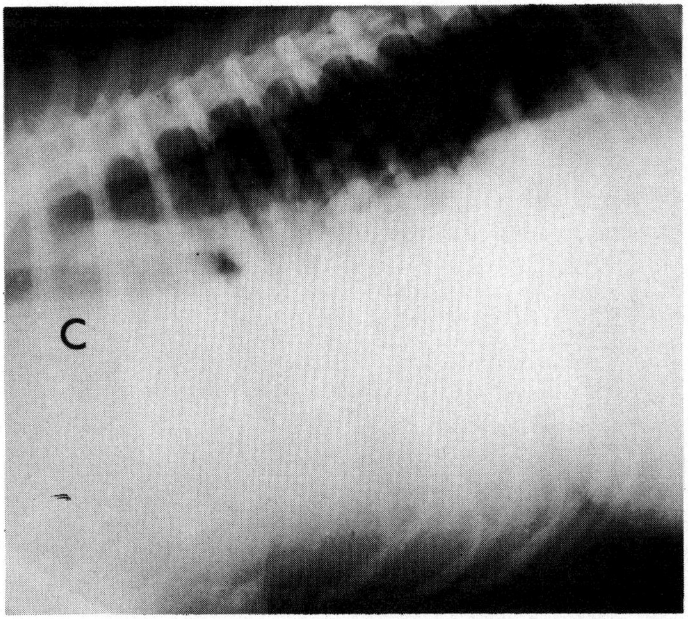

FIG. 8.33.

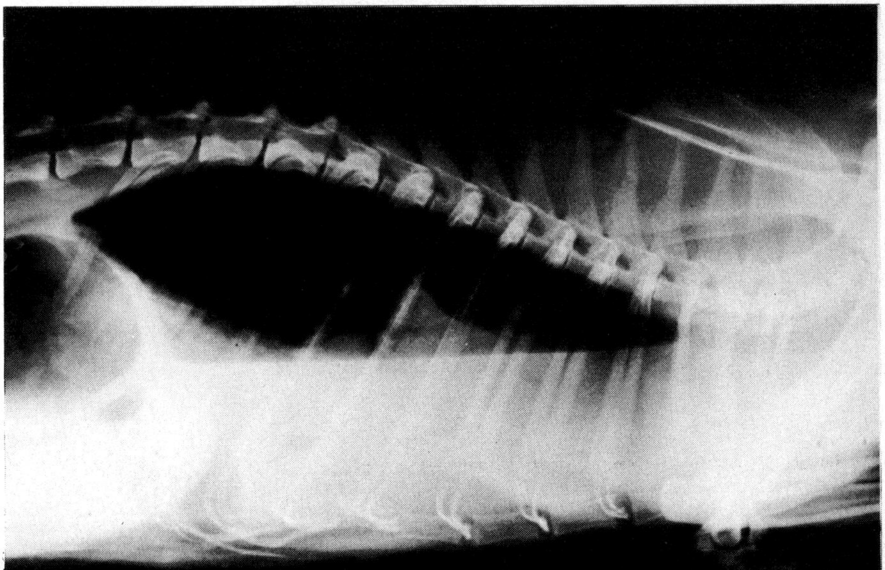

FIG. 8.34. A well-defined fluid level in the thorax of a cat due to an accidental pneumothorax occurring during paracentisis.

Obviously the radiological findings cannot be pathognomonic of haemorrhage, but where the clinical findings suggest that this has occurred, radiography can prove of assistance in confirming its presence and extent. Haemorrhage into the pleural cavity was mentioned in the previous section and films will show the characteristic features of fluid in this area. Bleeding into the lung substance will be reproduced as areas of opacity which may be localised or extensive, discrete or diffuse.

Where the condition is due to trauma radiography may reveal evidence of other injuries (fractured ribs or pneumothorax).

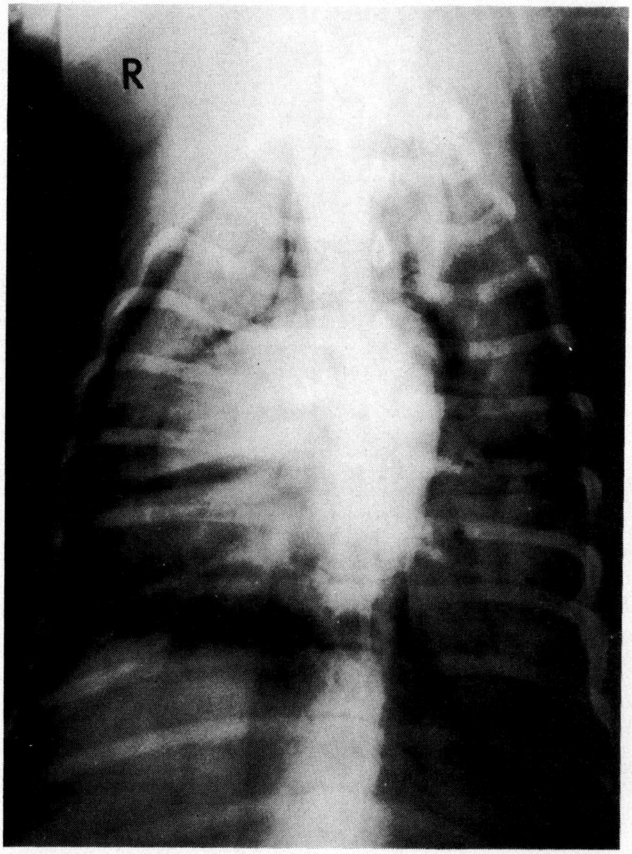

FIG. 8.35. Increased density of lung lobes due to intrapulmonary haemorrhage. A slight degree of pneumothorax is also present.

Diaphragmatic Hernia

The radiological appearance of this condition can vary considerably, depending on the site and extent of the hernia, on the length of time it has been present, and on which of the abdominal viscera have been displaced into the chest.

The most typical feature is the disappearance of the normal diaphragm line. This occurs as a result of the abdominal contents passing into the chest, displacing the lungs, and producing an increased density which no longer permits differentiation between chest and abdomen. However, if the diaphragmatic rent is small and the

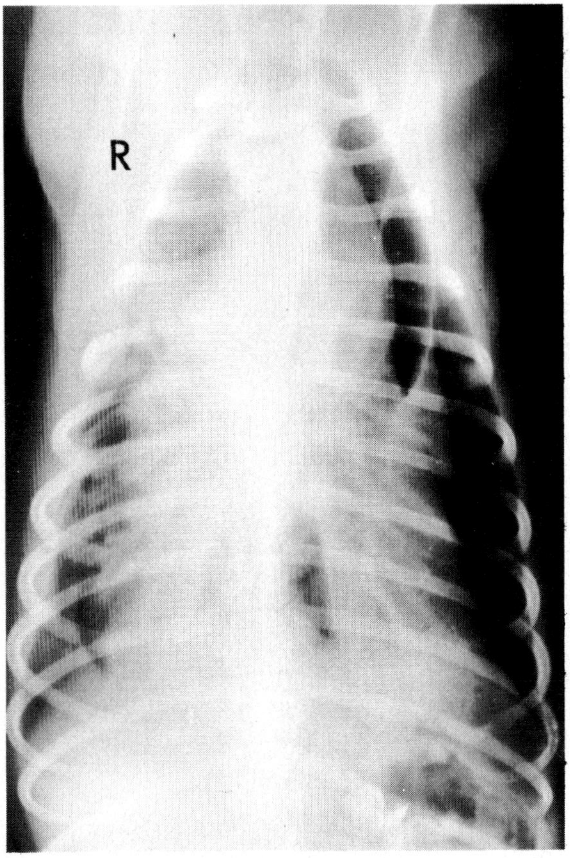

FIG. 8.36.

FIGS. 8.36 and 8.37. Rupture of diaphragm occurring on the right side of chest. Note the gas filled loops of bowel on right of chest (but extending into left apical region), the stomach (containing foreign material) still in normal position and the presence of fluid.

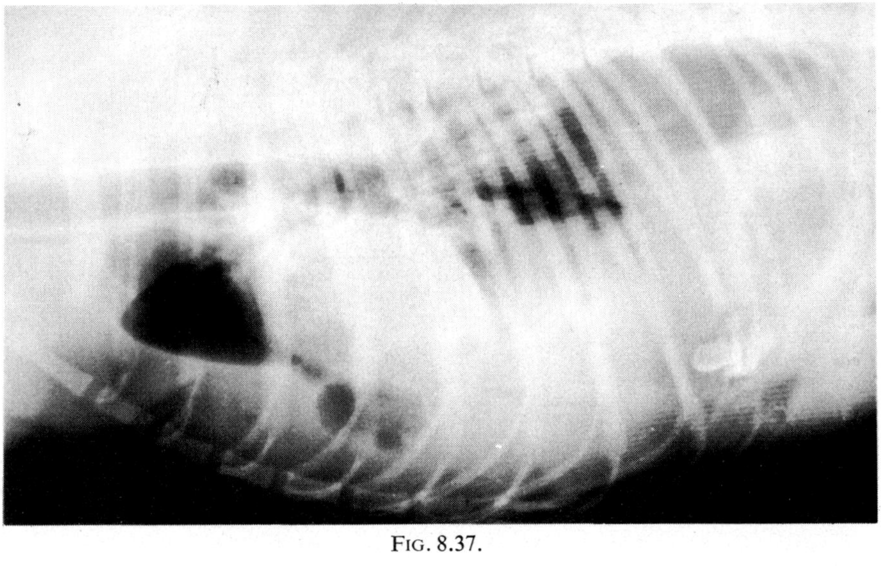

FIG. 8.37.

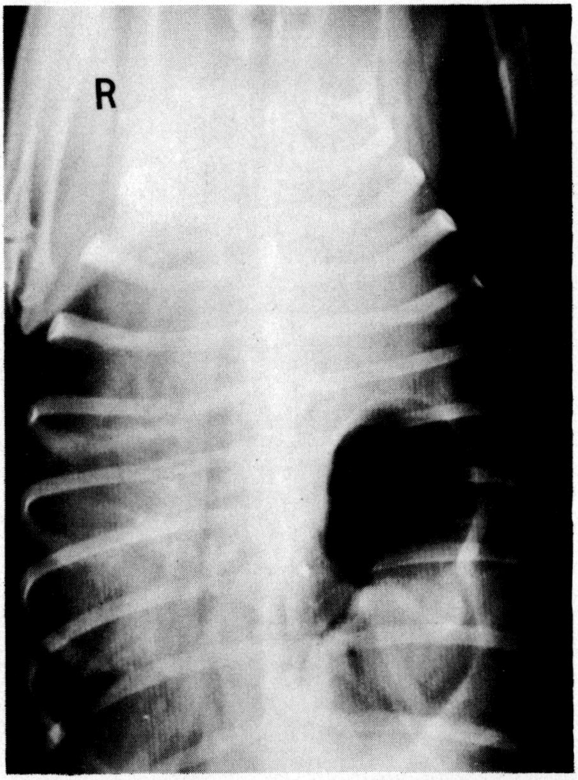

FIG. 8.38.

FIGS. 8.38 and 8.39. Left-sided rupture of the diaphragm in a Collie dog with displacement of stomach into chest.

FIG. 8.39.

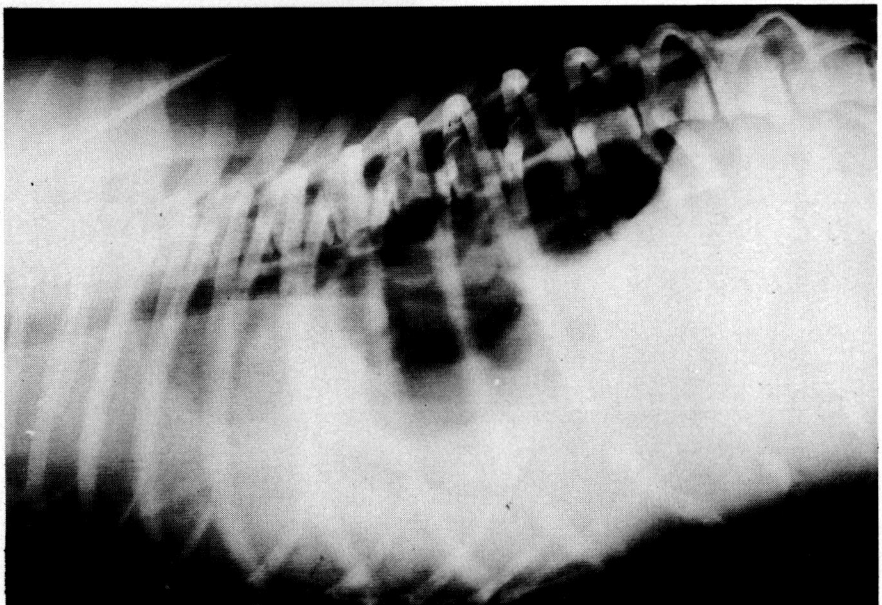

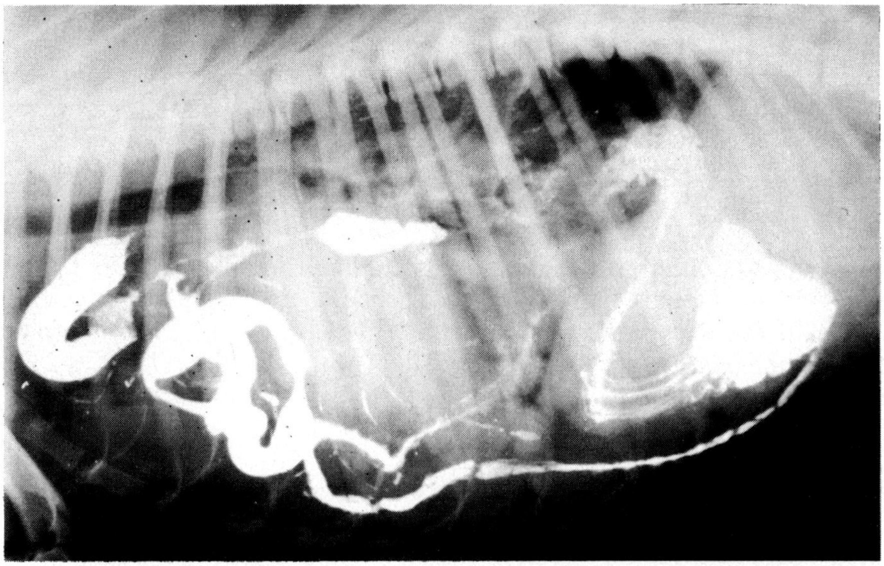

FIG. 8.40. Ruptured diaphragm in a Terrier. Displacement of small bowel into chest demonstrated by administration of barium.

liver is not appreciably displaced, the major portion of the diaphragm line may still be perceptible.

Since herniation tends to occur into one half of the chest, dorso-ventral views are most informative, and permit comparison of the two sides. The significant radiological features to be seen in such films are:—

(a) On the affected side—loss of the line of the diaphragm, the presence of a comparatively dense area extending forward from the diaphragm and filling much of that half of chest, and associated displacement and compression of the lungs.

(b) On the unaffected side—normal aeration of lungs, and some mediastinal protrusion away from the affected side.

If the hernia occurs in the central area of the diaphragm this typical contrast between the two halves of the chest may be less obvious.

Other significant features are the demonstration of a portion of the gastro-intestinal tract within the chest, and evidence of anterior displacement of the liver. The herniated stomach or bowel may be recognised if it contains sufficient gas to outline it but may need to be identified by administration of barium. The use of choleocystography to demonstrate displacement of the liver has been advocated (Frost, 1956). This displacement may also be inferred by noting an associated shift of the stomach (outlined with barium if necessary).

If the condition has been present for some time there may be sufficient fluid present to obscure detail.

A congenital form of diaphragmatic hernia is occasionally encountered. The hernia is situated in the mid-line and comprises the passage of some abdominal contents through a patent foramen of Morgagni into the pericardial sac. Radiologically this should be visualised by considerable enlargement of the cardiac outline, suggesting the possibility of pericardial effusion. However, the presence of a hernia is likely to be associated with a more irregular shape and density of the heart and, in some circumstances, the presence of gas-filled loops of bowel may be recognised within the pericardium.

Neoplasia

Neoplasia of the chest appears to be less common in dogs and cats than in man, but it does occur and may be primary or secondary, maglinant or benign, and may involve any of the structures comprising the thoracic cavity. Tumours of the ribs, heart and oesophagus are dealt with in the appropriate chapters. Here, consideration will be limited to neoplasia involving the lungs, which will occur in one of two forms.

(*1*) *Multiple Lesions*

This form is always associated with secondary neoplasia which may arise from malignant lesions elsewhere (commonly in bone or in mammary gland) or be associated with generalised lymphosarcomatous conditions.

The commonest type is the so called "cannon ball" secondary tumours which occur as multiple masses irregularly spread throughout lung tissue. The fact that the lesions are particularly dense, comparatively circumscribed, and not related to the lung or bronchial pattern, helps to differentiate them from density's due to infective causes.

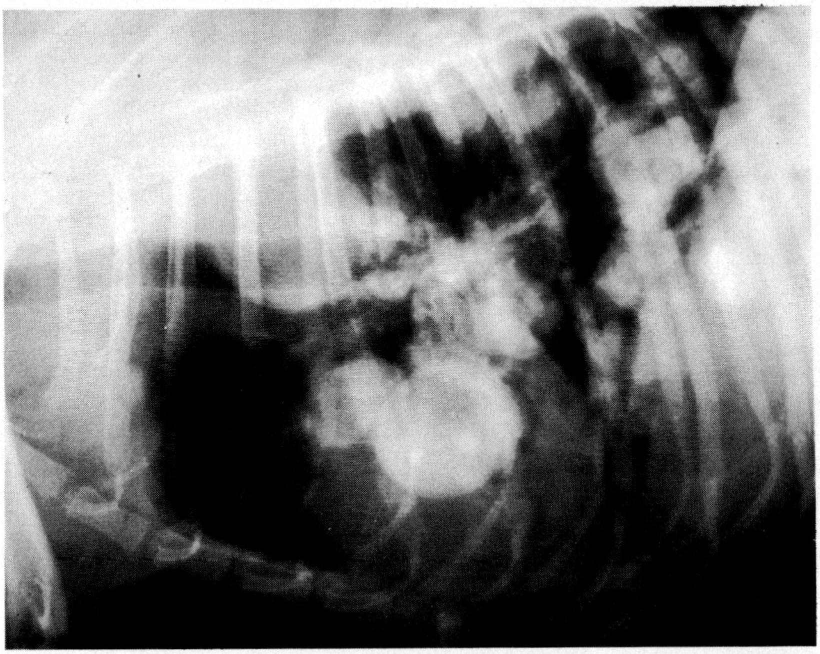

FIG. 8.41. Multiple secondary neoplastic foci in lungs (associated with an osteosarcoma of the tibia).

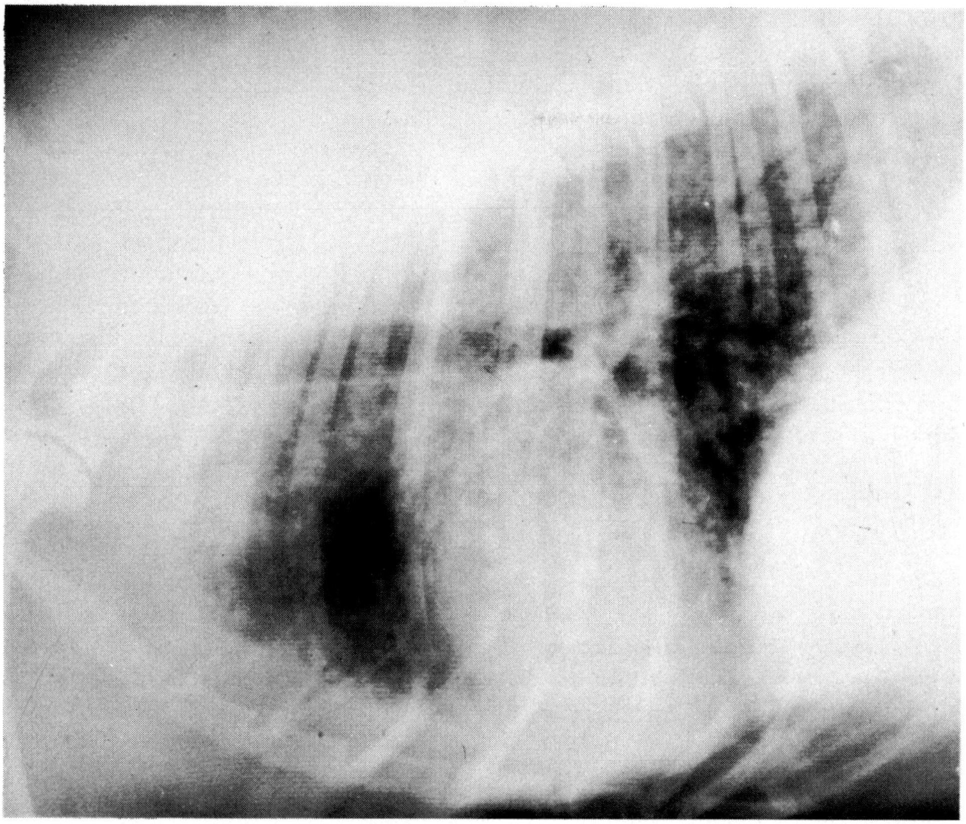

FIG. 8.42. Miliary secondary neoplasia spreading from a reticulum cell sarcoma arising in the mammary gland of a Spaniel.

Less commonly, secondary neoplasia takes a more diffuse form and appears as a reticular or miliary density extending through the entire lung fields.

Associated enlargement of the mediastinal lymphatic glands will usually be demonstrated in a lateral radiograph by upward displacement of the trachea and by the development of dense masses around the base of the heart. In particularly advanced cases consolidation of considerable areas of lung can occur, and the recognition of detail may be masked by the development of secondary fluid within the pleural cavity.

(*2*) *Solitary Lesions*

Single tumours arising in lung tissue are not often encountered but may be either primary or secondary. They will be recognised as localised areas of density in lung parenchyma and, in general, can be distinguished from similar pneumonic lesions by the fact that they are solitary, and by their marked density and discrete outline. However, such differentiation is not always easy.

Osteolytic rib tumours which have extended into the thorax can appear as neoplasms within the lung substance. When lesions of this nature are situated at the edge of the thorax the outline of the adjacent ribs should be closely examined for any evidence of involvement in the mass.

Intrathoracic neoplasms can become surprising large before their presence is suspected and the use of radiography may demonstrate such lesions before the animal is showing any clinical symptoms. For this reason, it is a wise precaution to make a routine radiographic examination of the chest when assessing the prognosis and treatment of any potentially malignant neoplasm. A lateral radiograph is usually adequate for the purpose and recognition of either enlargement of the mediastinal lymphatic glands or of the presence of neoplastic foci, would be a contra-indication for operation on the original neoplasm. Since it is important to recognise such foci at an early stage, good radiographic technique with the minimum of respiratory blur is essential. It must be pointed out however, that negative radiographic findings do not completely eliminate the possibility of neoplastic lesions being present. Such foci have to reach a small but definite size (0·5–1·0 cm.), before they can be visualised in a film. In doubtful cases it is worth repeating radiography after a lapse of a few weeks, as these lesions can develop quite rapidly.

Pneumonia

Pneumonia in animals is usually diagnosed clinically and, for a number of reasons (e.g., the risk of contagious disease), the patient is not often subjected to radiographic examination. Because of this and the practical difficulties involved in obtaining good chest films, the radiological features of pneumonia have not been studied as thoroughly in animals as in man. The following comments are based on practical experience, but it should be borne in mind that there can be considerable variation between individual cases.

The viral interstitial pneumonia which occurs in association with canine distemper is likely to produce a slight but diffuse increase in the density of the entire lung parenchyma. This can, in some circumstances, be associated with denser and more localised lesions of bacterial broncho-pneumonia.

In the more typical bacterial pneumonia radiography will demonstrate irregular but poorly defined areas of increased density which tend to spread outwards from the hilum of each lobe of lung. These areas of increased density may follow the course of the bronchial tree, or be confined to individual lobes of lung. Characteristic features are the fact that the affected areas tend to merge with the surrounding lung tissue and cannot be clearly defined, and the fact that the increased density of the lung parenchyma obliterates the vascular markings but intensifies the air-filled outline of the bronchi.

Radiography is employed to a greater extent in the investigation of the more chronic lung infections (e.g., nocardia, Friedlander's bacillus) since the clinical symptoms are far less typical. Radiology should again demonstrate areas of increased density which may extend outwards from the hilar area or be dispersed as small lesions throughout the lung substance. In general, the opacities associated with the more chronic infections are particularly dense and discrete in outline and can closely resemble the appearance of neoplastic lesions.

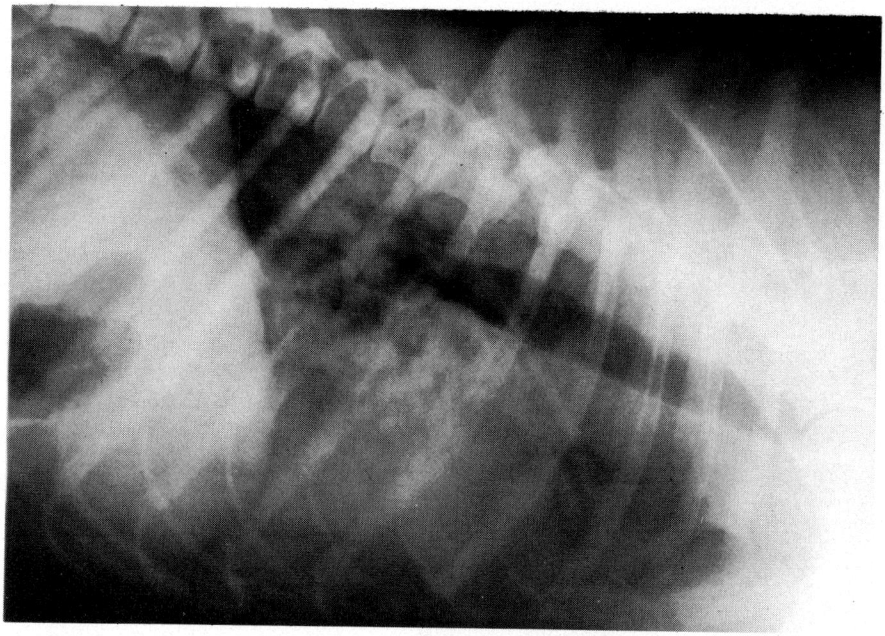

FIG. 8.43 (a). Patchy increased density of lung parenchyma in a dog due to pneumonia.

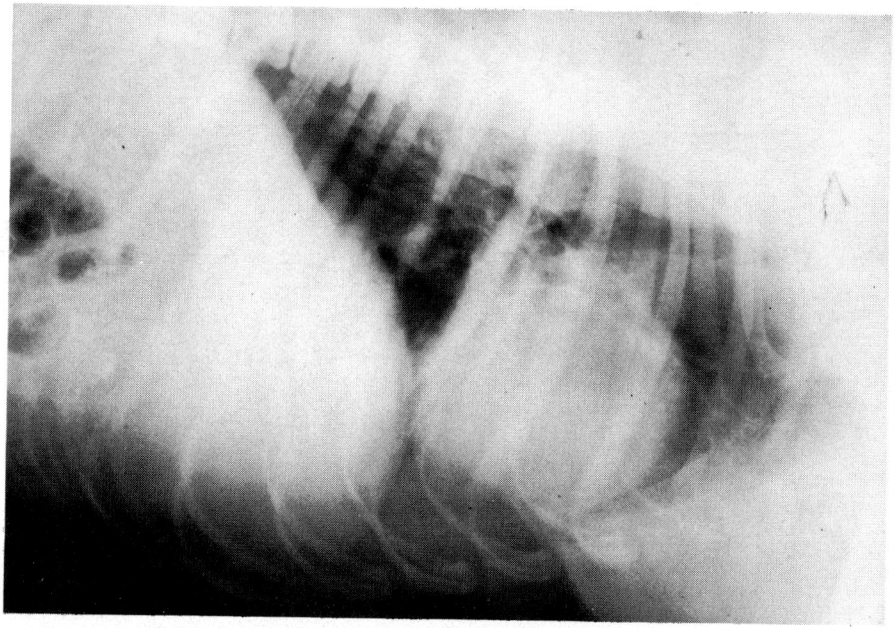

FIG. 8.44 (b). Clearing of the pneumonia following antibiotic treatment.

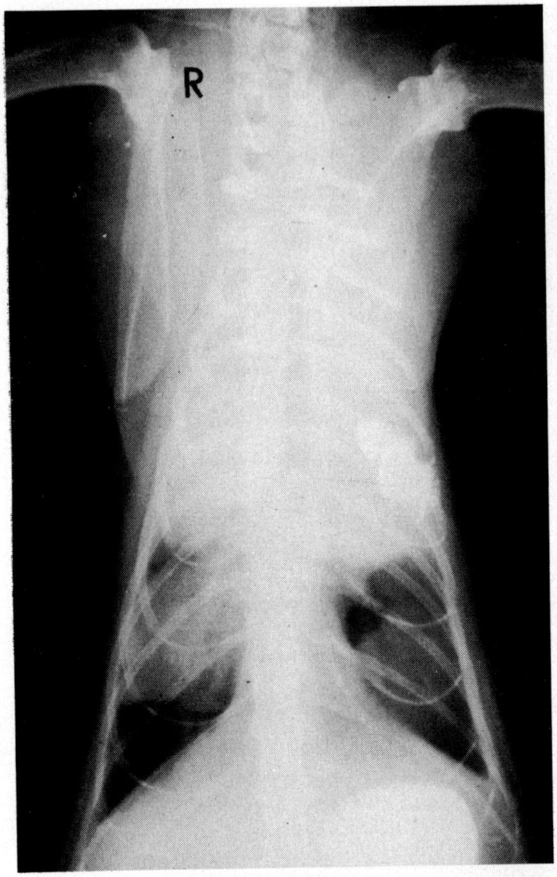

FIG. 8.45.

FIGS. 8.45 and 8.46. Lateral and dorso-ventral projections of a cat suffering from chronic pneumonia due to Friedlander's bacillus. The area of greatest density in the dorso-ventral projection is due to barium which had been administered as the animal was also showing symptoms of oesophageal obstruction.

FIG. 8.46.

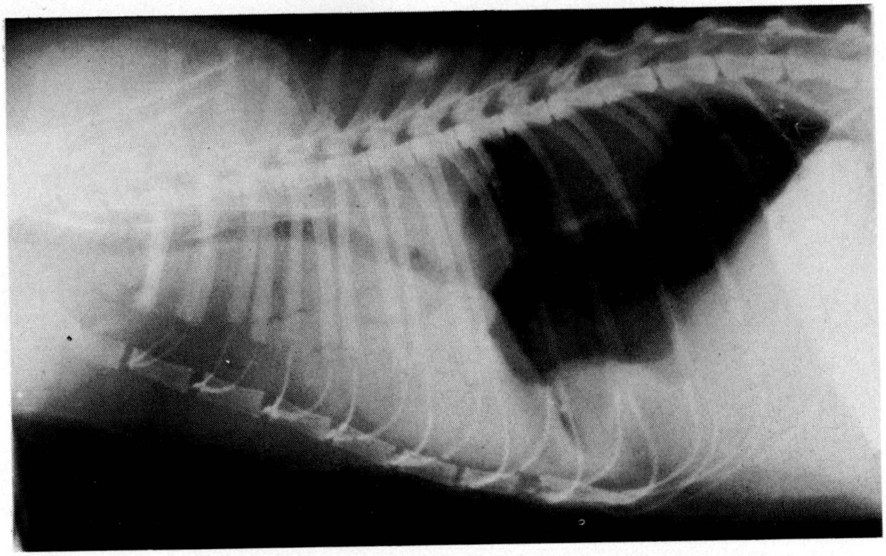

Tuberculosis

This condition is now extremely rare in small animals in this country, and the fullest radiological description of the respiratory form of this disease is that given by Olsson (1957). The principle findings were, lymphatic enlargement, areas of opacity in lung parenchyma, and the presence of pleural fluid, although these did not necessarily all occur in the same case. Similar findings are recorded by Lauder and Lawson (1959). These writers report the recognition of cavitation and of calcified nodules on the pleura as a less common feature of the condition.

It is worth pointing out that tuberculosis is still a common cause of respiratory disease in exotic animals (particularly primates) and that radiography can be of value in demonstrating this.

REFERENCES

Burriss, W. M. (1961), J. Am. vet. med. Ass., **138,** 139.
Carlson, W. D. (1967), Veterinary Radiology. Second Edition. London: Bailliere, Tindall and Cassell.
Douglas, S. W., and Hall, L. W. (1959), Vet. Rec., **71,** 901.
Frost, R. C. (1956), Vet. Rec., **68,** 1014.
Lauder, I. M., and Lawson, D. D. (1959), Vet. Rec., **71,** 1096.
O'Brien, J. A., Buchanan, J. W., and Kelly, D. F. (1966), J. Am. vet. Radiol. Soc., 7, 12.
Olsson, S. E. (1957), Cornell Vet., **47,** 193.
Reif, J. S. and Rhodes, W. H. (1966) J. Am. vet. Radiol. Soc., **7,** 5.

CHAPTER 9

THE CARDIO-VASCULAR SYSTEM

The detailed investigation of this system which is undertaken in human radiology depends very largely on the employment of contrast media techniques and on the availability of highly specialised X-ray apparatus. Similar studies have been undertaken in animals by those having access to suitable facilities, but obviously this is seldom practicable in general practice. It is probably for this reason that the importance of simple radiography in the examination of the heart is sometimes underestimated, although it can be of considerable value.

In this chapter it is proposed to concentrate on considering the information which may be obtained from the examination of plain films of the heart and major vessels, and then to refer more generally to the use of contrast media (references are given for those who wish to pursue this aspect in greater detail).

Radiography

The need for precise positioning for radiography of the chest has been stressed in the previous chapter. This is even more important when this region is being positioned for demonstration of the heart. Ventro-dorsal positioning will lead to displacement of the heart and variations in the cardiac contour. Dorso-ventral projections result in a more consistant radiographic image and should be used routinely. When positioning in this plane however, care must be taken to avoid lateral tilting of the chest which can cause distortion of the cardiac outline and a false effect of one-sided enlargement.

The size and position of the heart (particularly in dorso-ventral projections) will inevitably result in some enlargement of the cardiac image as recorded on the film. For this reason the longest film-focal distance which is compatible with the use of brief exposure times should be employed.

NORMAL RADIOLOGICAL ANATOMY

The major problem encountered in simple radiology of the heart is the fact that one is attempting to visualise an organ which is of relatively large size in all three dimensions and which also has an important internal structure, solely by means of films which can demonstrate only the silhouette, size and position of the heart. It is, therefore, important to appreciate the relationship of the cardiac silhouette to the position of the chambers of the heart. This is shown in the accompanying radiographs and diagrams obtained during the passage of contrast medium through the

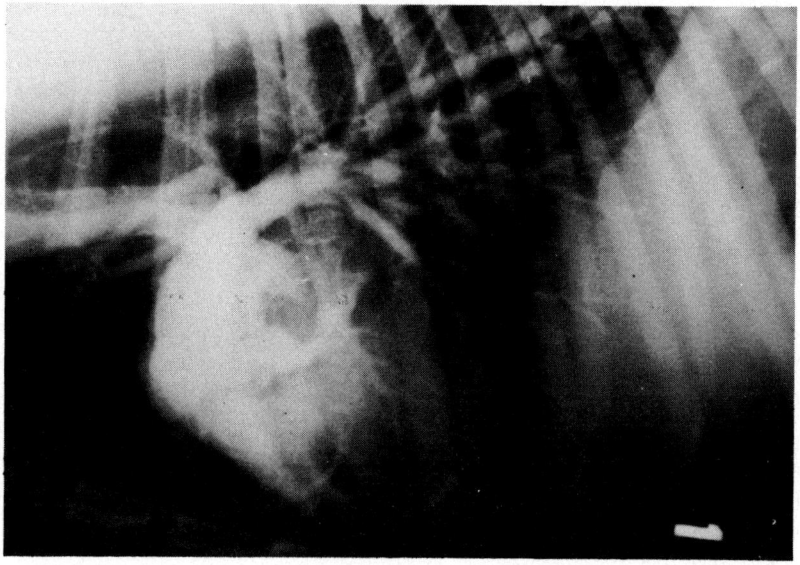

FIG. 9.1.

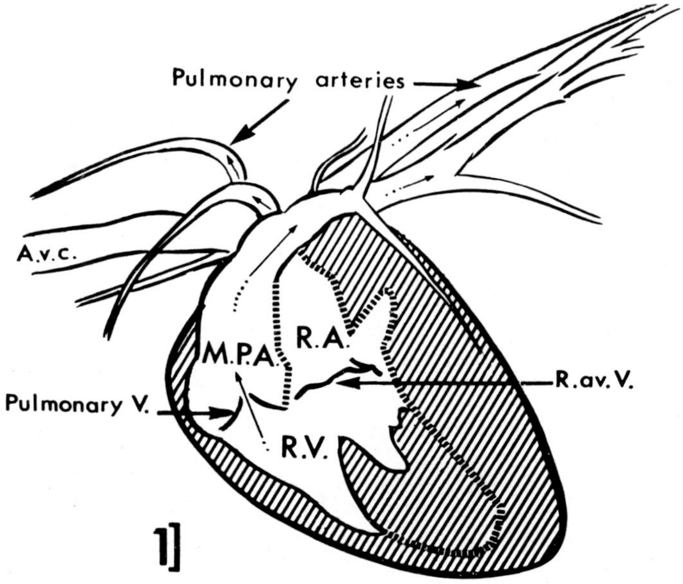

FIG. 9.2.

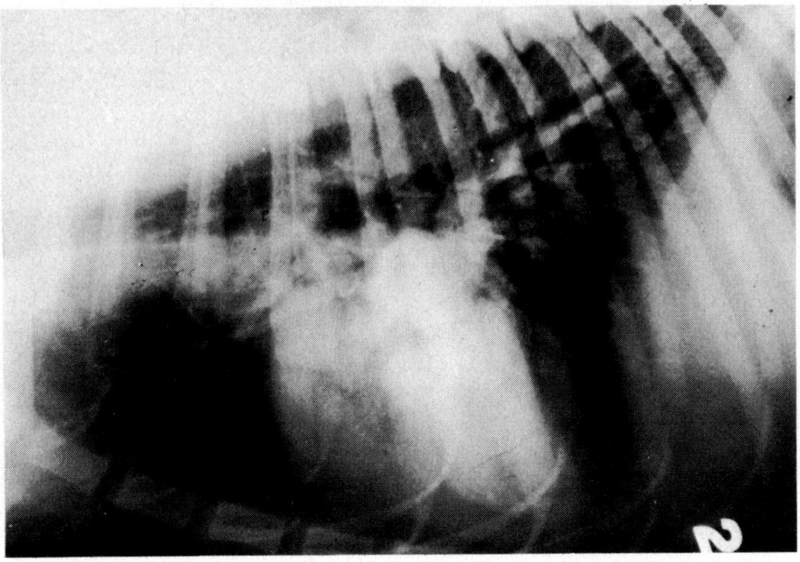

FIG. 9.3.

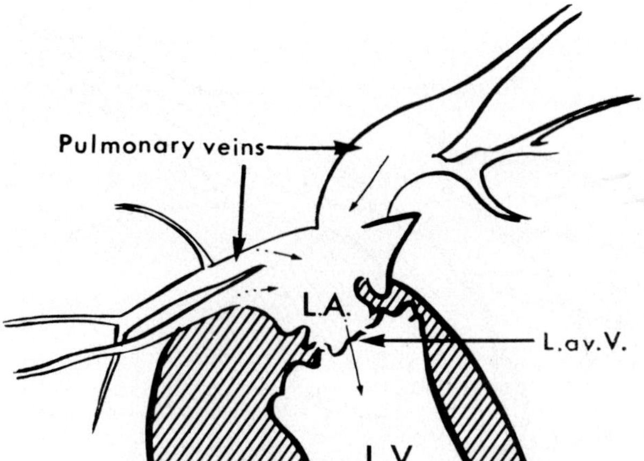

FIG. 9.4.

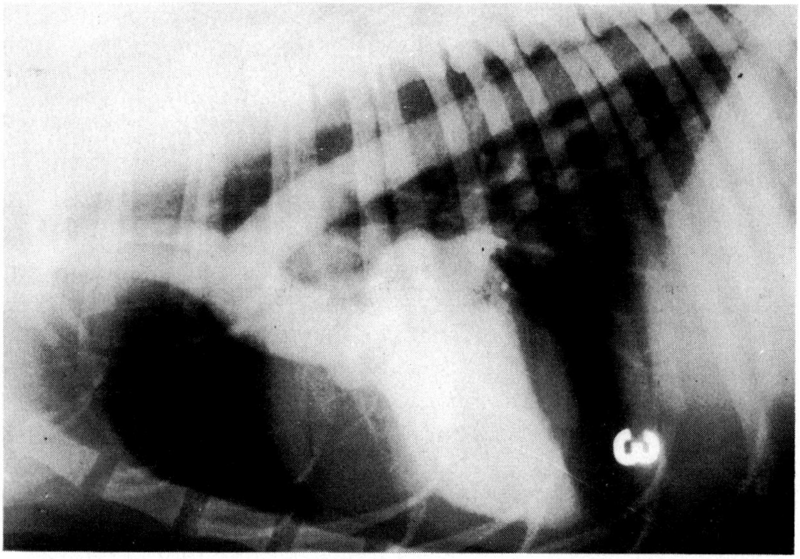

FIG. 9.5.

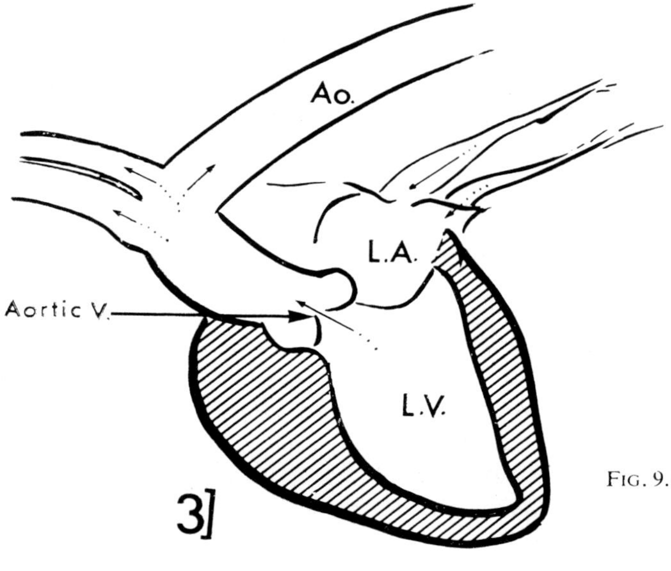

FIG. 9.6.

FIGS. 9.1 to 9.6. Lateral cardio-angiograms demonstrating the passage of contrast medium through the chambers of the normal canine heart.

Ao. Aorta
A.v.c. Anterior vena cava
L.A. Left atrium
L.av.V. Left atrial-ventricular valve
L.V. Left ventricle
M.P.A. Main pulmonary artery
R.A. Right atrium
R.V. Right ventricle
R.av.V. Right atrial-ventricular valve

chambers of the normal canine heart. Such visualisation of the internal structure also helps to emphasise the fact that in the dog and cat, the use of the terms "right" and "left" to describe the atria and ventricles is not really correct. The right chambers are in fact situated more anteriorly and the left chambers more posteriorly, than laterally. However, since these adjectives are still generally employed and understood, they will be used throughout this chapter.

The Lateral Silhouette of the Heart

In lateral projections the heart appears roughly ovoid in outline and is located between the third and seventh ribs. The long axis of the "egg" is directed backwards at a slight angle to the vertical, but the actual slope varies between different breeds of dogs. In the deeper chested dogs (Greyhounds, Collies) the heart is relatively long and narrow with its long axis nearly vertical, while in those dogs possessing a shallow chest the cardiac outline is wide and short and directed backwards at a greater angle.

Owing to the considerable variation in the shape of the heart and chest which occurs normally in different breeds, no precise ratio of thoracic to cardiac measurements can be established to indicate the limits of normality. However, it can be taken as a rough general guide, that the vertical height of the heart should be almost three quarters of the depth of the thorax at the level of the fifth rib.

The lateral silhouette of the heart can be considered to comprise four borders:

(a) The anterior border, which commences dorsally with the root of the aorta and extends downwards over the wall of the right atrium and also includes part of the wall of the right ventricle. This border often shows a slight indentation or notch at the junction of the aorta and right atrium.

(b) The ventral border, which runs roughly parallel with the sternum and consists of portions of the walls of the right and left ventricles.

(c) The posterior border may merge with the line of the diaphragm (particularly at expiration) and comprises the wall of the left ventricle.

(d) The dorsal border is less clearly visualised because it tends to be masked by the major vessels, trachea and bronchi. It is made up anteriorly by the wall of the right atrium and posteriorly by the left atrium.

A second notch may often be recognised at the junction of the posterior and dorsal borders (or the junction of the left atrium and left ventricle). This, together with the notch described on the anterior border, can give a "waist-like" effect to the cardiac outline.

The Great Vessels and Associated Structures (Lateral Projection)

The aorta arises from the upper portion of the anterior border of the heart and arches posteriorly, running parallel with the vertebral column. It is usually clearly perceptible as its density contrasts with normal lung tissue.

The posterior vena cava should also be perceived as a dense, straight shadow which arises in the region of the left atrium and passes posteriorly through the diaphragm. It is best seen in films taken at full inspiration.

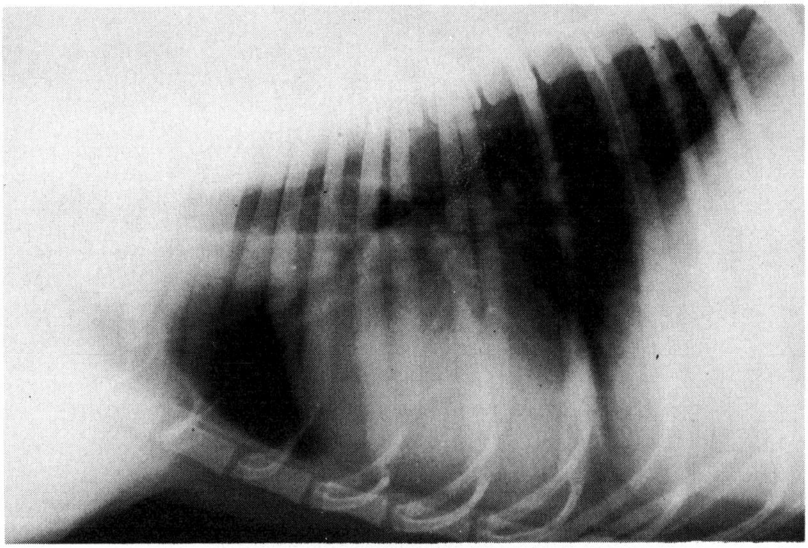

FIG. 9.7.

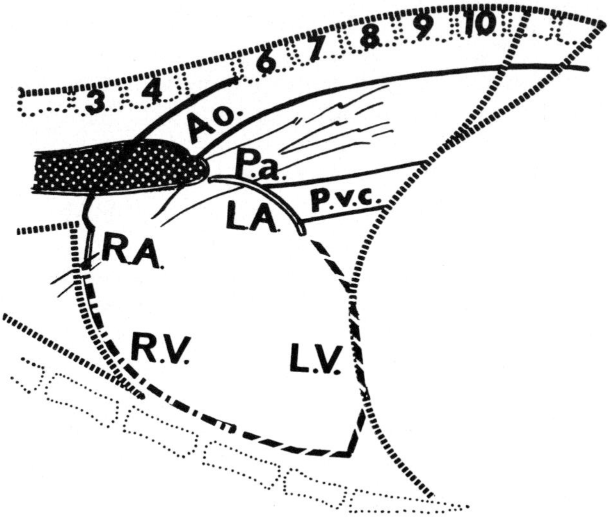

FIGS. 9.7 and 9.8. Lateral silhouette of the normal canine heart.

Ao. Aorta
L.A. Left atrium
L.V. Left ventricle
P.a. Pulmonary arteries
P.v.c. Posterior vena cava
R.A. Right atrium
R.V. Right ventricle.

FIG. 9.8.

The pulmonary vessels are unlikely to be clearly distinguished but they help to make up the area of density situated immediately above the dorsal border of the heart.

The air-filled trachea should also be easily perceived and recognition of its normal downward curve to the carina helps to identify the level of the dorsal border of the heart.

The Dorso-ventral Silhouette of the Heart

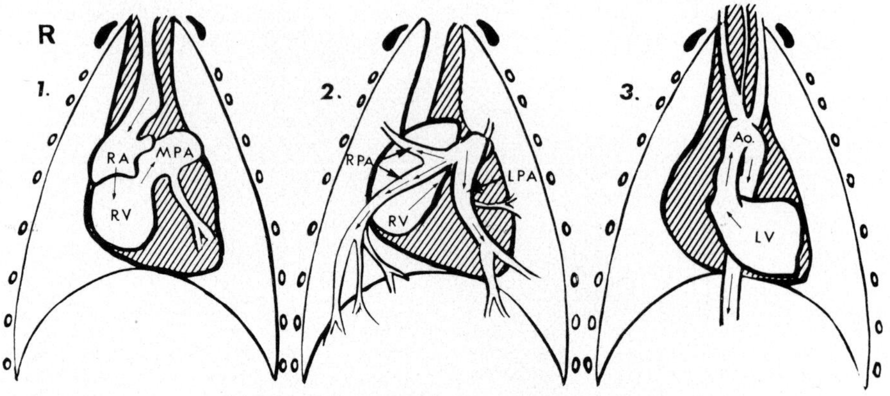

FIG. 9.9. Diagrammatic representation of dorso-ventral cardio-angiograms of the normal canine heart.

Ao.	Aorta
LPA	Left pulmonary arteries
LV	Left ventricle
MPA	Main pulmonary artery
RA	Right atrium
RPA	Right pulmonary arteries
RV	Right ventricle

The significance of the dorso-ventral cardiac contour is more difficult to appreciate because of superimposition of the major vessels, the atria and the ventricles. The above diagrams obtained from angio-cardiograms in this plane indicate the approximate positions of the chambers of the heart (owing to superimposition the left atrium cannot be distinguished from the other chambers, but it is situated centrally and does not normally contribute to the cardiac outline).

For the purposes of description the dorso-ventral silhouette is best considered as though it were divided into two unequal halves by a line drawn longitudinally through the centre of the chest.

The outline of the smaller right half corresponds with a segment of a circle and consists very largely of the right ventricular wall on which the right atrium is superimposed anteriorly.

The left half of the heart is shown as a distorted curve which extends further laterally and posteriorly than the right half. The curve of the aorta (the aortic arch) may overlap and contribute to the cardiac silhouette at its extreme anterior end, but this is a variable feature usually most obvious in dogs with a narrow long (in the antero-posterior direction) heart. The portion of the cardiac silhouette immediately lateral and posterior to the aortic arch is known as the pulmonary segment and comprises the pulmonary artery and its main branches. The rest of this half of the heart is made up of the left ventricular wall.

The relationship of cardiac to thoracic measurements can again vary considerably with different breeds and types of dog. The greatest width of the heart is usually

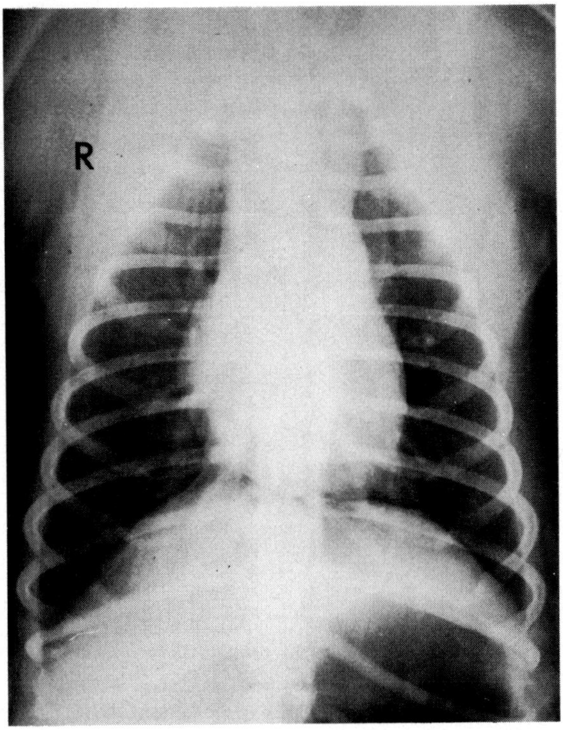

FIG. 9.10.

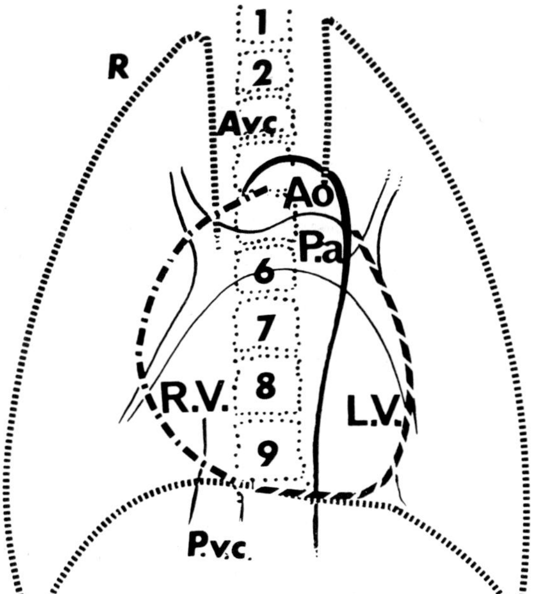

FIGS. 9.10 and 9.11. Dorso-ventral silhouette of the normal canine heart.

Ao. Aorta
A.v.c. Anterior vena cava
L.V. Left ventricle
P.a. Pulmonary arteries
P.v.c. Posterior vena cava
R.V. Right ventricle.

FIG. 9.11.

equal to one half to two-thirds of the width of the chest at the level of the fifth pair of ribs. However, this ratio is not very precise and only marked variations outside it can be assumed to be of pathological significance.

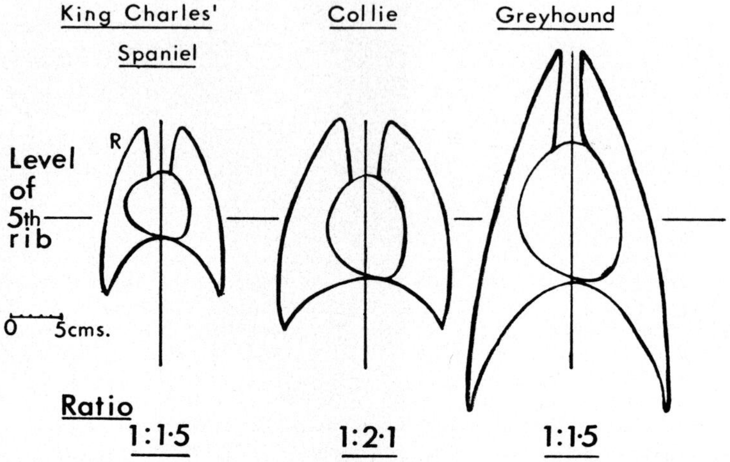

FIG. 9.12. Tracings obtained from radiographs to show the variation in the ratio of cardiac/thoracic measurements encountered in different breeds of dog.

The Great Vessels and Associated Structures (Dorso-ventral Projection)

Recognition of these structures in this plane is rendered difficult by superimposition of the heart and vertebral column. It is likely that the air-filled trachea, and main bronchi will contrast sufficiently with the dense background to be just perceptible in this plane. The particularly dense outline of the aorta may also be just recognisable as it arises at the anterior limit of the heart, curves sharply to the right, and then is continued posteriorly where it tends to be masked by the vertebral column, and the pulmonary vessels.

PATHOLOGICAL CHANGES

The evidence of cardiac abnormality which can be recognised in plain films is best considered under four separate headings.

1. Changes Involving the Whole Heart

Essentially the change which occurs is an increase in size of the cardiac silhouette. This may take one of two forms.

(*a*) **Cardiac enlargement**

The enlargement may be due either to hypertrophy of cardiac muscle or to dilatation of the chambers of the heart, but these cannot be distinguished radiologically without the use of contrast media.

As already mentioned, it is not possible to define precise normal limits of cardiac size by relating this to measurements of the thorax. Thus only the more advanced

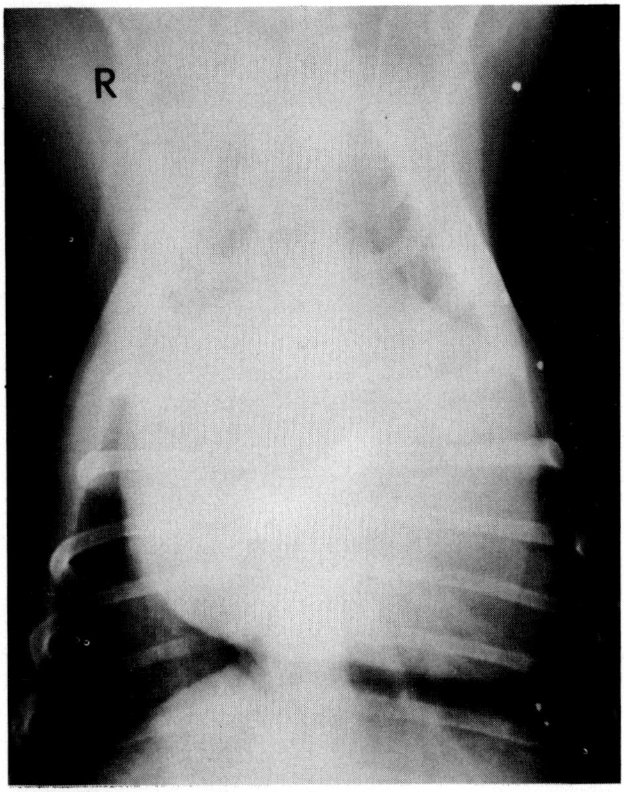

FIG. 9.13.

FIGS. 9.13 and 9.14. Gross cardiac enlargement in a one year old Labrador dog.

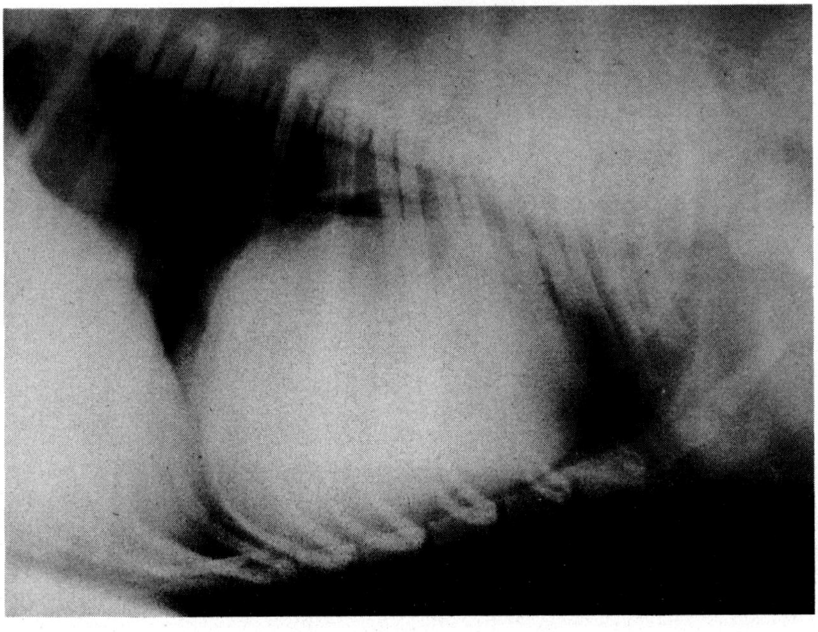

FIG. 9.14.

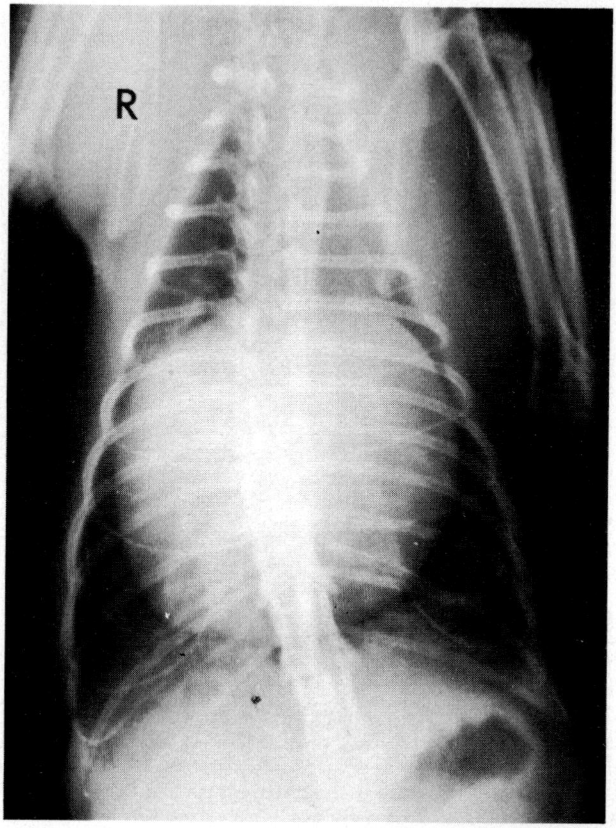

FIG. 9.15.

FIGS. 9.15 and 9.16. Marked enlargement resulting in posterior displacement of the heart of the cat.

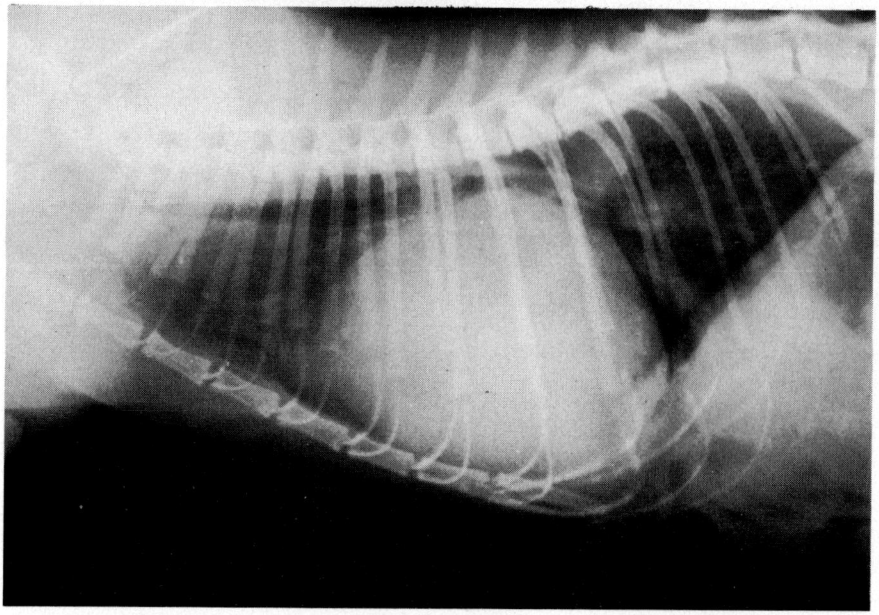

FIG. 9.16.

FIG. 9.17.

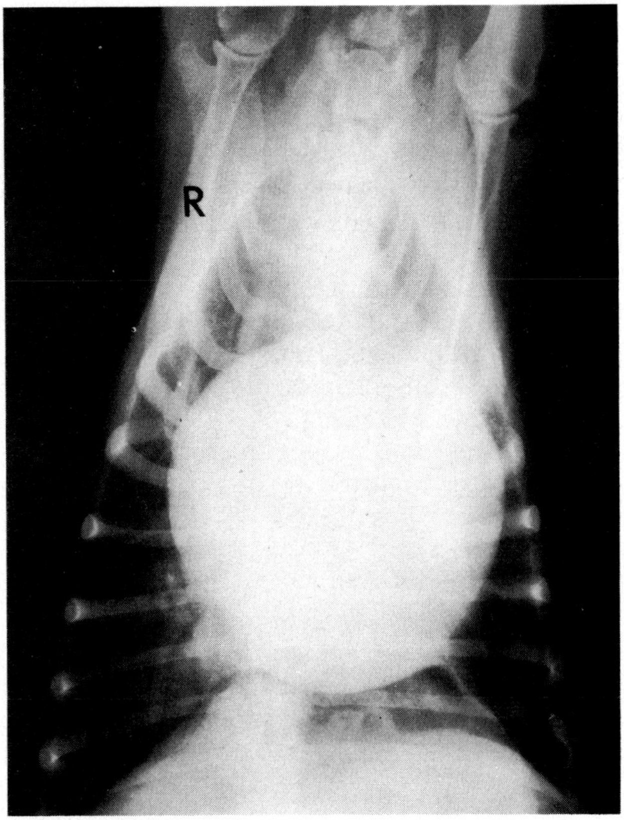

FIGS. 9.17 and 9.18. Pericardial effusion in a Sheepdog. Note the typically distinct cardiac outline.

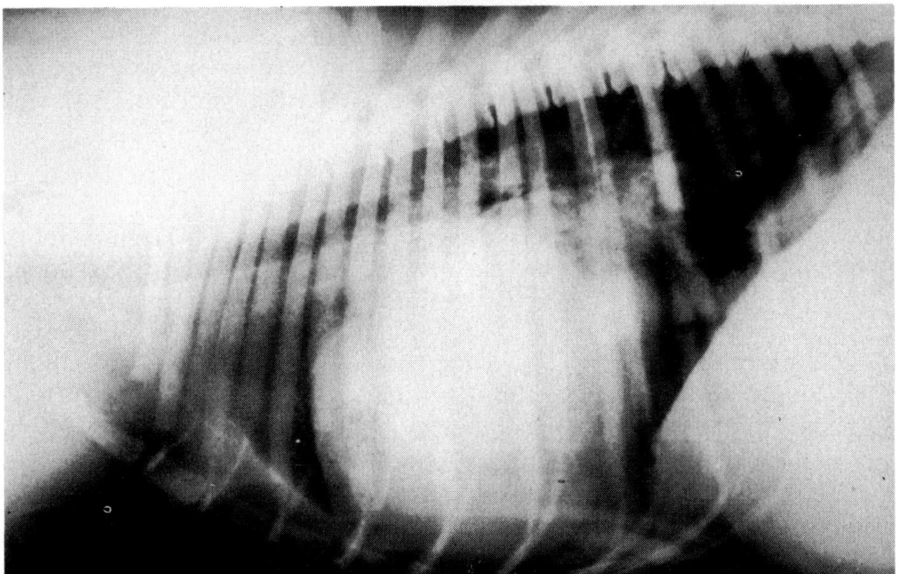

FIG. 9.18.

cases of cardiac enlargement can be definitely identified. The two characteristic features are that, the outline of the heart becomes more rounded when seen in either plane, and it obviously occupies a much larger area of the thorax. In lateral projections the effect of a "waist" is lost and the posterior border of the heart becomes straighter and tends to overlap the diaphragm line. The trachea and major blood vessels are seen to be displaced dorsally. In dorso-ventral views the cardiac silhouette approaches the thoracic walls and may be displaced posteriorly into the wider portion of the chest.

The most likely cause of such changes is generalised valvular insufficiency leading to congestive heart failure. In such cases radiography may also demonstrate vascular congestion within lung tissue.

General cardiac enlargement can also be associated with a patent ductus arteriosus, but here the enlargement is likely to be more marked on the left side. Furthermore, in the dorso-ventral projection associated enlargement of the pulmonary arteries is likely to cause a protrusion of the cardiac outline in the region of the pulmonary segment.

(*b*) Pericardial Effusion

It is not always easy to distinguish enlargement of the cardiac shadow associated with the presence of pericardial effusion from that described above. The most characteristic features are that the shape of the heart becomes even more spherical and of a uniform density. In addition, owing to masking of heart movement by the presence of fluid, the outline is particularly sharply defined.

2. Changes Involving Individual Cardiac Chambers

Again the only change which can be appreciated is an enlargement, whether this be due to hypertrophy or dilatation. While more than one cardiac chamber may be involved at the same time it is simplest to describe the particular features of each individually.

(*a*) Enlargement of the Left Atrium

Enlargement of this chamber is shown in lateral projections by a prominence of the region which results in the posterior border of the heart meeting the dorsal border at right angles, rather than in the form of a curve. An increase in the depth of the heart will be shown by upward displacement of the trachea. In particularly detailed films it may be possible to appreciate that the outline of the two main bronchi are no longer confluent as a result of upward displacement of the left bronchus by the enlarged atrium.

Enlargement of this chamber can seldom be recognised in dorso-ventral projections but in severe cases there may be evidence of an area of increased density extending towards the right posterior cardiac border.

Evidence of enlargement of the left atrium is commonly associated with mitral insufficiency.

FIG. 9.19.

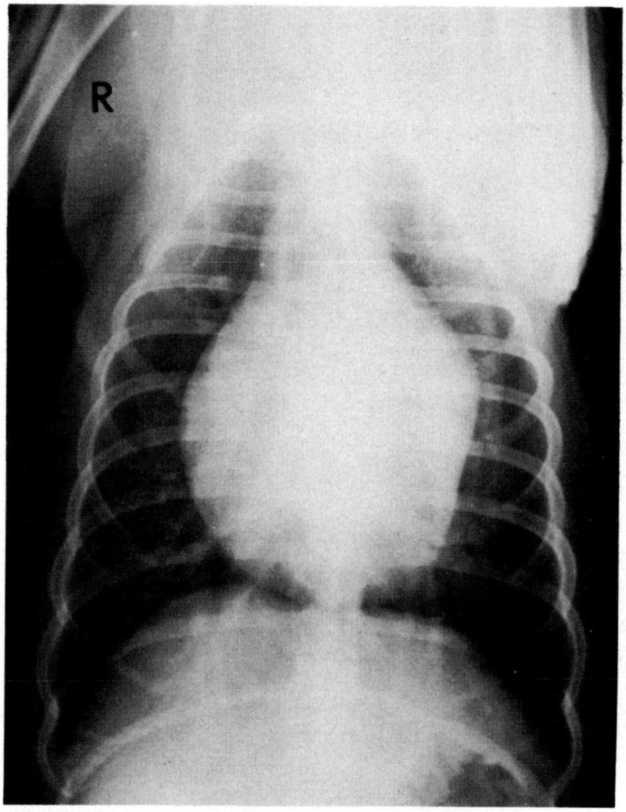

FIGS. 9.19 and 9.20. Left-sided enlargement of the heart of a Miniature Poodle dog.

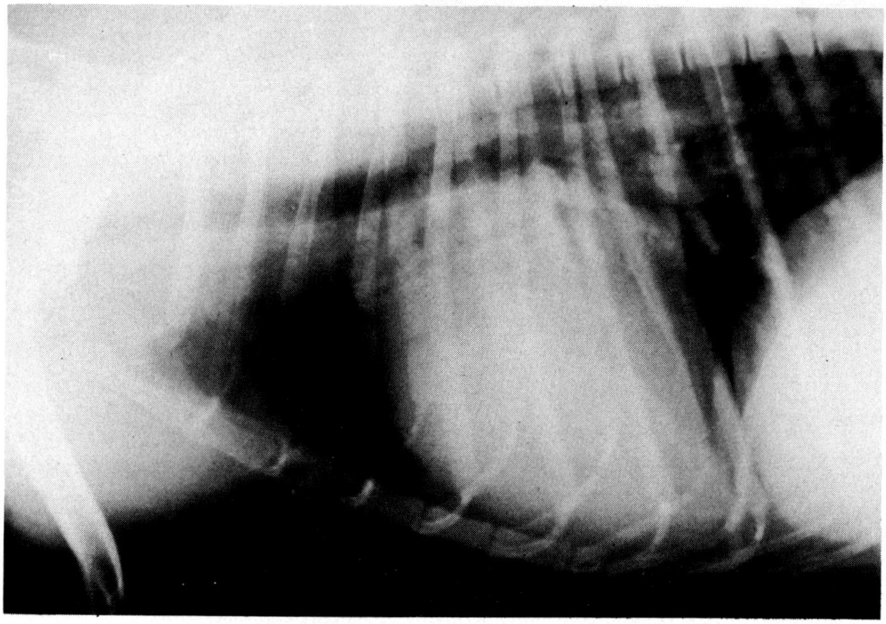

FIG. 9.20.

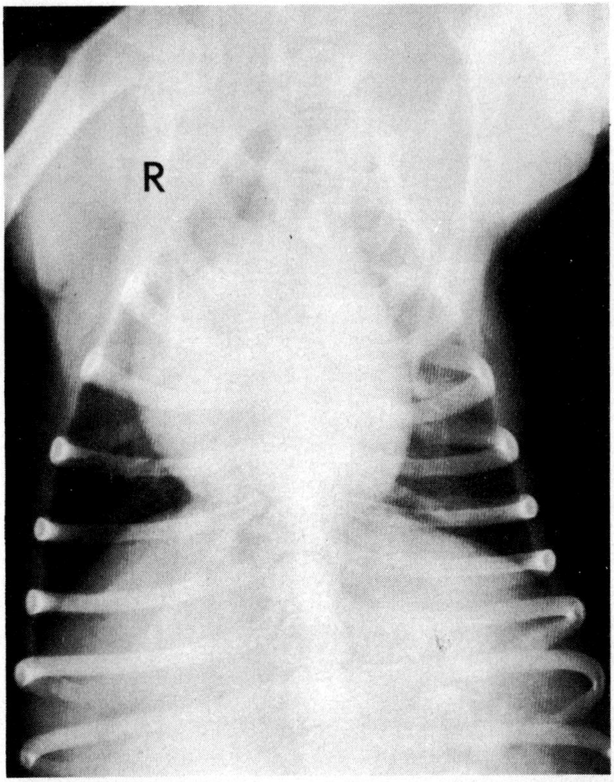

FIG. 9.21. Dorso-ventral projection showing right-sided cardiac enlargement in a Fox Terrier.

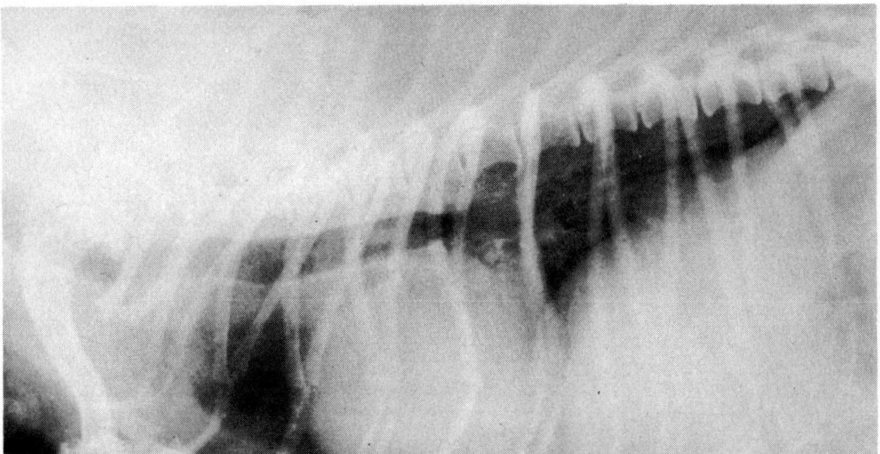

FIG. 9.22. Lateral view of right-sided enlargement of the heart in a Dachshund.

(*b*) Enlargement of the Left Ventricle

In lateral films enlargement of the left ventricle is shown by a straightening of posterior border of the heart which approximates and often overlaps, the line of the diaphragm (it is important to note the stage of respiration, as full expiration may create a false effect of such overlap).

Dorso-ventral films will show enlargement of the left posterior region of the heart, together with a decreased distance between the cardiac silhouette and the left thoracic wall and the diaphragm.

The radiographic appearances described above may be seen in association with mitral insufficiency, aortic stenosis and patent ductus arteriosus.

(*c*) Enlargement of the Right Atrium

Right atrial enlargement is likely to show similar changes in lateral films to those described for the left atrium (an increased depth to the heart, upward displacement of the trachea, and tilting of the two main bronchi) but it should be apparent that the main increase in the cardiac silhouette is occurring at the anterior rather than the posterior end of the dorsal border.

Dorso-ventral projections may demonstrate a protrusion on the right anterior region of the heart and also show some deviation of the trachea to the left.

Enlargement is seldom restricted to this chamber alone but is usually associated with similar changes in the right ventricle.

(*d*) Enlargement of the Right Ventricle

Enlargement of this chamber of the heart is shown in lateral projections as an increase in the size of the anterior cardiac border. It is usually associated with right atrial enlargement and the combination produces a straightening of the normally convex anterior border.

Right ventricular enlargement is usually associated with enlargement of the pulmonary arteries. Therefore the first change noted in dorso-ventral projections is likely to be an increase in the pulmonary segment of the cardiac silhouette. As the changes proceed further enlargement of the right side of the heart will also be recognised.

Recognition of the above changes may be associated with a number of cardiac conditions including: tetralogy of Fallot, septal defects, pulmonary stenosis, patent ductus arteriosus and tricuspid insufficiency.

3. Changes Affecting the Great Vessels and Associated Structures

The vessels and structures which can be involved in these changes will be considered separately.

(*a*) Pulmonary Arteries

The main change which can be appreciated is an enlargement of the common pulmonary artery. This will be visualised in dorso-ventral radiographs as a protrusion of the pulmonary segment which is commonly associated with enlargement of

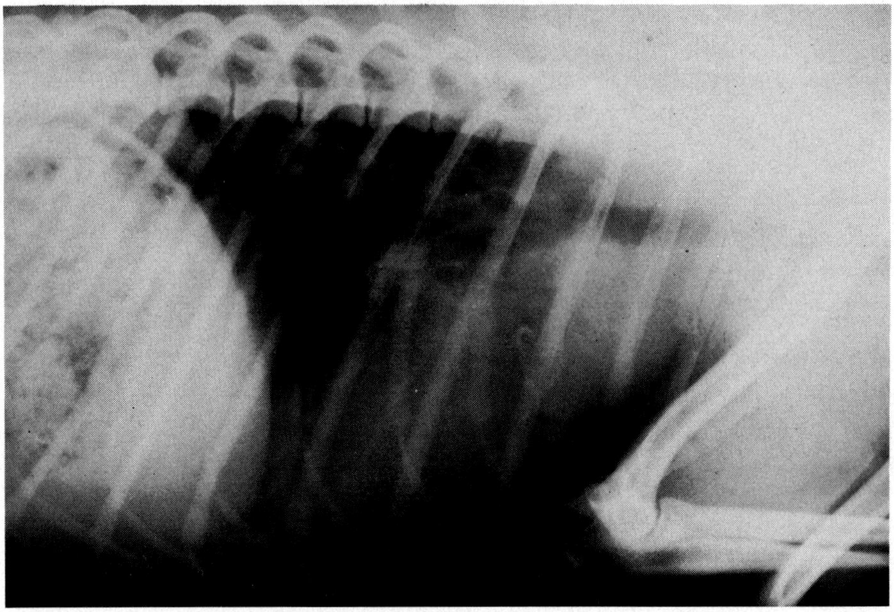

FIG. 9.23. Marked enlargement of the aortic arch in a Poodle associated with stenosis and incompetence of the aortic valve.

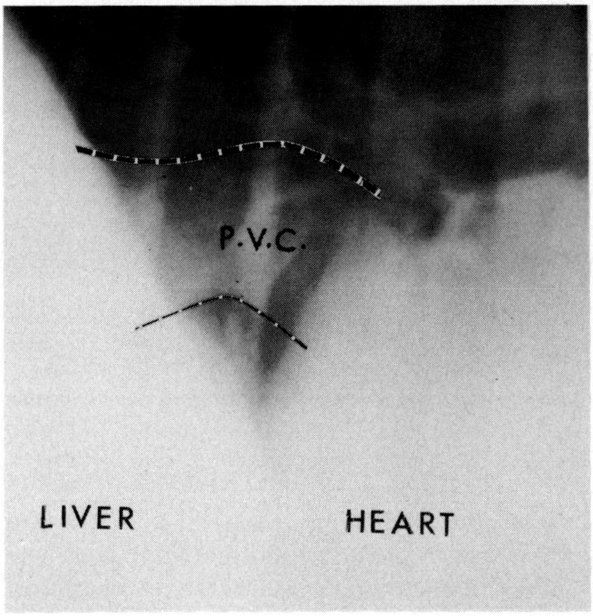

FIG. 9.24. Enlargement and bending of the posterior vena cava in a dog showing ascites and a chronic cardiac defect.

the right ventricle. These changes can be associated with pulmonary stenosis, patent ductus arteriosus, and septal defects.

(*b*) The Aorta

Enlargement of the aortic arch may be recognised in lateral projections as a prominence in the right atrial region of the lateral silhouette. In the dorso-ventral plane it may be possible to appreciate a protruberance at the most anterior point of the cardiac silhouette.

This feature is commonly associated with left sided cardiac enlargement and may be due to aortic stenosis.

(*c*) The Posterior Vena Cava

Enlargement of this vessel may be sufficiently severe to be appreciated in a radiograph (particularly in the lateral projection).

This feature is likely to be associated with pulmonary venous congestion, and its detection can be of value in differentiating between ascites of cardiac origin and that of hepatic origin.

(*d*) The Trachea and Main Bronchi

As already mentioned, the recognition in the lateral radiographs of the position of the carina indicates the level of the dorsal border of the heart. Recognition of dorsal displacement of this or of the trachea, provides definite evidence of an increase in the length of the heart (unless the ventral border is also displaced).

While the main bronchi are more difficult to identify accurately they are normally superimposed in lateral radiographs. Recognition of divergence of these bronchi can indicate tilting caused by enlargement of either the left or right atrium.

4. Changes in Other Organs

There are at least three significant features involving other organs which can be demonstrated radiologically and which can provide additional evidence of cardiac abnormality.

(*a*) Enlargement of the Liver

Hepatic enlargement can be due to a number of causes, one of which is generalised vascular congestion and recognition of this feature can help to confirm other evidence of severe cardiac disease. Furthermore, if it is possible to radiograph an affected animal at intervals of weeks or months, comparison of the films may show variations in the size of the liver which can act as a rough guide as to improvement or deterioration in the degree of congestion.

(*b*) Pulmonary Vascular Congestion

This feature, which is best appreciated in lateral projections of the chest, is shown by an increased density in the vascular pattern in the lobes of the lung. However some increase appears normally with age, and it is only in severe cases that it can be definitely identified.

The development of pulmonary oedema as a further stage of vascular congestion may occasionally be recognised. Radiologically this is likely to appear as dense patchy areas extending through the lungs but following the general vascular pattern.

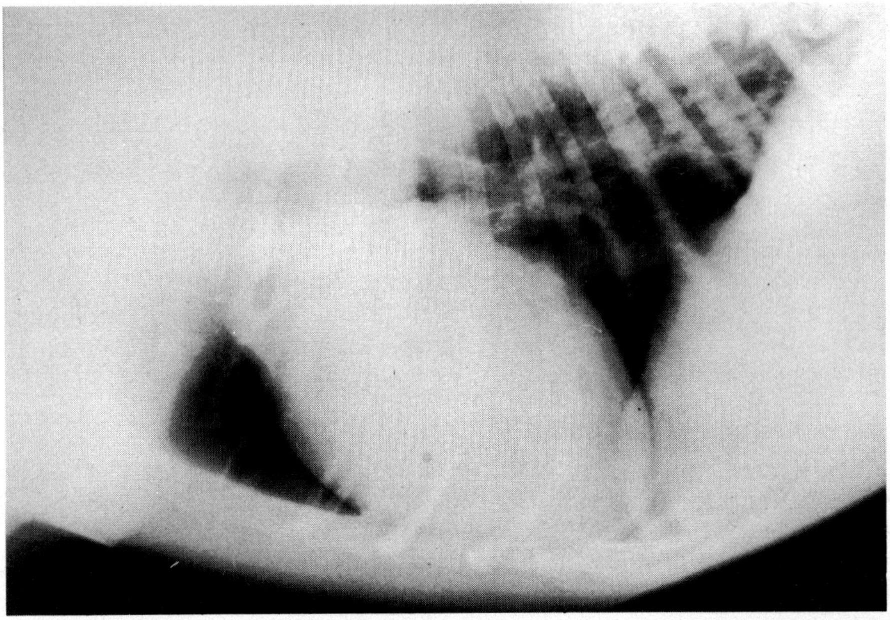

FIG. 9.25. Pulmonary vascular congestion associated with a suspected interventricular septal defect in a Boxer dog.

(*c*) Dilation of the Anterior Oesophagus

This condition will be discussed further in Chapter 11 but its recognition when investigating the cause of persistent vomiting in a young puppy, can be the first evidence of persistence of a "vascular ring", i.e. a congenital anomaly of the left and right aortic arch system which encircles and constricts the oesophagus. The exact anatomical composition of the vascular ring can vary considerably from case to case.

This form of oesophageal dilation terminates abruptly at the level of the vascular constriction and it is important to differentiate it from a second congenital form of dilatation which can involve the entire oesophagus. The administration of barium is usually necessary to distinguish the two forms.

Investigation of the precise type of vascular abnormality present would require angiographic techniques (Walker & Littlewort, 1964).

CONTRAST MEDIA TECHNIQUES

The introduction of a contrast agent (usually an aqueous solution of an organic iodine compound produced specifically for the purpose) into the cardio-vascular system can permit radiographic demonstration both of the flow of blood and of the internal structure of the heart and blood vessels. Unfortunately once injected, the contrast medium is rapidly diluted by the circulating blood and will be carried past any one point of the vascular system within a period of a few seconds. Thus, if sufficient visualisation is to be obtained, it is necessary to introduce the medium rapidly, and in sufficient volume and concentration, directly into the part to be demonstrated (this will usually require the introduction of a catheter into particular portions of the major vessels or into individual cardiac chambers). Furthermore, the passage of the contrast agent can only be accurately recorded if some form of mechanical device is available which permits exposure of a series of films within a very short period of time.

The above observations explain why contrast radiography of the vascular system is an involved technique and can seldom be performed in general practice. Nevertheless, a large number of angiographic techniques have been used in clinical veterinary investigation by those possessing suitable facilities and may be summarised as follows.

Cardioangiography

This procedure permits visualisation of the internal silhouette of the heart and major vessels and recognition of dilatations or strictures of the vascular lumen. It also visualises the actual flow of blood through the heart and demonstrates "shunts" or other abnormalities of this flow.

Comparatively simple techniques involving the direct injection of contrast agent into the jugular vein or into the left or right ventricles and its observation by exposure of a single film has been reported (Hamlin, 1959, 1960). However, the use of a single film limits the information that can be obtained from such an examination and, in the authors' opinion, the use of direct ventricular puncture is somewhat uncertain and not without risk in the clinical case.

If a thorough examination of the heart is to be undertaken by this method a more detailed technique (Tashjian et al, 1959, Tashjian and Albanese, 1960) will be required. A catheter is introduced into the vascular system and is manipulated into the appropriate portion of the major vessels or cardiac chambers, so that contrast agent may be injected directly in to this area. In order that the passage of the medium may be accurately recorded a series of films are exposed at intervals of a fraction of a second by means of a mechanical film changing device.

Cerebroangiography

This procedure visualises the vascular pattern of the brain and thus permits demonstration of abnormalities in this pattern due to the presence of neoplasia or other lesions. The technique which has been employed in the dog (James and Hoerlein, 1960) involves the surgical exposure of the carotid vessels. Injection of the contrast agent is made into the common carotid artery after temporary occlusion of the external carotid artery so that the medium is concentrated in the internal carotid circulation. The vascular pattern can usually be satisfactorily recorded by means of films exposed at approximately 2 and 6 seconds after the injection of the medium but the exposure of a larger number of films by means of a film changing device is preferable.

Other Techniques

The use of contrast media to demonstrate arterial thrombosis has been reported (Imhoff and Tashjian, 1961, Nims, 1962). Essentially this technique involves the introduction of contrast medium on the cardiac side of the suspected obstruction (this may require catheterisation) and demonstration of failure of the medium to pass beyond the obstruction.

Another region in which significant obstruction to the vascular flow may occur is the portal vessels. A lesion of this nature has been demonstrated following the injection of contrast medium into the spleen and observation of its subsequent passage through the portal system by radiography (Owen and Hall, 1962).

Angiography is sometimes employed in man to demonstrate the vascular pattern of a neoplastic lesion, since the presence of malignancy may show characteristic changes in this pattern. The use of a similar technique has been reported to be of value in animals (Imhoff and Ewald, 1961).

REFERENCES

Hamlin, R. L. (1959), J. Am. vet. med. Ass., **135,** 112.
Hamlin, R. L. (1960), J. Am. vet. med Ass., **136,** 265.
Imhoff, R. K., and Ewald, B. H. (1961), J. Am. vet. med. Ass., **139,** 1293.
Imhoff, R. K. and Tashjian, R. J. (1961), J. Am. vet. med. Ass., **139,** 203.
James, C. W. and Hoerlein, B. F. (1960), Vet. Med., **55,** 12, 45.
Nims, R. M. (1962), J. Am. vet. med. Ass., **140,** 668.
Owen, L. N., and Hall, L. W. (1962), Vet. Rec., **74,** 220.
Tashjian, R. J., Hofstra, P. C., Reid, C. F. and Newman, M. M. (1959), J. am. vet. med. Ass., **135,** 94.
Tashjian, R. J. and Albanese, N. M. (1960), J. Am. vet. med. Ass., **136,** 359.
Walker, R. G., and Littlewort, M. C. G. (1964), Vet. Rec., **76,** 215.

CHAPTER 10

THE ABDOMINAL CAVITY

This chapter is concerned with the radiology of the abdomen as a whole, rather than with the detailed investigation of the alimentary, urinary and genital systems, which is dealt with in Chapters 11, 12 and 13. For convenience, those abdominal organs which are not specifically included in those chapters (the liver, spleen and pancreas) are also considered here.

Radiography

The principle factors which hinder accurate visualisation of the abdominal cavity and its contents are:—

(1) The lack of radiological contrast between the various soft tissue structures involved.
(2) The superimposition of these structures.
(3) Respiratory movement.
(4) The presence of food, faeces, or gas within the alimentary tract.
(5) The presence of free fluid in the abdominal cavity.

The effect of these factors may be minimised by adopting some, or all, of the following precautions.

(1) The use of a grid.
(2) Employment of ventro-dorsal, rather than dorso-ventral projections. The former will extend the abdomen, while the latter will compress it and lead to increased superimposition of abdominal organs and of the hind limbs.
(3) The use of localised or generalised compression (with a wooden spoon or a compression band) to thin the area to be examined and to eliminate the effect of respiratory movement.
(4) Suitable preparation of the patient to empty the alimentary tract or urinary bladder, or the aspiration of any abdominal fluid.
(5) The use of contrast media (either within particular organs or around them, e.g. pneumoperitoneum).

Ideally, radiography should be undertaken with the patient in the standing position. This would ensure that the intra-abdominal structures were in the normal position, and would facilitate demonstration of any significant fluid levels (within bowel or within the abdominal cavity). In practice, however, such positioning is seldom feasible on account of the difficulty of restraining the animal under these conditions, and because the patient cannot be applied so closely to the film. Inevitably radiography in the lateral and ventro-dorsal planes and the use of a compression band will lead to some displacement of the mobile abdominal organs, but it usually results in considerably better definition.

While the employment of pneumoperitoneum can assist greatly in visualising the abdominal cavity and the organs which it contains, this technique can lead to distortion of the abdominal outline and to displacement of abdominal organs.

It should also be appreciated that fat can act as a natural "contrast agent" as it causes slightly less absorption of X-rays than other tissues. This can assist in demonstrating organs which are likely to be surrounded by fat (e.g. the kidneys) and one can often obtain better definition of the abdomen in an obese animal than in a thin patient (young puppies and kittens can be particularly difficult subjects for abdominal radiography).

Radiology

THE ABDOMINAL CAVITY

The bounds of the abdominal cavity as seen in a radiograph, are approximately: the diaphragm anteriorly, the abdominal muscles laterally and ventrally, the lumbar

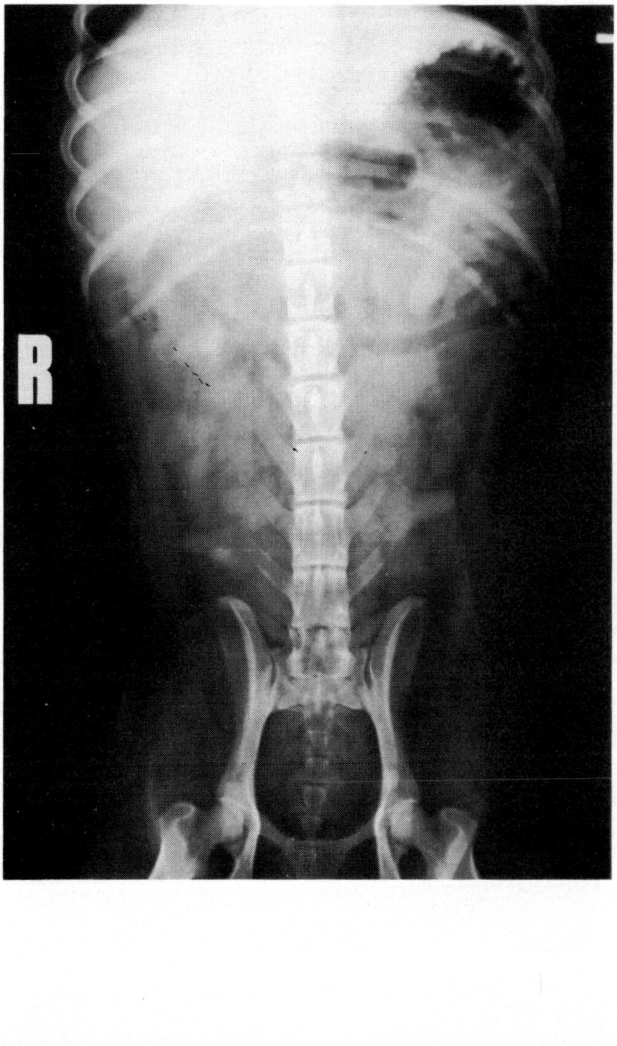

FIG. 10.1. Normal ventrodorsal abdominal radiograph.

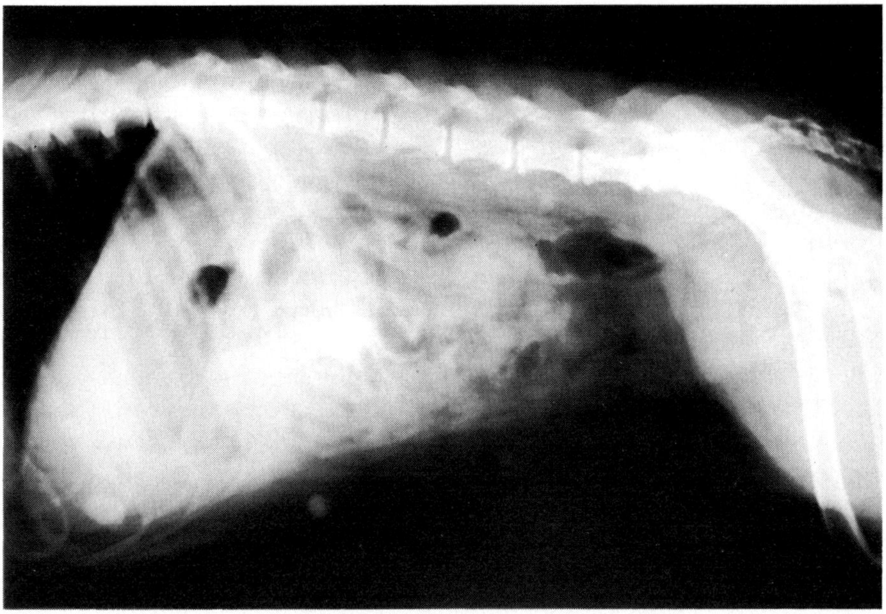

FIG. 10.2. Normal lateral abdominal radiograph.

muscles dorsally, and the anterior edge of the pelvis posteriorly. The structures and detail which can be appreciated within this area will vary considerably with the circumstances and technique of radiography. In the normal animal and under ideal conditions it should be possible to identify at least a portion of the liver, spleen, kidneys, bladder and alimentary tract (stomach, small and large bowel). It is unlikely that one will be able to recognise the pancreas, uterus, ovaries or abdominal lymph nodes.

Abdominal radiography in the ventro-dorsal plane can result in a particularly dense projection of the penis and testicles (the latter over the pelvic, rather than the abdominal region) which can cause confusion if not accurately identified.

Extraneous lines due to skin folds or muscle outlines can occur in this region, as in the thorax, but can be similarly identified because they extend outside the abdominal cavity.

Pathological Conditions

The only conditions involving the whole abdominal cavity which would show typical radiological features would be the accumulation of either free fluid or free gas within that cavity.

Abdominal Fluid

The above term is used in preference to "ascites" since, on radiological evidence alone, it is not possible to distinguish other causes of abdominal fluid (e.g. rupture of the chyle duct, or tuberculous exudative peritonitis).

The actual radiological appearance of this condition will vary with the amount of fluid which is present in the abdominal cavity, but all films should show two characteristic features. The first of these is blurring and obliteration of the detail which can normally be appreciated in an abdominal radiograph, and the second is increased radio-opacity of the whole area. However, both these features can also result from errors or limitations in the radiographic technique employed (e.g., movement of the patient, scattered radiation, under-exposure of the film) and such factors should be eliminated as far as is possible. The blurring and increased density will become more obvious as the quantity of fluid increases and there is little difficulty in the radiological diagnosis of the more advanced cases of ascites, which also show obvious distension of the abdominal cavity.

Definite diagnosis of the presence of small amounts of abdominal fluid may be more difficult and is usually aided by taking lateral projections with the animal in the standing position. Such films should demonstrate a ventral dense area of fluid and a dorsal area of more normal abdominal detail. A horizontal "fluid line" denoting the upper border of the fluid is often described as a typical feature of the condition. However, in practice, there is usually some merging of the two areas and a distinct line is seldom seen, unless pneumoperitoneum is also present. Another feature of films taken in the standing position is the fact that gas-filled portions of bowel tend to rise and are located dorsally (the presence of gas within the alimentary tract is the one feature which contrasts with the homogeneous density of the fluid and soft

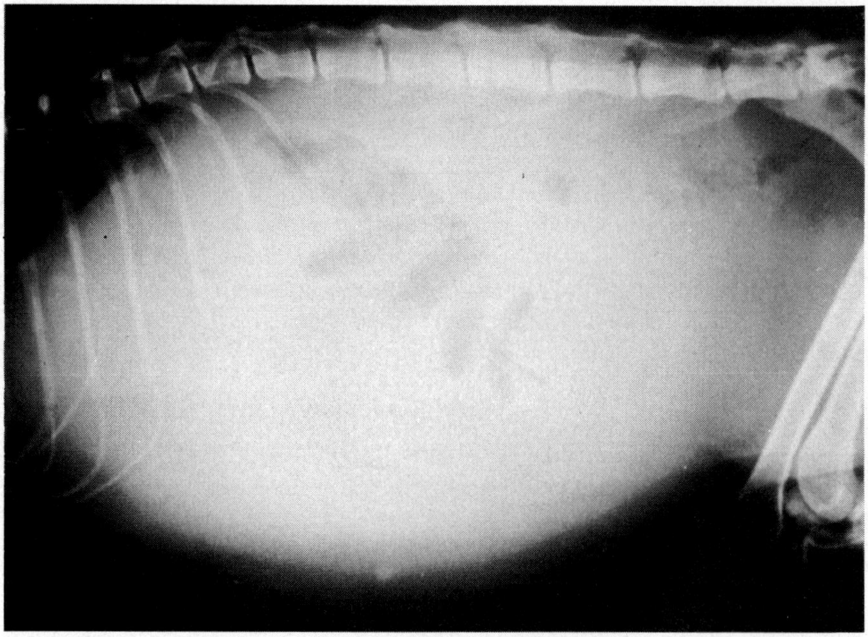

FIG. 10.3. Severe distension of the abdomen of a cat with fluid (over 1,000 ml. of ascitic fluid was subsequently aspirated).

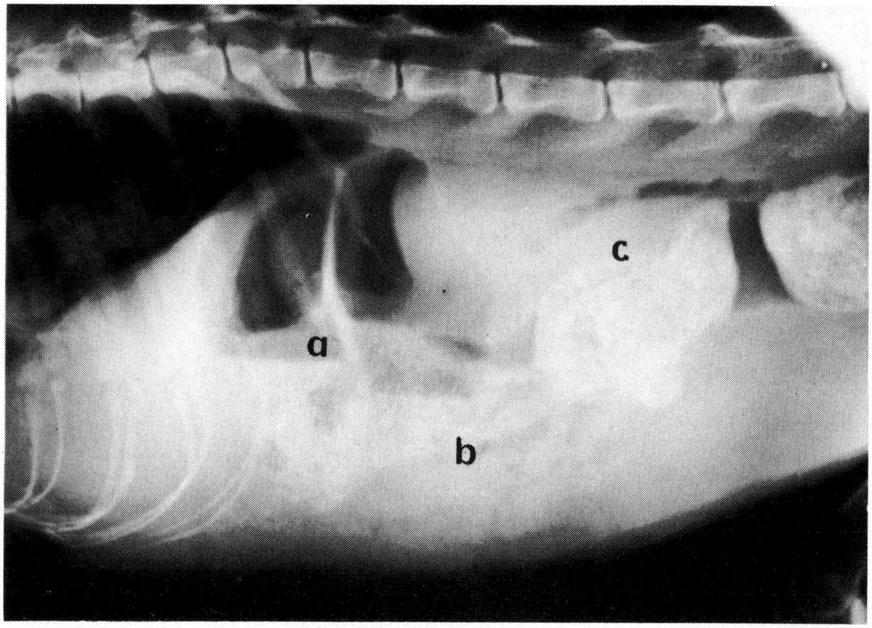

FIG. 10.4. The abdomen of a cat radiographed in the standing position to demonstrate fluid levels.

a—fluid levels and gas within stomach and large bowel.
b—abdominal fluid in the ventral abdomen.
c—absence of fluid in the upper abdomen.

tissues, and this can usually be recognised in all but the most severe accumulations of abdominal fluid).

Since many cases of accumulation of fluid are associated with other abdominal pathology (e.g., enlargement of the liver or of the mesenteric lymph nodes) it may be necessary to repeat radiography after aspiration of the fluid in order to investigate such lesions.

Abdominal Gas

The demonstration of free gas or air within the abdominal cavity could be associated with, the presence of gas-producing organisms, with penetrating wounds of the abdomen, or with perforation of a lesion of the wall of the alimentary tract. It is also to be expected for a few days after a laparotomy has been performed.

The radiological findings are identical with those of pneumoperitoneum, i.e. a darker appearance of the whole abdomen and better definition of the edge of the abdominal organs. Small quantities of gas may not be very obvious and are best demonstrated by using a horizontal X-ray beam and showing that the gas has concentrated in the dorsal part of the abdomen.

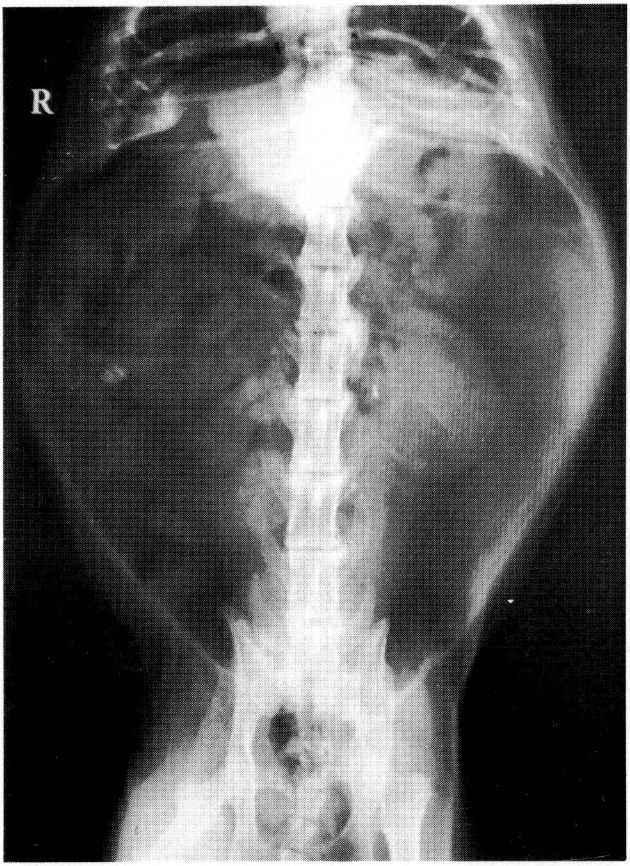

FIG. 10.5. Abdominal gas which developed spontaneously in a cat.

INDIVIDUAL ABDOMINAL ORGANS

The Liver

The position of the liver will be recognised as an area of considerably increased density, but the precise outline of this organ is seldom clearly demarcated.

In lateral radiographs the liver occupies a roughly triangular area between the line of the diaphragm and the ventral wall of the abdomen. The point of a lobe or lobes of liver are usually seen more clearly protruding a short (but variable) distance behind the curve of the last ribs. This protrusion can merge with, and be difficult to distinguish from, the outline of the spleen. Dorsally, the posterior border of the liver tends to merge with the density of the stomach shadow and the particularly dense area of the gastric pylorus can sometimes suggest a liver mass or tumour. Anteriorly a small amount of the diaphragmatic lobes of the lungs will overlie this organ but can seldom be appreciated because of the much greater density of the liver.

In ventro-dorsal projections the liver is seen as a dense area occupying almost the entire concavity of the curve of the diaphragm but not clearly demarcated posteriorly. The main bronchi and pulmonary vessels of the diaphragmatic and intermediate

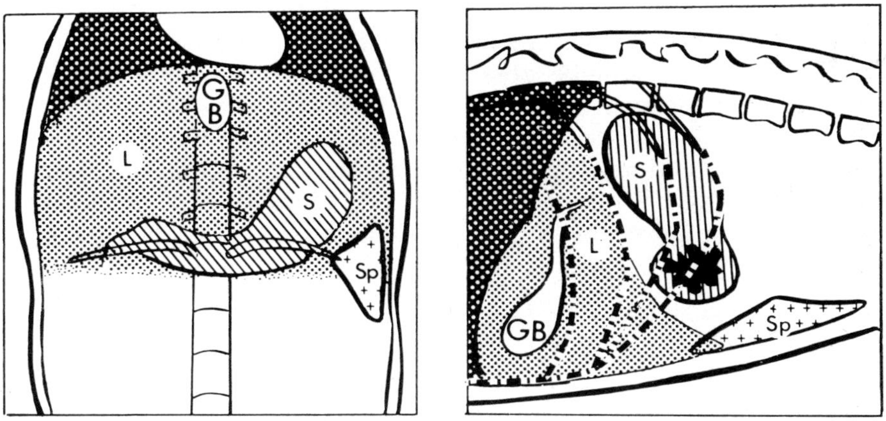

FIG. 10.6. Diagrammatic representation of approximate position of the liver and adjacent structures.

GB — Gall bladder
L — Liver
S — Stomach
Sp — Spleen

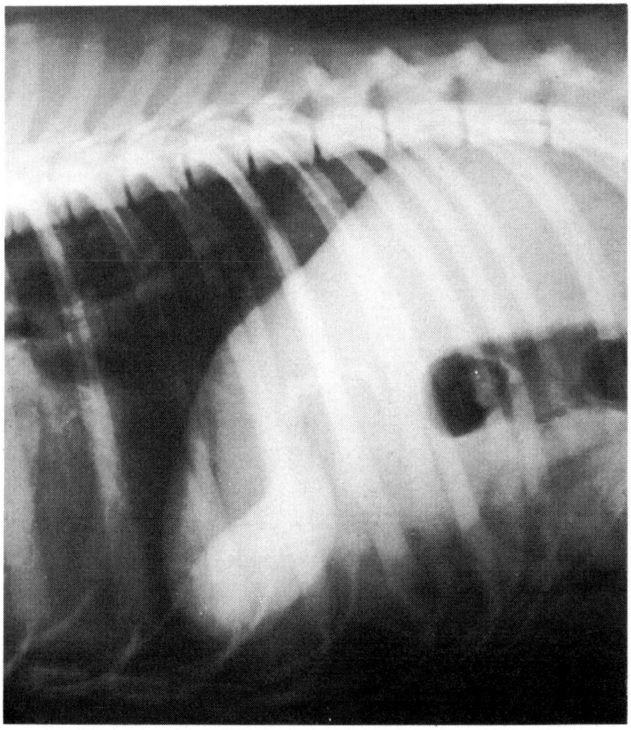

FIG. 10.7. Normal cholecystogram in a dog.

lobes of the lungs can usually be recognised superimposed on the anterior edge of the liver.

In obese animals the liver may be displaced upwards and partly outlined by fat, but the best delineation will be obtained by employing pneumoperitoneum and positioning the liver dorsally.

Cholecystography is of little assistance in demonstrating the whole liver, but it can be of considerable value in outlining the gall bladder. This is best seen in lateral radiographs at the antero-ventral angle of the liver. In the other plane the gall bladder is located near the mid-line but is poorly visualised because of the superimposition of dense tissues.

Pathological Changes

Changes in the contour of the liver have to be comparatively gross before they can be appreciated radiologically and are most easily recognised in those lobes which in lateral abdominal radiographs protrude behind the last ribs. In the young animals

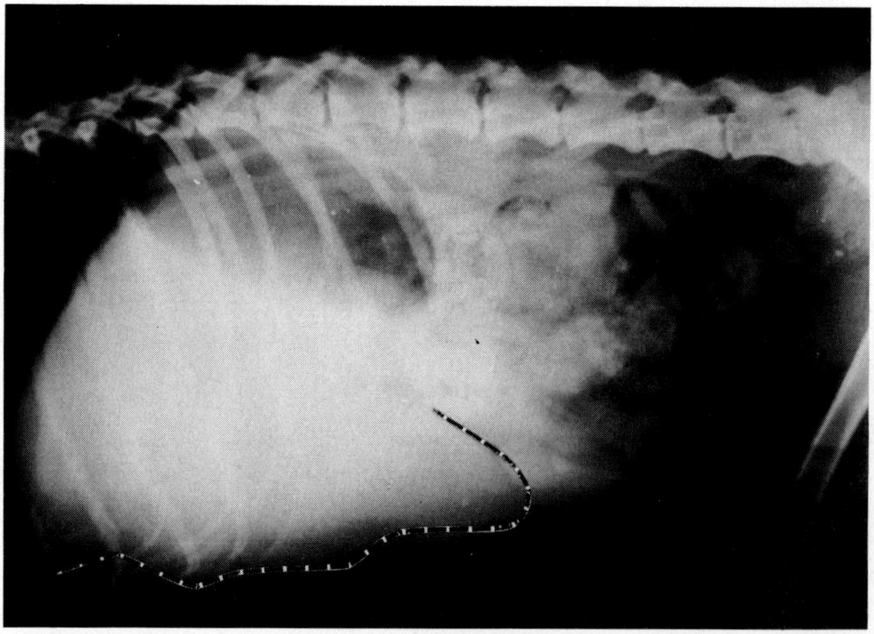

FIG. 10.8. Diffuse enlargement of the liver with associated displacement of the stomach.

these lobes will be seen to terminate in a relatively acute point, while with age and in association with fatty and proliferative changes this point becomes round or even flattened. Associated enlargement of the whole liver would be shown by the fact that lobes of liver extend considerably further back into the abdomen than normal.

However, since the liver can be displaced by movement of the diaphragm or by thoracic masses, it is not possible to fix a precise point indicating the limit of the "normal" liver, and, in general, there has to be gross enlargement of this organ before it can be recognised radiologically.

Similarly, while the liver is a common site of neoplasia, this has to be comparatively advanced before the irregular outline of tumour masses can be appreciated in a radiograph.

Anterior displacement of the liver into the thoracic cavity can occur in association with rupture of the diaphragm. Under these circumstances it can again be difficult to demonstrate this organ precisely but such displacement should be suspected if liver lobes can no longer be recognised behind the ribs and an associated particularly dense area can be demonstrated in the posterior chest. Frost (1956) has suggested that in doubtful cases cholecystography might be employed to visualise the associated displacement of the gall bladder.

Cholecystography can be used to visualise the larger bile ducts and the gall bladder and to demonstrate the passage of bile into the duodenum. The clinical indications for this procedure, however, appear to be extremely limited in animals. The technique is used in man, principally for the visualisation of non-radiopaque gall stones, which are rare in animals.

The veterinary radiologist may well be consulted concerning the use of cholecystography in investigations into the etiology of particular cases of jaundice in animals. In general, where jaundice is severe and likely to be associated with considerable damage to hepatic cells, it is unlikely that the contrast agent will be excreted and reach and outline the biliary system. Under these circumstances the technique is unlikely to be of any assistance at all and its use might involve some risk. In chronic cases showing mild jaundice (where it is likely that some excretion of bile is still occurring) it is possible that sufficient contrast agent would be concentrated in the gall bladder and bile ducts to outline these and demonstrate, or eliminate, the presence of calculi, neoplasia or other causes of partial obstruction of the biliary system.

Another contrast media technique which may be mentioned here, is the use of portal venography to demonstrate interference with venous drainage of the abdomen by the liver or other structures, when investigating the cause of a case of ascites.

The Spleen

The normal spleen can vary considerably in size (e.g., it is likely to be considerably enlarged if barbiturate anaesthesia is employed) and a small spleen may be imperceptible in a radiograph. But in the majority of lateral abdominal radiographs the spleen will be visualised as a narrow, roughly diamond-shaped, dense area extending from the liver to the mid point of the ventral abdominal wall (a large spleen will extend considerably further than this).

In ventro-dorsal projections the spleen is less clearly outlined, but the left tip of the spleen can usually be recognised in the angle between the stomach and left abdominal wall. The other end of the spleen is seldom visible as it extends to the mid-line and merges with the denser lumbar muscles and vertebral column.

Pathological Changes

Diffuse splenic enlargement can usually be demonstrated radiologically and, in general, the larger the spleen the more distinctly it will be shown. However, as already stated, the use of barbiturate anaesthesia is likely to result in an increase in the size of this organ and this "normal" change must be allowed for. Where there is a particularly marked increase in splenic size the outline of the organ will no longer be confined to the floor of the abdomen in a lateral radiograph but will extend dorsally, and displacement of abdominal viscera may also be demonstrable.

Localised enlargement of the spleen (e.g., due to neoplasia or haematoma formation) may be more difficult to demonstrate precisely but the radiological evidence is likely to comprise loss of the distinct splenic outline and the presence of an associated diffuse mass.

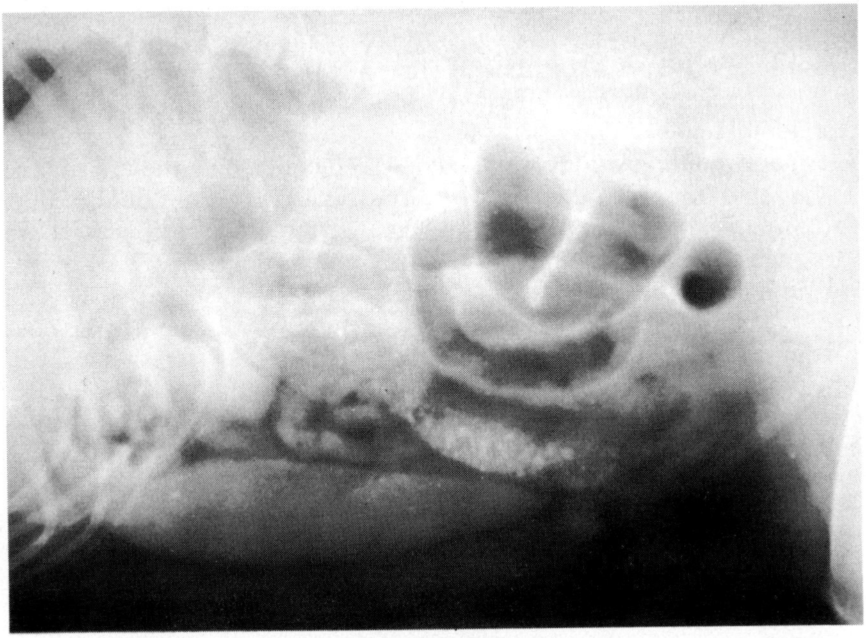

FIG. 10.9. Splenic enlargement in a dog.

The Pancreas

Since this organ is not normally demonstrable radiologically, any neoplastic changes would have to be particularly severe before they could be recognised and then could only be expected to show as a dense mass in the region of this organ (just ventral and posterior to the pylorus of the stomach in a lateral radiograph), which could not be identified precisely. It is probable that the associated changes in the function of this organ could be shown more accurately by laboratory methods.

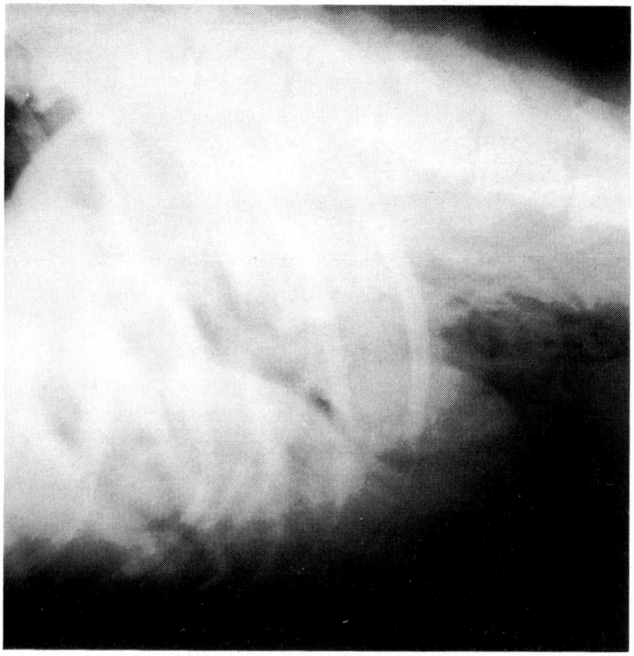

FIG. 10.10.

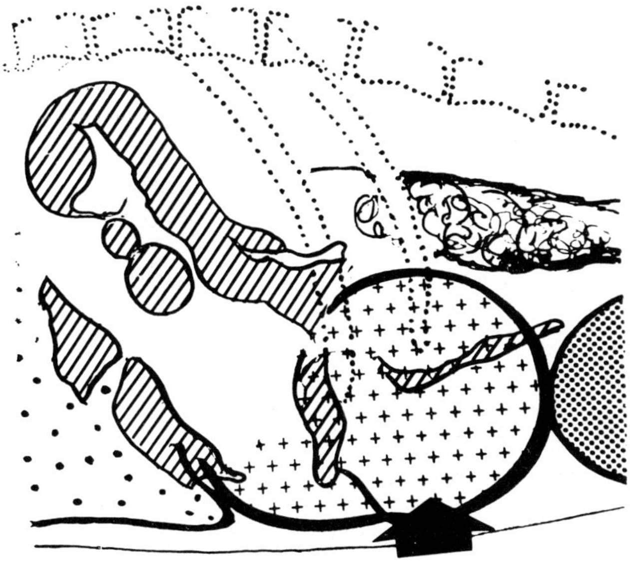

FIG. 10.11.

FIGS. 10.10 and 10.11. Irregular enlargement of the spleen due to haematoma formation.

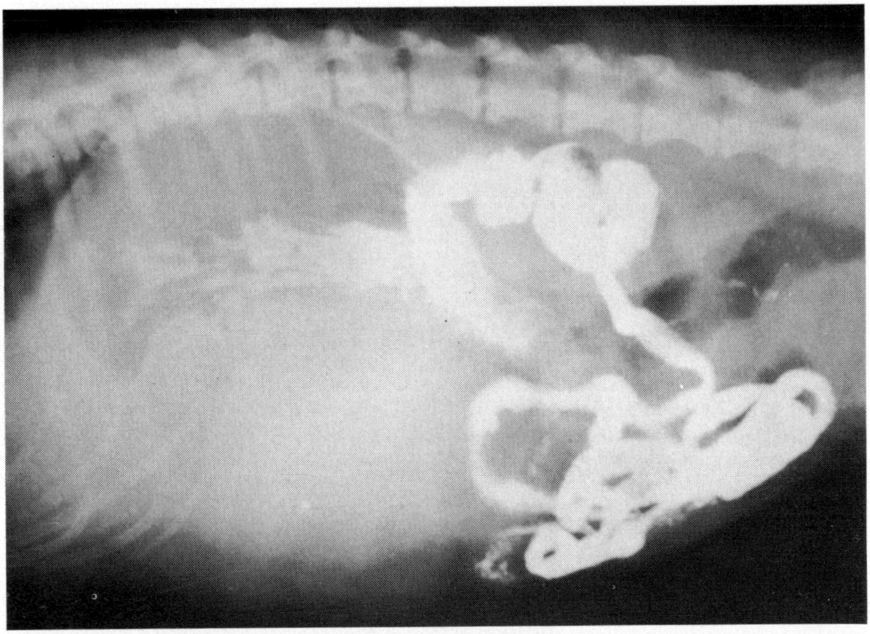

FIG. 10.12. Abdominal mass (pancreatic tumour) causing displacement of stomach (containing gas) and of intestines (containing barium).

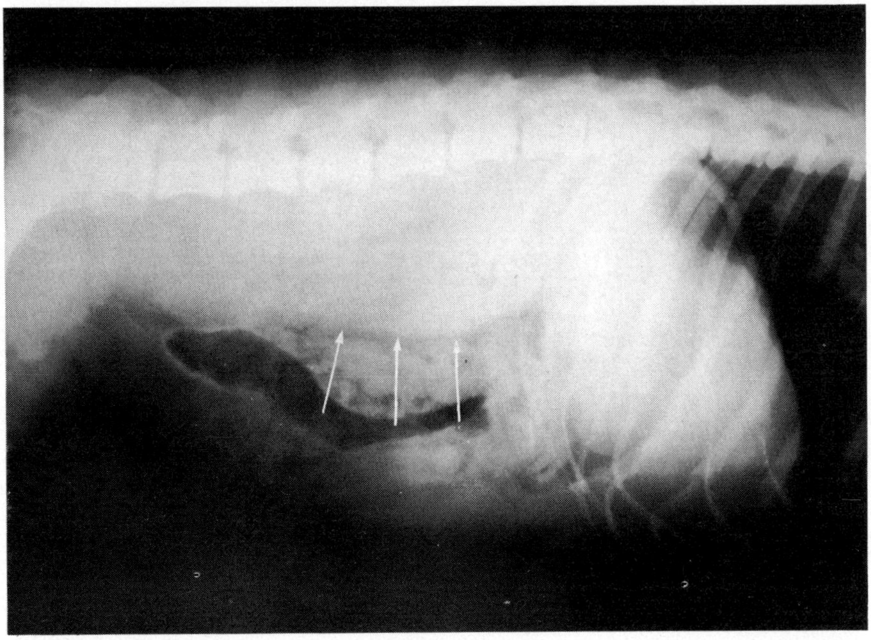

FIG. 10.13. Ventral displacement of the abdominal contents as a result of marked enlargement of the anterior and posterior mesenteric lymphatic glands (a case of generalised lymphosarcoma).

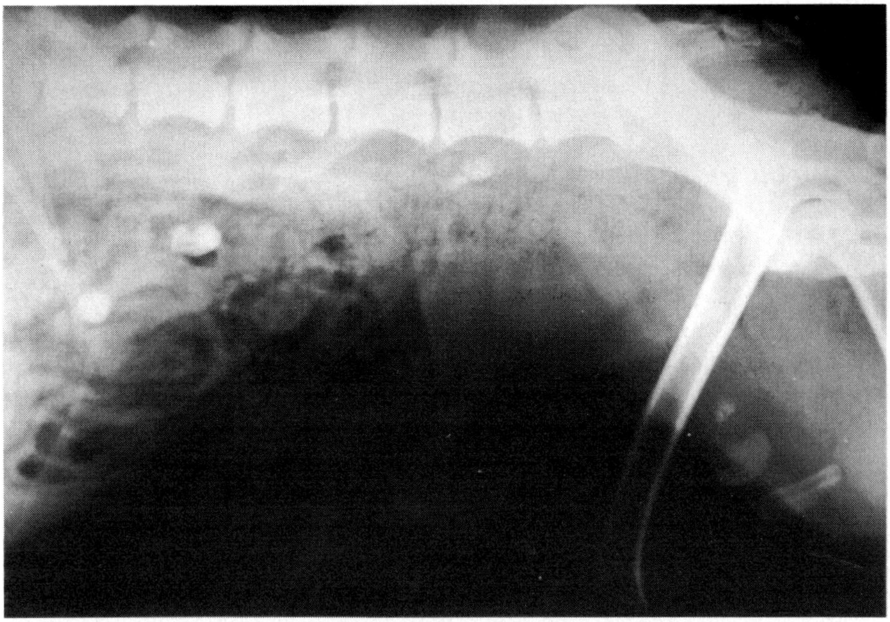

FIG. 10.14. Calcification within lymphatic nodes and glands.

The Abdominal Lymph Nodes

Marked enlargement of these nodes (usually due to neoplasia) should be recognised in lateral abdominal radiographs as irregular dense masses situated behind the kidney area (anterior mesenteric lymph nodes) or just anterior to the pelvis (posterior mesenteric lymph nodes). Such masses may extend ventrally into the abdomen and result in displacement of the alimentary tract. Calcified changes in these nodes are not common but may occasionally be recognised in radiographs.

Pathological changes in other intra-abdominal organs will be considered in the appropriate chapters.

REFERENCE

Frost, R. C. (1956), Vet. Rec., **68,** 1014.

CHAPTER 11

THE ALIMENTARY TRACT

Radiography provides a useful and important method of investigating the structure and function of the alimentary tract of the dog and cat. However, the radiographic technique employed for such an investigation will vary considerably, both with the nature of the pathological condition suspected, and with the particular portion of the tract being investigated. Thus, with acute conditions (e.g., obstruction of the small intestine) immediate radiography may be all that is practicable and necessary to demonstrate the lesion, but for visualisation of more chronic abnormalities (e.g., neoplasia of the gastric wall) careful preparation of the patient and a detailed radiographic technique is essential.

Because of the wide variation in procedure associated with the circumstances and site of radiography, generalisations concerning the radiographic technique and radiological features of the alimentary tract are of little value. These subjects will therefore be considered only in relation to the various divisions of the system. There are however certain general aspects of the use of contrast media which can be usefully discussed at this stage, before considering the detailed investigation of the different sections of the alimentary tract.

CONTRAST MEDIA TECHNIQUES

The use of a contrast agent (usually barium sulphate) to outline and visualise the soft tissues of the alimentary tract greatly extends the scope of radiography in the investigation of this system. At the same time it is important to appreciate the limitations involved in the use of barium meals in animals, compared with the specialised development of this technique in man.

In human radiology the radiologist normally observes the passage of barium through the portion of the alimentary tract in which he is interested by fluoroscopy. This enables him to assess the active functioning of the part and, at the appropriate moment, he will have radiographs taken so that he may make a more detailed examination of the structure of the area. In such examinations the cooperation of the patient and the availability of intricate apparatus (usually incorporating image intensification) permit the concentration of the contrast agent in the portion of the digestive system under investigation and also allow the procedure to be carried out with the minimum risk of irradiation of those taking part.

Theoretically the alimentary tract of animals should be studied by similar fluoroscopic methods, but the difficulties involved are obvious. The major problem is the restraint of the patient. The use of general anaesthesia or heavy sedation slows or completely arrests the passage of barium and is usually contra-indicated. Restraint of the conscious patient by assistants will involve a very serious risk of irradiation of those assistants, particularly if attempted with simple screening apparatus. The authors have experimented with the use of various shaped boxes and containers designed to prevent movement of the conscious patient during such examinations. While such devices are of some assistance, they are not always tolerated, and it is usually necessary to design or adapt the container for each individual animal examined if movement is to be prevented. Other difficulties include the problem of inducing the patient to swallow a sufficient quantity of barium and the expense of suitable apparatus which would permit safe screening of the abdomen at a variety of angles.

Despite these problems, there is much advantage in being able to observe and assess the dynamic function of the alimentary tract and further effort must be made to overcome the difficulties and to extend the use of such techniques in animals. However, considerations of human safety must be paramount and such procedures should only be permitted when modern apparatus incorporating image intensification is available, when adequate shielding of assistants can be provided, and when monitoring of the amount of radiation received by all concerned is carried out.

Thus, in practice, giving a barium meal to a dog involves administering barium sulphate by mouth, and then recording the passage of the medium through the alimentary tract by taking a series of radiographs at varying intervals. Such a technique is of considerable value but it does have certain disadvantages which must be borne in mind. The first of these is that, owing to wide variation in the rate at which contrast medium passes through the system even in the normal animal, a large number of films will need to be exposed if the whole tract is to be examined or if concentration of the medium in a particular region is not to be missed. An even more important problem arises in relation to the interpretation of films. Radiographs are likely to show various indentations and distortions of the column of barium which usually result from peristaltic activity, but can easily be mistaken for neoplastic or other lesions of the bowel wall. Thus considerable caution must be exercised in interpreting individual films of barium meals and significance should be attached only to those lesions which can be recognised consistently in a series of radiographs.

If the maximum assistance is to be obtained from barium meal investigations in animals it is important that the procedure should be planned carefully before it is carried out. Except for the demonstration of gross lesions (oesophageal dilatations, complete obstruction of the bowel, etc.) it is essential that the alimentary tract should be completely emptied (by withholding food and by the administration of laxatives and enemas) before giving barium. If this is not done, the presence of food or faecal material will arrest or distort the barium outline.

Similarly if the clinical history or other investigations suggest that the lesion is situated in a particular portion of the alimentary tract, it is advantageous to plan both the positioning of the patient and also the amount and form of barium sulphate administered so as to promote the demonstration of that particular region. These two points will be considered in greater detail under the separate divisions of the alimentary system.

To a lesser degree the presence of "gas" within portions of the alimentary tract can also act as a contrast agent. Whether it is in fact swallowed air or other gases is open to argument but is immaterial for radiological purposes. The term "gas" will be used throughout this chapter.

THE MOUTH AND PHARYNX

Only limited use is made of radiography in the investigation of this region. One reason for this is the fact that general anaesthesia, which is usually necessary to permit suitable restraint and accurate positioning, also facilitates direct visualisation of the area and may render radiographic examination unnecessary.

Accurately positioned lateral projections of the skull (using half the usual mAS to give good soft tissue detail) will demonstrate the extent of the oral cavity and give some idea of the size and position of the soft palate. It is not normally feasible to record actual swallowing of barium and thus assess the functioning of this region.

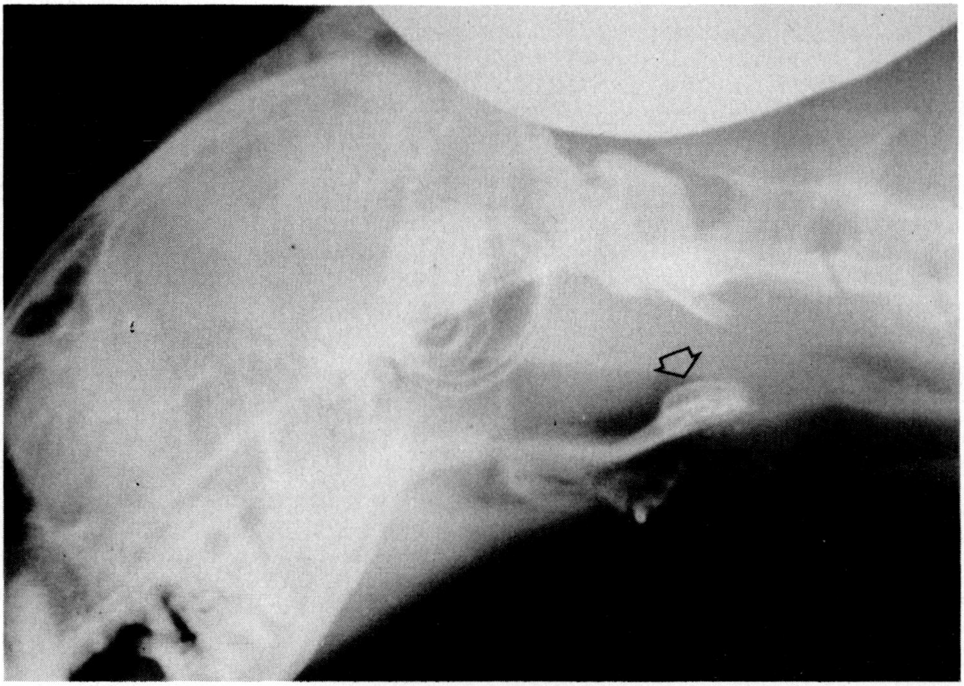

FIG. 11.1. A foreign body (fish bone) in the pharynx of a cat.

Radiography may be required for the demonstration of foreign bodies in this area. While usually obvious, small objects of low radio-density (e.g., small fish bones in the pharynx of the cat) can easily be confused with the hyoid apparatus, or missed altogether if blurred by movement of the patient.

Conditions of the teeth and jaws have been considered in Chapter 4.

The Salivary Glands will not be distinguishable in a plain radiograph of the region and when salivary cysts are present films are only likely to show soft tissue swelling of the appropriate areas. Salivary calculi appear to be rare in animals and are usually small and of poor radio-opacity and therefore unlikely to be distinguished radiologically from the surrounding soft tissues.

Contrast media techniques have been employed to visualise the salivary ducts (Cawley and Sorrell, 1959). This is a fairly simple procedure—one of the more viscous preparations of contrast material is introduced through the orifice to fill and outline the duct. However, false breaks can occur in the column of contrast material, because it is particularly thin, and do not necessarily indicate an obstruction.

THE OESOPHAGUS

Radiography

Lateral projections of the neck and chest are normally employed for radiography of the oesophagus. Owing to the superimposition of denser structures, films taken in the other plane are of little value unless considerable lateral deviation of this organ has occurred. In most instances it is necessary to use contrast media to visualise the oesophagus. While the usual watery suspensions of barium sulphate will accumulate in and demonstrate any marked dilations of this organ, they will pass through and be eliminated from the normal oesophagus almost immediately. The thicker paste-like suspensions of barium sulphate do tend to adhere to the mucous membrane of the oesophagus for a slightly longer time and may be preferable for the visualisation of the normal organ or of comparatively minor lesions.

If the act of swallowing can be observed by means of fluoroscopy it will be appreciated that peristaltic action carries food material through the oesophagus at an extremely rapid rate, and that all ingested material is passed into the stomach within a few seconds. This is in complete contrast to the lack of tone, and even paralysis, of the organ which is a feature of some pathological conditions of the oesophagus.

Radiology

Normal Appearance

In the cervical region the oesophageal wall cannot be distinguished from the surrounding soft tissues but the lumen of the organ may be indicated by a thin column of gas which contrasts with adjacent tissues.

Within the chest it is seldom that the oesophagus can be positively identified but the radiologist should be familiar with its approximate position. In a lateral chest radiograph the oesophagus is situated slightly dorsal to, but overlapping, the trachea at the entrance to the chest. It is superimposed on the trachea as it passes backwards and then traverses the base of the heart just under the curve of the major vessels. In the posterior half of the chest it is situated immediately dorsal to the vena cava.

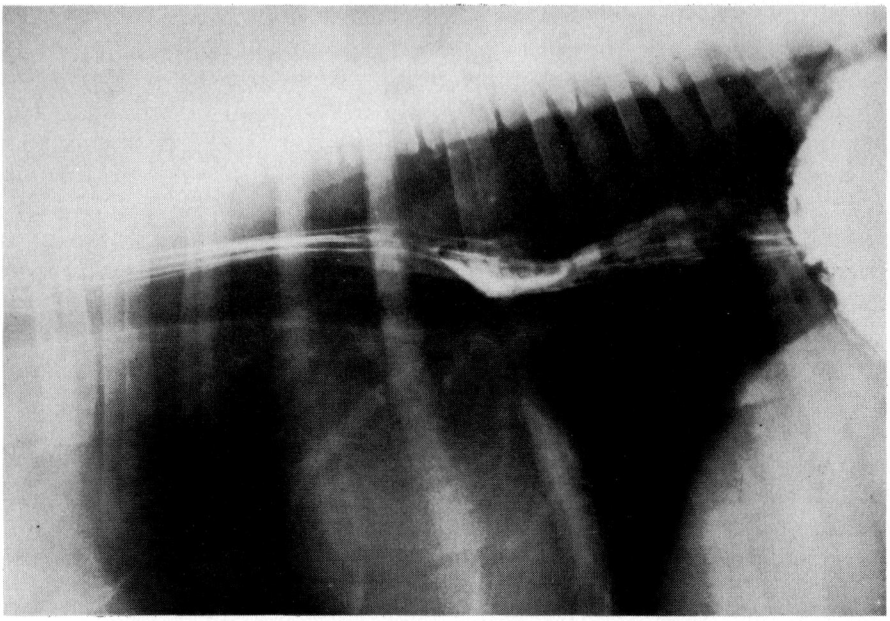

FIG. 11.2. The position of the normal oesophagus outlined by thin streaks of barium.

Pathological Conditions

Dilation of the Oesophagus (Achalasia)

The term "dilation" is used here as it is the main radiological feature of the conditions described. However it is usually assumed that the enlargements are a compensatory dilation and atony occurring anteriorly to constructions of the oesophagus caused by vascular abnormalities or by spasm of the cardia.

When the condition is associated with a vascular ring the dilation terminates at the base of the heart and the posterior portion of the oesophagus is of normal diameter. The term "achalasia" is usually restricted to the second form in which the enlargement extends to the diaphragm.

It is possible to recognise the more severe forms of this abnormality in radiographs without the use of contrast media. Since the enlarged oesophagus usually contains a considerable quantity of gas, the oesophageal wall is more clearly demarcated and the distended organ can be appreciated occupying the upper half of the chest in lateral films, and possibly projecting beyond the shadow of the spine in dorso-ventral projections. In the more insidious forms of achalasia which are occasionally encountered in the adult animal food material may accumulate within the dilated structure and help to demonstrate it.

In the less severely affected cases, or if the films are blurred by respiratory movement, it will not be possible to diagnose the condition without the use of contrast media and this is probably always advisable if the full extent of the dilation is to be visualised. Both the watery suspensions and the thicker pastes of barium sulphate

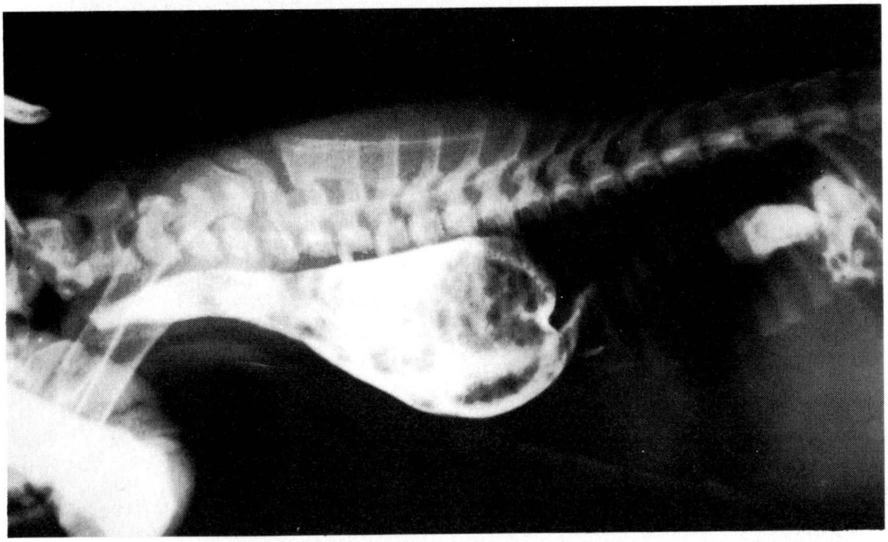

FIG. 11.3. Dilation of the anterior oesophagus associated with a vascular ring abnormality in a kitten.

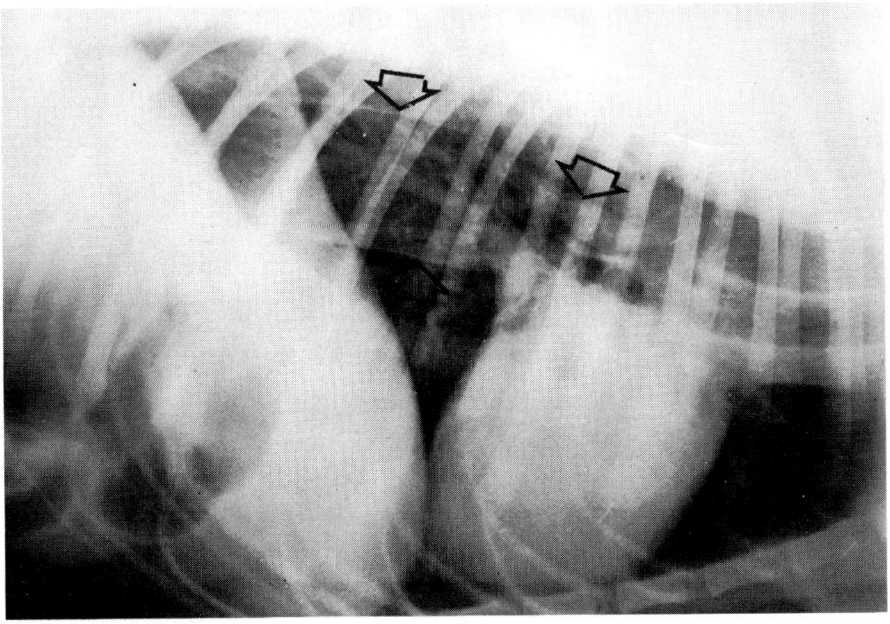

FIG. 11.4. Achalasia—the wall of the dilated oesophagus can be recognised without the use of contrast media.

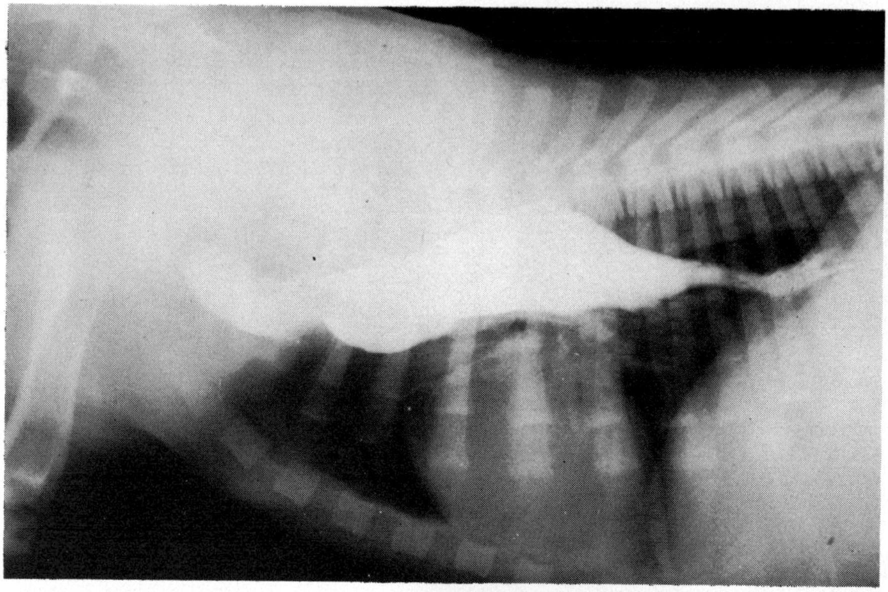

FIG. 11.5. Achalasia in an Alsatian dog.

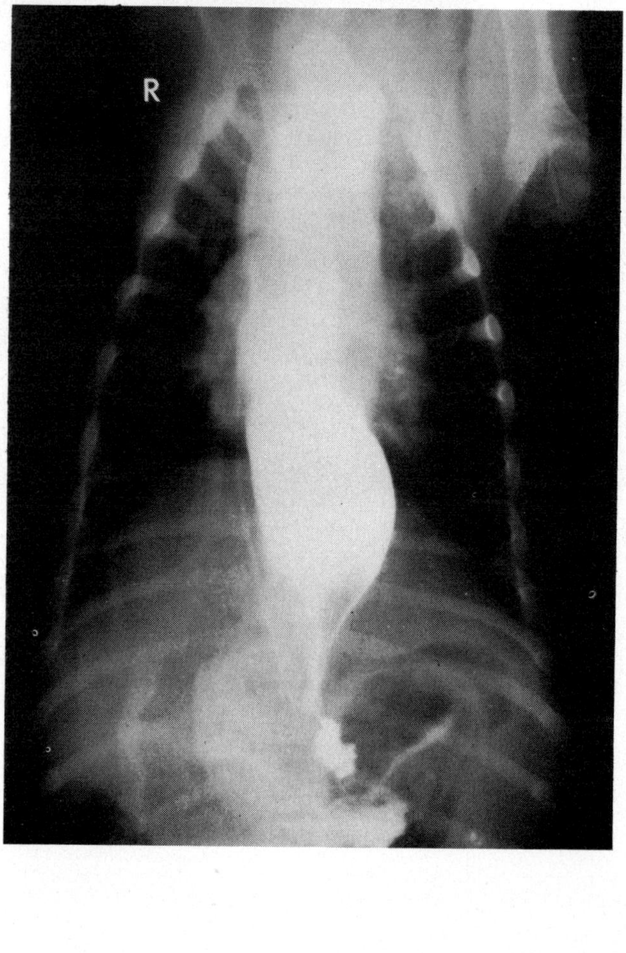

FIG. 11.6. Dorso-ventrical projection of the same dog—taken subsequently and showing more complete filling of the posterior oesophagus.

are satisfactory but time must be allowed for the thicker forms to permeate through the oesophageal folds of the more severely affected cases.

If fluoroscopic facilities are available it is possible to appreciate that the condition is associated with a complete flaccidity of the oesophageal wall.

Oesophageal Foreign Body

The radiological demonstration of a foreign body within the oesophagus can be very typical and apparent, but in some circumstances it is less obvious and can be overlooked by the inexperienced. The reason for this is that the swallowed object (usually a portion of bone or a piece of gristle) is seldom of dense radio-opacity and its outline is frequently blurred by respiratory movement. Furthermore such objects are commonly located just anterior or posterior to the heart, and in this region the surrounding vascular and bronchial markings are comparatively dense and permit of less contrast with the foreign body. Thus, if the presence of an obstruction is not obvious, films should be carefully examined for otherwise unexplained areas of increased density corresponding with the estimated position of the oesophagus. In doubtful cases the administration of small amounts of a thick suspension of barium sulphate may either outline the obstruction or demonstrate its absence.

Once a foreign body is located it is important to make a careful examination for evidence of inflammatory or infected involvement of the surrounding tissues. If the object has been present for any length of time it is likely that some thickening of the

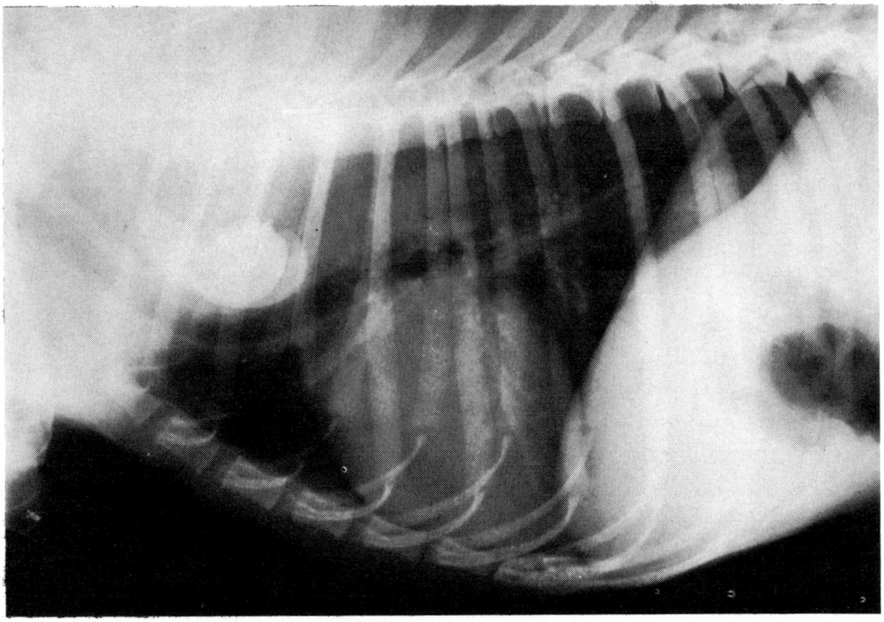

FIG. 11.7. A large bony foreign body situated in the anterior thoracic oesophagus and causing depression of the trachea.

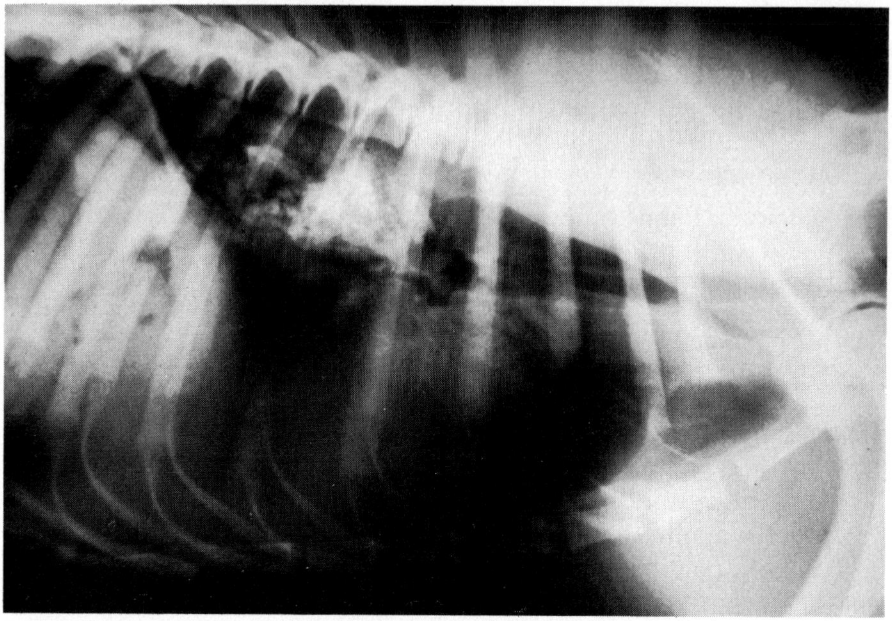

FIG. 11.8. A less radio-opaque foreign body (a piece of gristle) located in the oesophagus posterior to the heart.

oesophageal wall and increased density of the immediately adjacent lung parenchyma will be recognised in a radiograph. Should there, however, be evidence of pneumonic changes extending out from the affected area or of the presence of fluid within the chest, then perforation of the oesophagus by the foreign body must be suspected. Where there is the possibility of this complication having occurred considerable caution should be observed in administering barium sulphate as, if it leaks into the chest, it will not be absorbed or eliminated. In such circumstances the use of one of the organic iodine compounds designed for the demonstration of the alimentary tract is preferable as such preparations will be subsequently absorbed.

Neoplasia

Neoplastic lesions of the oesophageal wall appear to be rare but are encountered, particularly in cats, from time to time. While advanced lesions might be perceptible in plain films the use of contrast media is usually necessary for their demonstration. A small quantity of barium sulphate paste should outline the irregularity of the oesophageal wall caused by the tumour.

Other Causes of Oesophageal Compression

Symptoms of oesophageal obstruction can be due to compression by intrathoracic masses (e.g., mediastinal gland enlargement, neoplasia or other enlargement of the thymus, etc.) and are likely to be investigated by means of radiography. In these

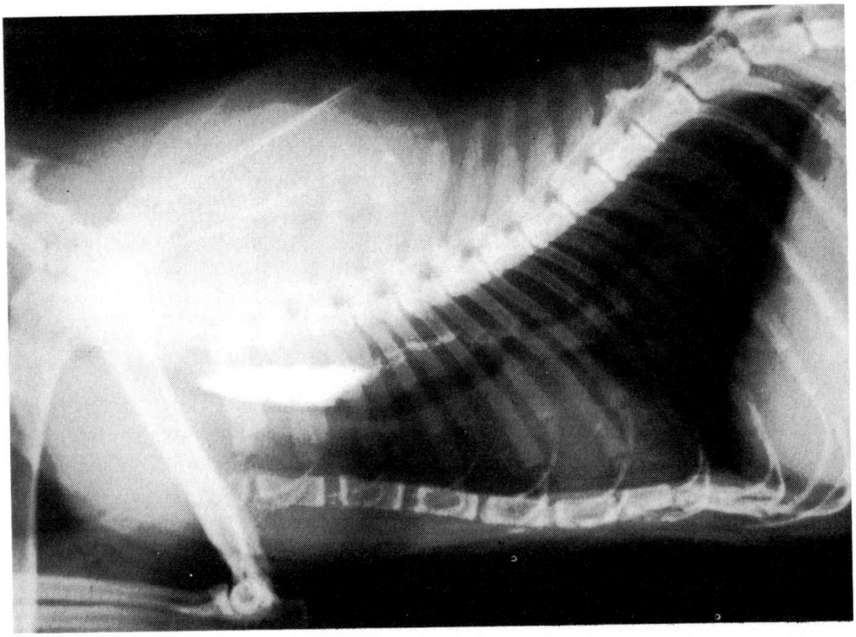

FIG. 11.9. Barium outlining the anterior and dorsal border of an oesophageal neoplasm in a cat.

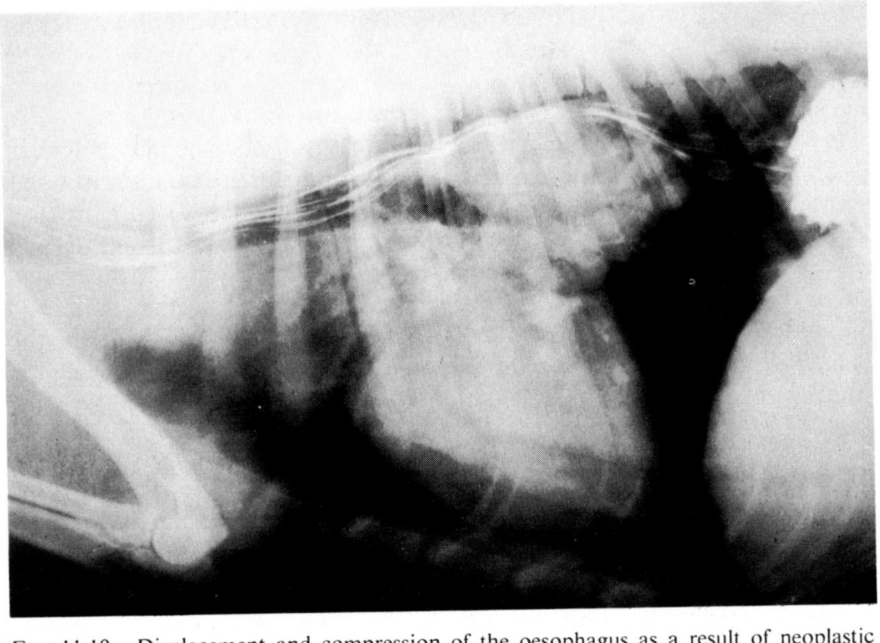

FIG. 11.10. Displacement and compression of the oesophagus as a result of neoplastic enlargement of the mediastinal lymphatic gland.

circumstances it is unlikely that the oesophagus can be identified in plain chest films but associated displacement of the trachea may be recognised. It is probable that the masses responsible for the compression will also be demonstrated. If barium sulphate is given it is possible that the more dilute suspensions may pass straight through and fail to reveal any abnormality. The use of the thicker pastes would be preferable and should demonstrate the displacement and compression of the oesophagus (bear in mind that, even in the normal animal, slight compression and displacement of the oesophagus can be expected at the level of the first pair of ribs and over the base of the heart).

THE STOMACH

Radiography

The presence of food within the stomach can distort this organ or obscure the recognition of lesions. Whenever possible food should be withheld for 12 hours before radiography and this is an essential precaution if contrast media are to be employed.

For most purposes a combination of lateral and ventro-dorsal projections provide adequate demonstration of the stomach, but in some circumstances dorso-ventral (and occasionally oblique) projections are also required.

Contrast media techniques are of considerable importance in the investigation of gastric lesions. The presence of gas within the stomach acts as a form of contrast agent and helps to identify the position of this organ. Such a gas shadow can be produced or increased by administering sodium bicarbonate solution immediately before radiography. Barium sulphate is the agent normally employed for contrast purposes and provides better demonstration of the gastric outline. However, because of its considerable radio-density, the administration of too large a quantity can obliterate small gastric lesions. For most purposes it is best to give a medium quantity (15–60 ml. depending on the size of the dog) of the 100 per cent. suspension and to carry out an examination of the stomach. Additional volume can be obtained by administering water or, more usually, further amounts of barium suspension if radiography indicates that this is necessary, or for subsequent examination of the intestines.

The effect that the positioning of the animal, prior to and during radiography, has on barium studies of the stomach is not always appreciated. The patient is normally held in an erect position during the introduction of barium and as this administration takes time it will be found that the contrast agent has concentrated in the pyloric region (and usually already entered the duodenum) before radiography is undertaken. For demonstration of the cardiac end of the stomach the dog should be placed on its back or on its left side as quickly as possible after administration of barium. It is kept in one of these positions for a few minutes and then radiography is undertaken in the ventro-dorsal and lateral (with the left side down) planes. Positioning is then reversed and radiography repeated some 5 minutes later in the dorso-ventral and lateral (with the right side down) projections for investigation of the pyloric end of the stomach.

Radiology

The radiological appearance of the stomach can vary considerably with the degree of distension of the organ and with the displacement caused by positioning, and no precise description can be given.

Although the administration of barium sulphate is probably always necessary for a full radiological examination of the stomach, it is important that the radiologist should first examine plain films of the gastric area. This will permit recognition of the more radio-opaque foreign bodies (which could be masked by the administration of barium) and of gross changes in the position and size of the stomach.

In ventro-dorsal projections the outline of the stomach is superimposed on the lumbar muscles and on the posterior edge of the liver and can seldom be distinguished. However there is usually an accumulation of air in the fundus and this should be apparent to the left of the mid-line and at the level of the last one or two ribs.

In lateral views a foreshortened view of the stomach is obtained and this tends to merge with the posterior edge of the liver. Usually the only features which can be recognised are the fundic air shadow, situated just above and behind the liver, and a relatively dense rounded area, which is an "end on" view of the pyloric region and is situated ventral to the air shadow in the curve of the posterior edge of the liver. This latter feature can appear particularly round and distinct in outline and can, on occasion, be difficult to distinguish from a rubber ball within the stomach.

The above appearance will be altered if the stomach contains food, and, if the animal has recently eaten a large meal, it may occupy a large area of the anterior third of the abdominal cavity. The rate of emptying of food from the stomach varies but will take some hours and is a much slower process than the passage of watery suspensions of barium.

Radiological demonstration of gastric enlargement and of the retention of swallowed material for long periods would suggest the likelihood of some obstruction at the pyloric outlet. Gross gastric distension, but containing gas, would indicate torsion of the stomach.

The administration of barium aids visualisation of the position and lumen of the stomach, particularly in ventro-dorsal and dorso-ventral projections. As already mentioned, the precise appearance will vary with, the amount of barium given, the positioning of the patient, and the stage at which films are exposed. Usually three regions can be recognised.

(1) The fundic area comprises the largest area and is situated to the left of the mid-line. The presence of gastric rougae result in a particularly irregular outline.

(2) A short constricted region corresponding with the base of the concavity of the lesser curvature. (Neither the lesser or greater curvature of the stomach are fully demonstrated in the projections normally employed.)

(3) The pyloric region is a more elongated area with a smoother outline which curves forward to unite with the duodenum at the level of the last ribs. A pointed tip to the column of barium in this region often identifies the actual position of the pylorus.

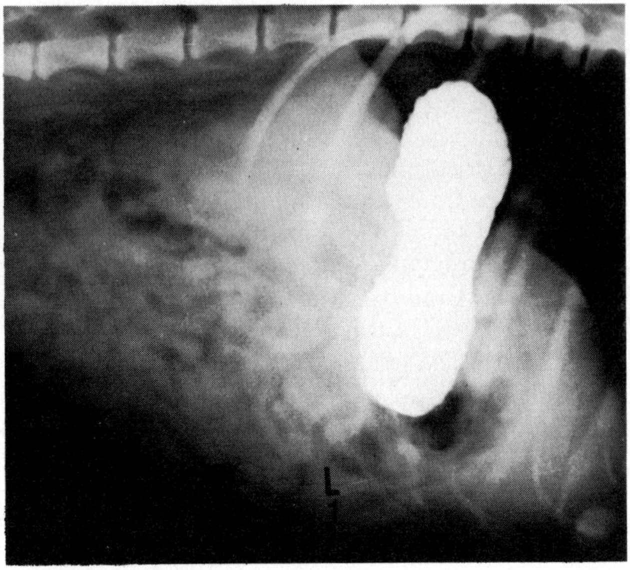

FIG. 11.11.

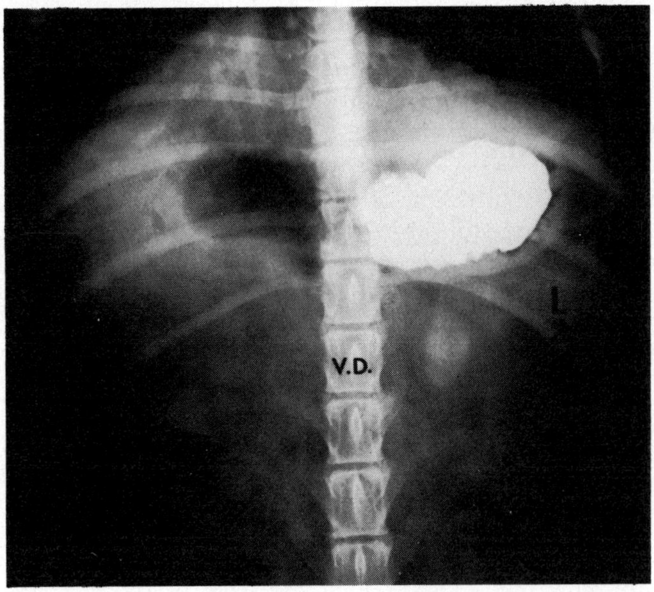

FIG. 11.12.

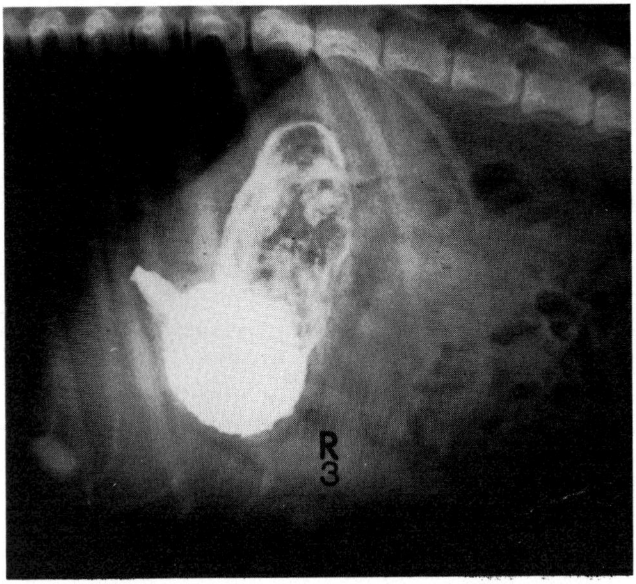

FIG. 11.13.

FIGS. 11.11 to 11.14. The effect of positioning on the outline of barium within the stomach.

1. with the left side down
2. ventro-dorsal
3. with the right side down
4. dorso-ventral.

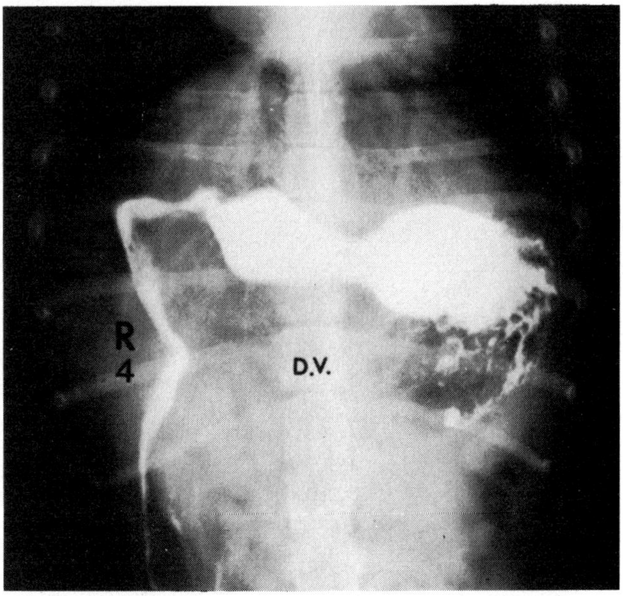

FIG. 11.14.

In lateral projections a foreshortened appearance of the stomach is again obtained. The fundic region is seen as an inverted pear-shaped mass situated dorsally while the pyloric area comprises a circular region beneath this.

Pathological Conditions

Gastric Foreign Body

Most gastric foreign bodies are of dense radio-opacity and are obvious in a radiograph (unless they are obliterated by over-enthusiastic administration of barium). Occasionally it will not be clear whether the foreign body is situated within the stomach or in an overlying portion of the small bowel. The problem can usually be resolved by comparison of films taken in two planes or by close examination of the associated gas shadows.

Foreign bodies of low radio-opacity (some rubber objects, portions of rag, hair balls, etc.) may be just perceptible in some high quality films but often cannot be definitely recognised. In these circumstances the administration of a small quantity of barium (8–30 ml.) is likely to be of assistance. The patient should then be rotated to distribute the contrast agent throughout the stomach, when immediate radiography may show the object outlined by the barium. If this is inconclusive

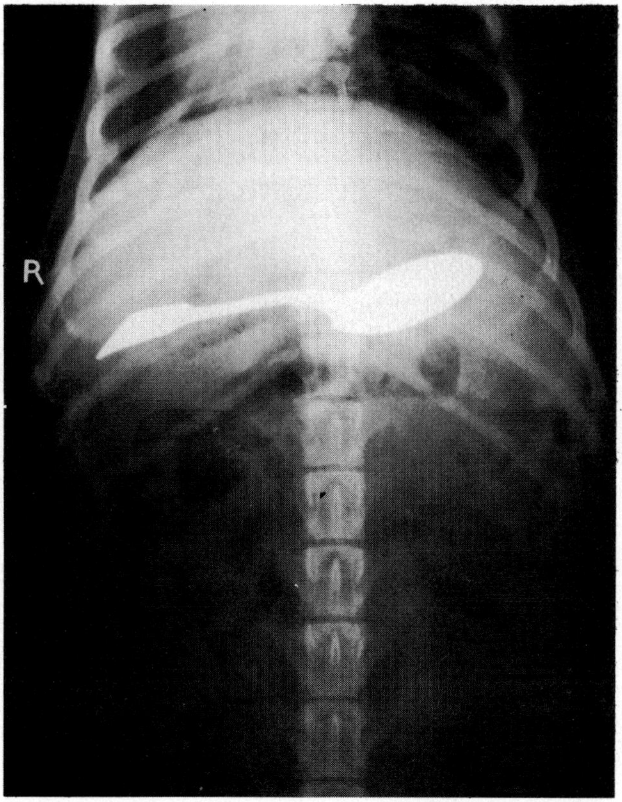

FIG. 11.15. An obvious gastric foreign body.

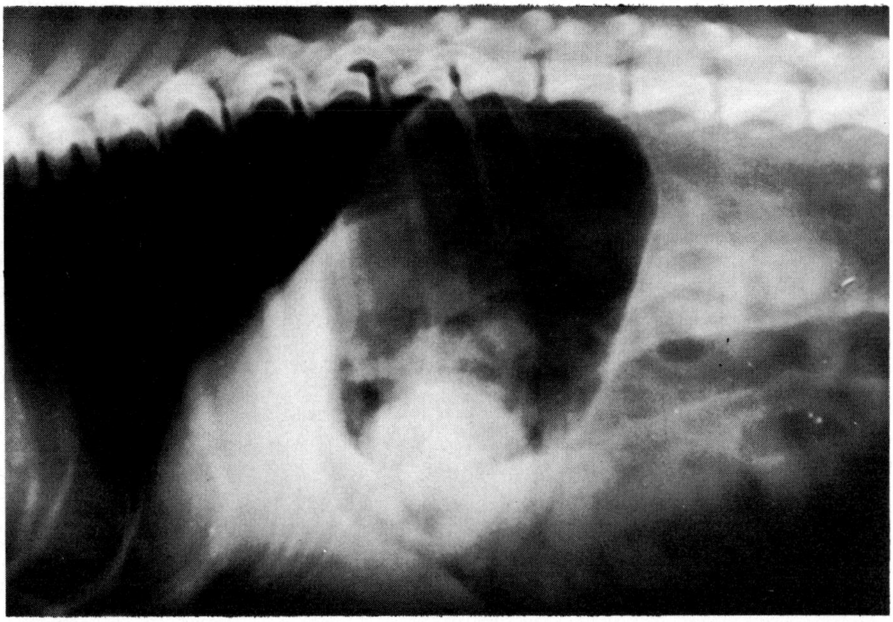

FIG. 11.16. A less obvious foreign body (a rubber ball) outlined by gas within the stomach.

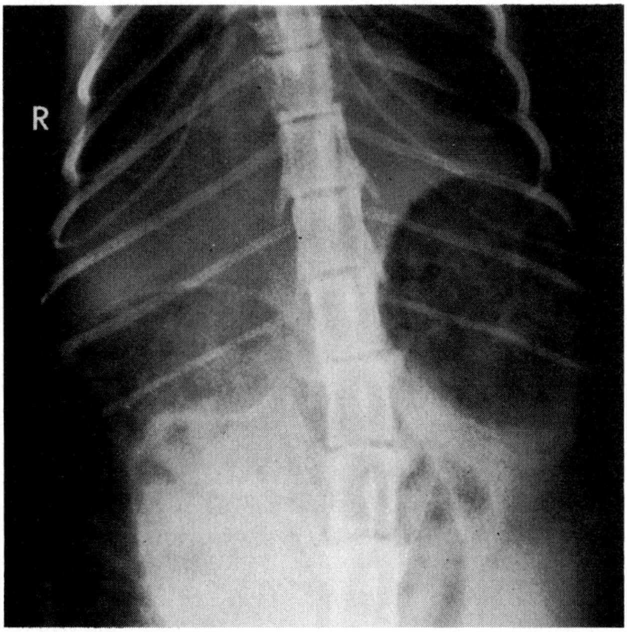

FIG. 11.17. A mixture of hair and gas distending the stomach and duodenum of a cat.

further barium can be given and a series of films taken to record the emptying of the stomach. Once the majority of the barium has passed into the small intestine, a residue may be demonstrated adhering to the foreign material. If no emptying of stomach occurs, this would suggest that the object is obstructing the pylorus (this is discussed further under "pyloric obstruction").

In the case of hair balls barium is likely to be irregularly distributed through an obviously distended stomach but in at least one case encountered the hair was so tightly packed that barium failed to enter the organ and was retained in the oesophagus.

Pyloric Obstruction

This general term is used for a number of clinical conditions involving the pyloric region (impaction of a foreign body, spasm of the pyloric sphincter, or the presence of hypertrophic or neoplastic thickenings in the area) which all show the common symptom of partial or complete obstruction of the passage of gastric contents into the duodenum. While radiography is the most satisfactory way of demonstrating this malfunction and its exact location, one will not necessarily be able to differentiate between the various causes from films alone.

In many instances of obstruction plain films of the gastric region will show no abnormality but in some of the more chronic cases enlargement of the stomach, or the retention within it of fluid or of material known to have been swallowed some time previously, will be recognised. The presence of excessive gastric fluid may be shown by an enlarged homegenous appearence of the stomach area, by the presence of a fluid line in the standing animal, or by the fact that barium mixtures are flocculated and irregularly dispersed after administration.

The administration of barium is essential if the passage of material through the pylorus is to be accurately demonstrated and recorded. However, differentiation between "normal" and "abnormal" passage is not always obvious.

The usual procedure is to withhold all food for at least 12 hours and then to administer a fairly large quantity (30–120 ml.) of barium. This is likely to take at least 5 minutes to give, and in most animals it will be found that by the time radiography can be undertaken some of the barium will have already entered the duodenum. With the more nervous dog however the barium may be retained in the stomach for several hours before passing through the pylorus. If such a delay is suspected of being due to the dog's nervous temperament, the procedure should be repeated a few days later after the animal has become more used to the apparatus and to being handled. Sedatives should not be administered in such cases, as they may temporary relieve any spasm of the pylorus and prevent its demonstration.

When a pyloric obstruction is present, radiography is likely to demonstrate that gastric peristalsis has caused the barium to accumulate in the pyloric end of the stomach but that little or none of the material has passed into the duodenum. The very forceful gastric movements which propel barium into this region are best appreciated if they can be observed by means of fluoroscopy. This can also be visualised in radiographs, because it results in a smooth "stretched" appearance of this area of stomach which, together with the prolonged gastric emptying time, are characteristic radiological features of this condition. The concentration of barium within this region can result in good deliniation of foreign bodies or of hypertrophic or neoplastic lesions if these are responsible for the obstruction. Where the condition results from pyloric spasm, temporary relief can usually be demonstrated if the procedure is repeated a short while after the oral administration of a suitable atropine preparation.

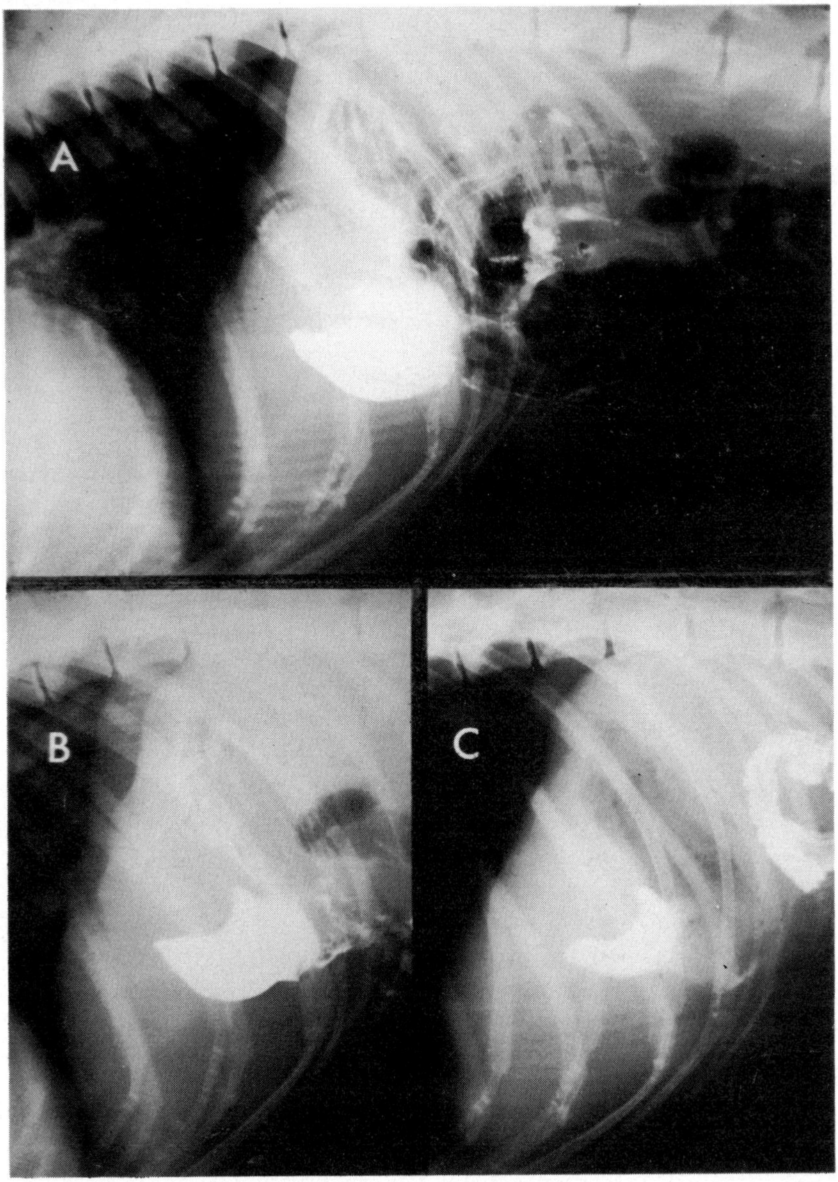

FIG. 11.18. Retention of barium within the pyloric region outlining a consistent filling defect (a carcinoma). Films were exposed at (A) 30 minutes, (B) 2 hours, (C) 24 hours after administration of the barium.

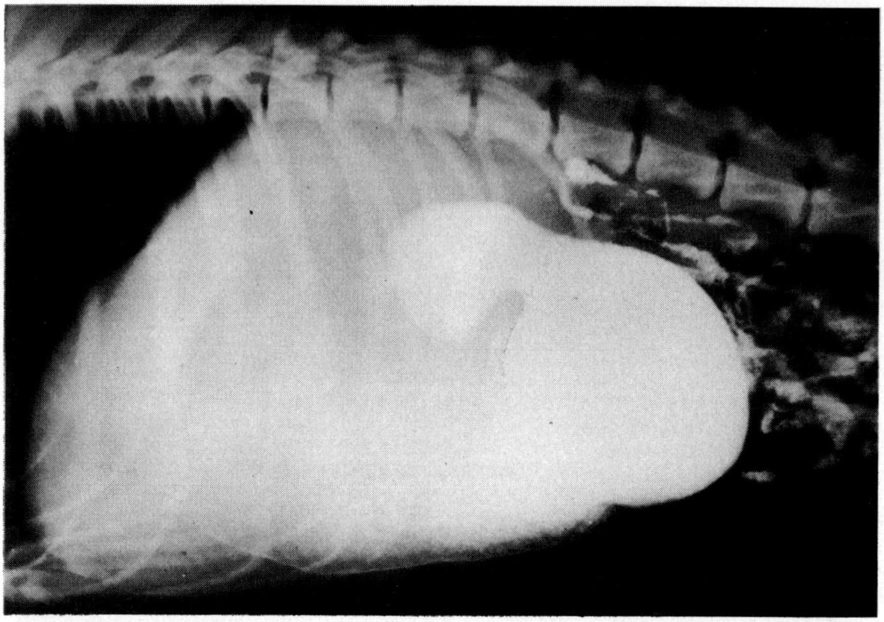

FIG. 11.19. Gross dilation of the stomach due to obstruction by hypertrophy of the pylorus.

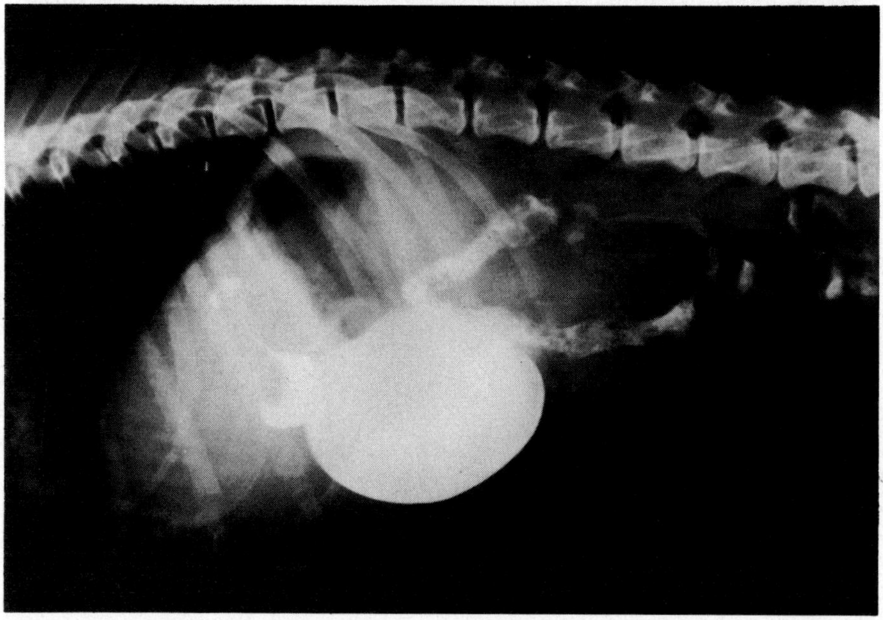

FIG. 11.20. Obstruction of the pylorus by a neoplasm (adenocarcinoma). Radiograph taken 4 hours after administration of barium. Note typical smooth distended outline of the pyloric region.

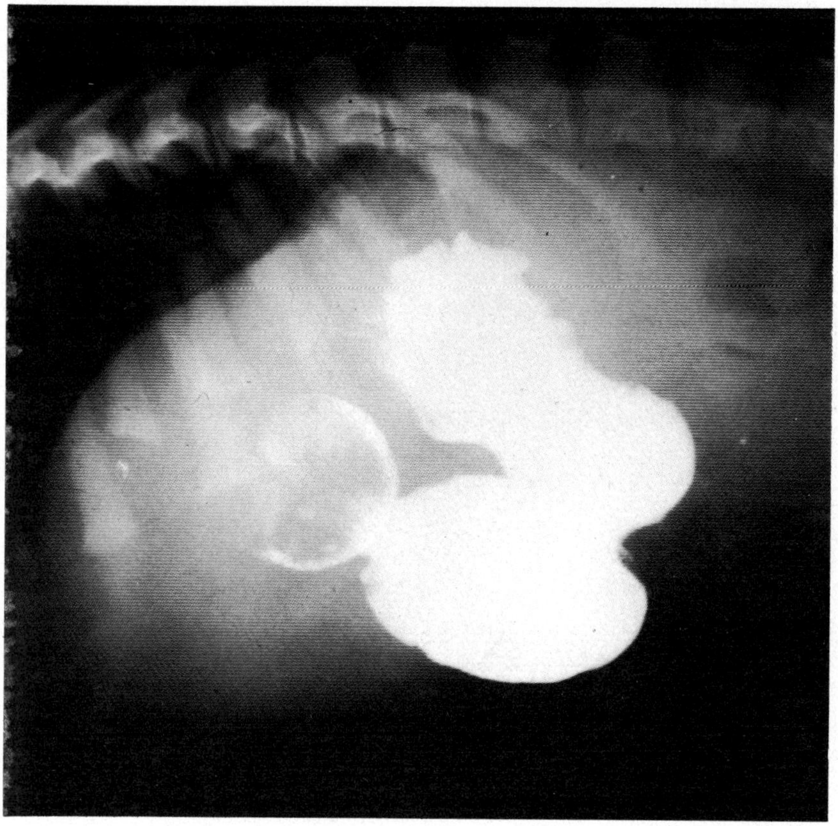

FIG. 11.21. Blockage of the anterior end of the duodenum by a potato (outlined by barium) resulting in pyloric obstruction.

Gastric Torsion (Gastric Tympany)

This condition is frequently diagnosed and treated on clinical symptoms alone. When radiography is employed it will show a greatly distended gas-filled organ filling the major portion of the anterior abdomen. The administration of barium is unnecessary and is in any case unlikely to enter the stomach.

Gastritis

Although frequently used, this is a rather vague term employed to describe any form of inflammation of the gastric mucosa. It is unlikely that it can be convincingly demonstrated by radiographic means. When outlined by barium the gastric rougae of the fundic portion of the stomach will, even in the normal dog, show a particularly irregular outline, which to the inexperienced can suggest "gastritis". If such an animal suffers from an actual gastritis it is likely that films will show enlargement of the rougae and a more rapid passage of barium through the stomach, but this is a comparative change and unlikely to be appreciated accurately in a particular case.

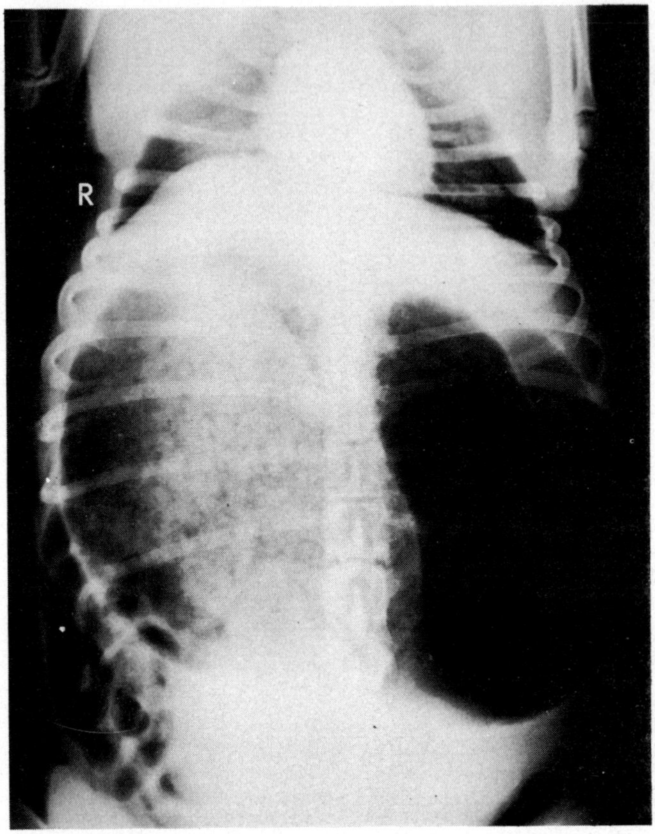

FIG. 11.22. Gastric torsion resulting in tympany.

Lesions of the Gastric Wall

While gastric neoplasms and ulcers appear to be relatively rare in animals and the radiographic techniques available for their demonstration are far less precise than in human radiology, such lesions can occasionally be shown. The demonstration of neoplastic lesions resulting in obstruction of the pylorus has already been discussed. Other tumours and ulcers may show either or both of the following features:

(a) A constant defect in the silhouette of an accumulation of barium within the stomach. If this is associated with a neoplasm the defect will extend into the barium, while in the case of an ulcer the barium is likely to bulge outwards into the region of the gastric wall. For recognition of this feature it is advisable to slightly distend the stomach with barium. If the defects are small it is probable that they will be obliterated by the contrast agent and not seen unless the X-ray beam happens to be directed at such an angle that the lesion is situated at the periphery of the barium. Thus in addition to the standard views, oblique projections of the stomach may be required.

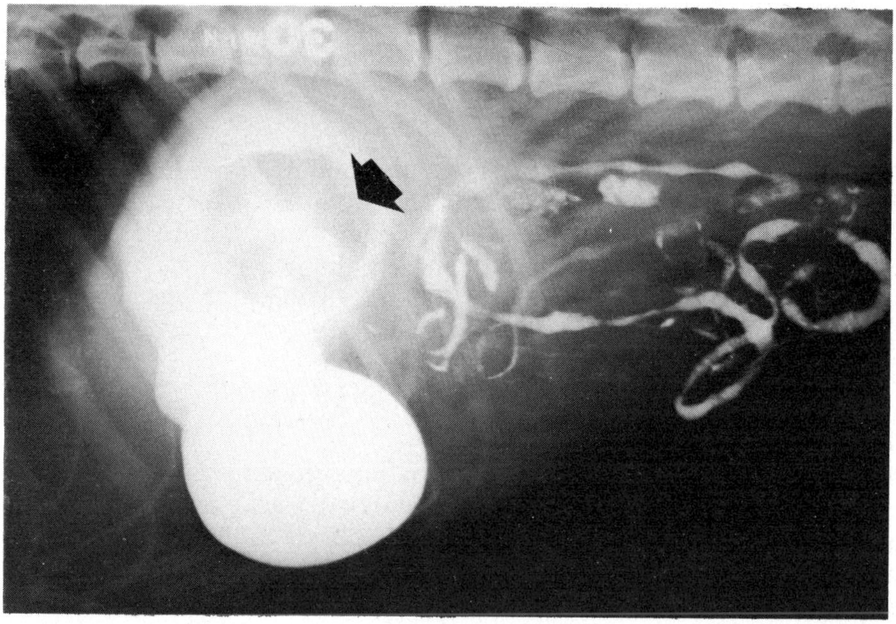

FIG. 11.23.

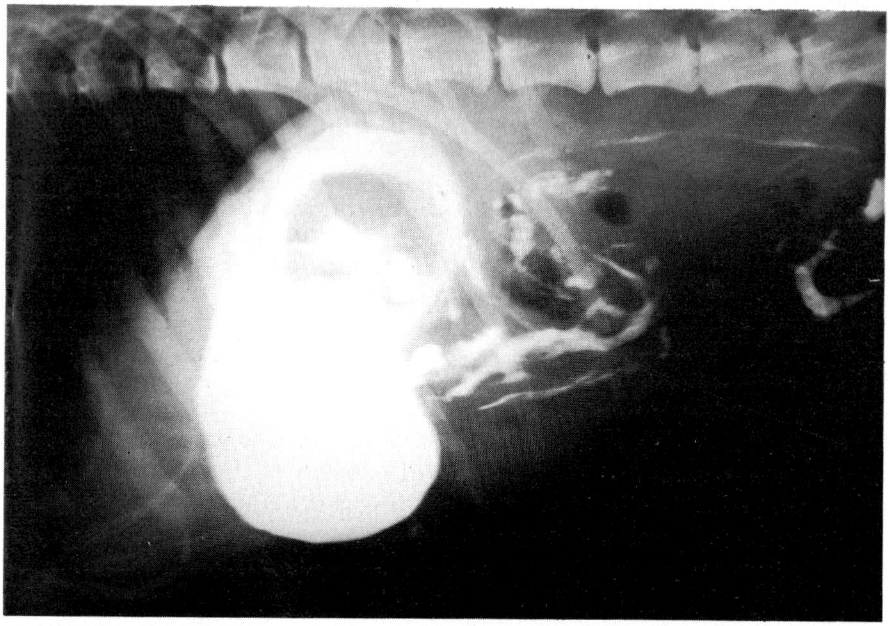

FIG. 11.24.

FIGS. 11.23 and 11.24. Consistent adhesion of barium to a small gastric tumour in the fundic region (2 examples from a series of radiographs).

(b) Adhesion of small quantities of barium to the surface of an ulcer or ulcerated neoplasm. This finding is most likely to be recognised when most of the barium has been removed by normal gastric emptying. Since perception of this feature does not depend on a "sky line" effect, positioning is less critical.

It must be stressed however that an irregular outlining or accumulation of barium due to normal gastric contractions can easily be mistaken for either of the above features. Attention should be paid to such findings only when they are seen as a consistent feature in a series of films. Similarly the fact that radiography has not revealed any lesion of the gastric wall should not be assumed to preclude its presence.

THE SMALL INTESTINES

Radiography

When investigating the small intestine it is important to use a film of sufficient size to permit inclusion of the entire abdominal cavity as, particularly if abdominal pressure is applied, significant lesions may be displaced to the periphery and missed in smaller radiographs. Lateral projections are usually the most informative but they may need to be supplemented by ventro-dorsal views (although the central area of these films is obscured by superimposition of the spine). The use of abdominal pressure to check the effects of respiratory movement and to thin the area being radiographed, improves definition with either projection. When practicable, and particularly if administration of barium is intended, the usual precautions should be taken to empty the bowel prior to radiography.

The actual amount of barium sulphate administered for the investigation of the intestines need not be very precise, although very small quantities may fail to fill the lumen and extremely large amounts may obscure detail in overlapping loops of bowel. If it is known that the radiographic examination is to be concerned only with this portion of the alimentary tract it is preferable to use a more watery form of barium (25 per cent. suspension) as this appears to pass more rapidly and smoothly. The position of the patient immediately previous to radiography does not appear to have any marked effect on the barium pattern.

Radiology

When examining abdominal radiographs particular portions of the bowel can be identified only if they happen to contain some material (e.g., gas, food or barium) which acts as a contrast agent and outlines the lumen of the tract. For this reason it is proposed to describe what may be seen in normal abdominal films after administration of barium. Some of these features may be recognised in plain films if particular portions of the alimentary tract can be identified because they contain gas or ingested material.

The duodenum may be identified, not only because it is the first portion of the intestines outlined with barium, but more particularly because it is fairly constant in position within the abdomen. Thus in dorso-ventral films it will be observed to

FIG. 11.25.

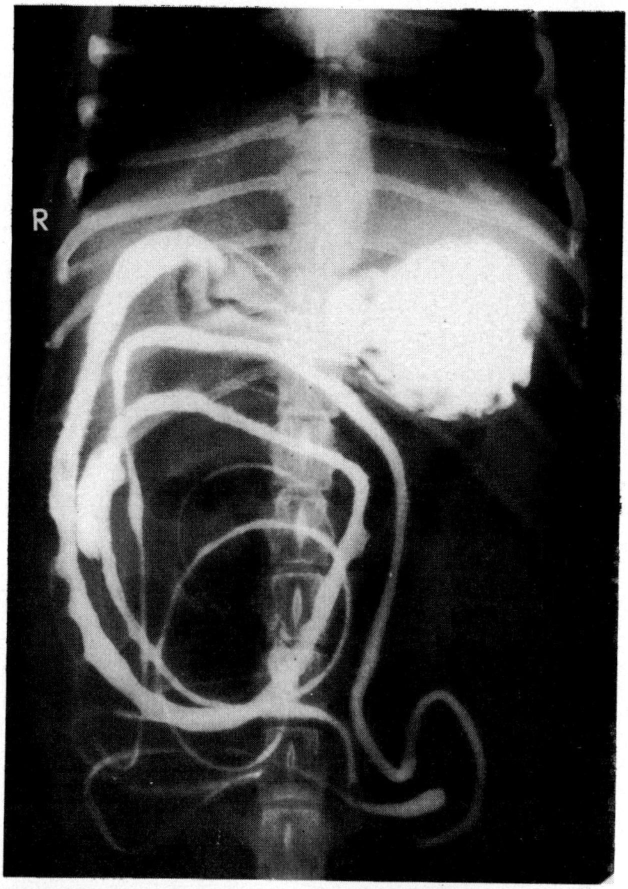

FIGS. 11.25 and 11.26. Ventro-dorsal and lateral projections of the abdomen demonstrating the position of the normal duodenum.

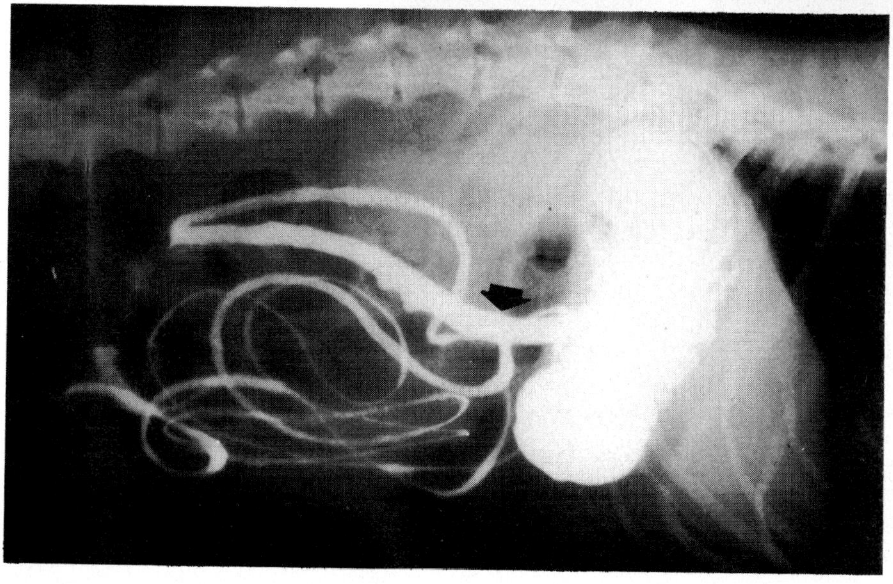

FIG. 11.26.

commence immediately anteriorly to the gastric pylorus and, curving sharply backwards, to follow the right abdominal wall until its takes a semicircular turn forward to end in the mid-abdominal region. In lateral films the position of the duodenum is less characteristic, but when barium is present, it can be identified by following the column of contrast agent backwards from the pylorus.

The remainder of the intestines are seen as overlapping loops of bowel occupying the central area of the abdomen. These loops may be displaced by other abdominal organs (e.g., a distended bladder or enlarged uterus).

The diameter of the column of barium is likely to appear irregular as a result of peristaltic contractions but there is no typical mucosal pattern as is seen in man.

The time taken for barium to pass through the intestines and reach the large bowel can vary considerably. This is usually anything from 1 to 4 hours but no particular figure can be taken as a limit of normality. All that can be said is that the rate of movement of barium will be increased by such conditions as acute enteritis, and slowed if the patient is heavily sedated or in a shocked or collapsed condition.

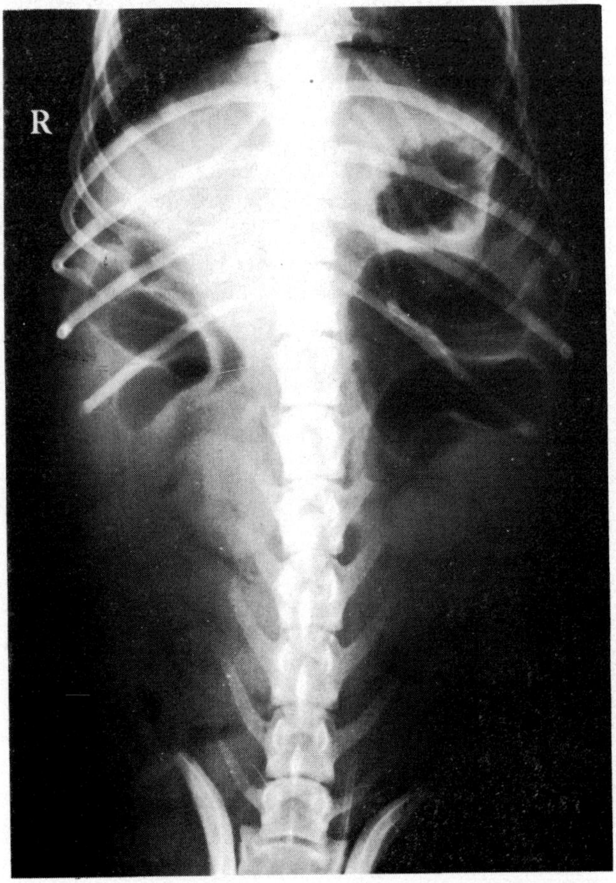

FIG. 11.27. Gas-filled loops of small bowel indicating intestinal obstruction and stasis.

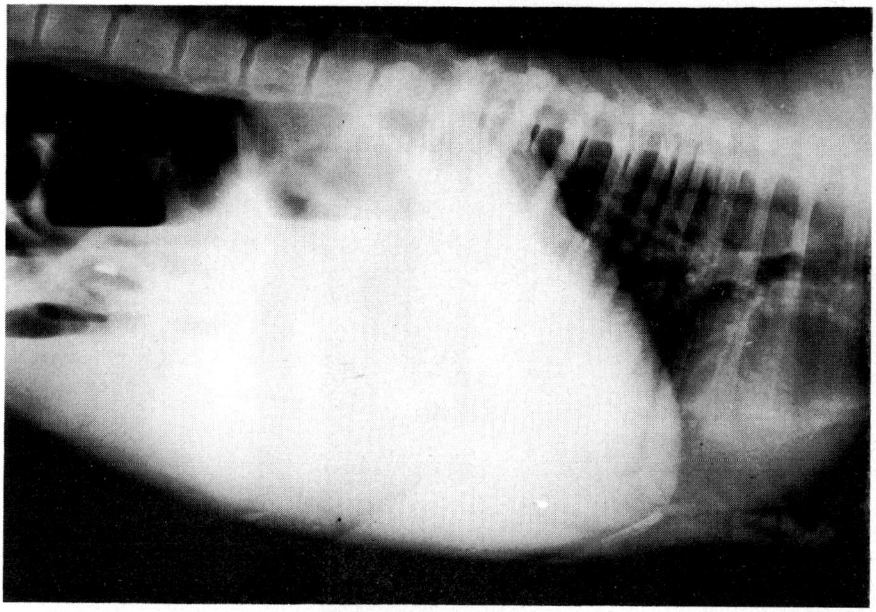

FIG. 11.28. Standing lateral radiograph to show fluid levels in the small bowel.

One of the most important reasons for investigating this portion of the alimentary tract is to determine if normal intestinal movement is occurring, or if there is an obstruction or a paralytic condition of the bowel present. This can be a difficult matter to decide if no obvious foreign body is present. In addition such a case is usually an acute one and there is little time available for (and the patient's condition will not permit) preparation for radiography.

In a plain film the fact that, either food or faecal material, or small accumulations of gas, could be recognised dispersed throughout the small and large bowel would suggest that normal intestinal action was proceeding. Large local accumulations of gas (or occasionally of ingested rubbish) within the small intestine would point to an obstruction (it is important to distinguish between a gas-filled dilated portion of small bowel and gas within "normal" large bowel). The fact that either of these appearances had changed in films taken an hour or so later would provide evidence that bowel movement was occurring—the converse would also be true. If radiography of the abdomen can be undertaken with the beam directed in the horizontal direction, it may be possible to show another feature indicative of bowel stasis. This is the demonstration of fluid levels within the bowel lumen (i.e., gas separates into the dorsal portion and fluid into the ventral portion of the intestinal loops).

If barium is administered and can be shown to pass normally and completely into the large bowel, an obstruction or intestinal stasis can be ruled out (in some circumstances barium may slowly pass lesions which are causing a partial obstruction). In contrast, any consistent arrest of the movement of barium which had commenced to pass normally through the intestines, would point to the presence of an obstructing

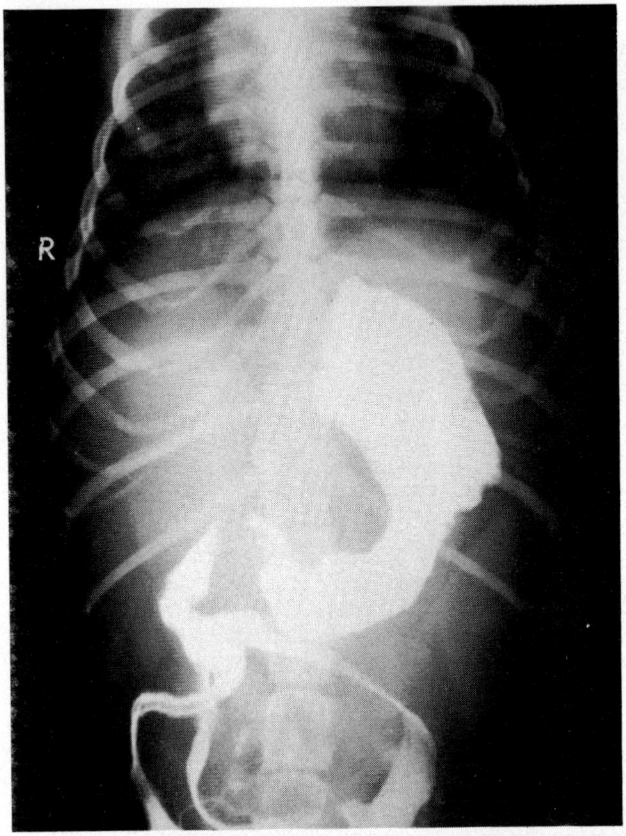

FIG. 11.29.

FIGS. 11.29 and 11.30. Displacement of barium-filled stomach and bowel by a mass in the anterior abdomen (pancreatic tumour and enlarged liver).

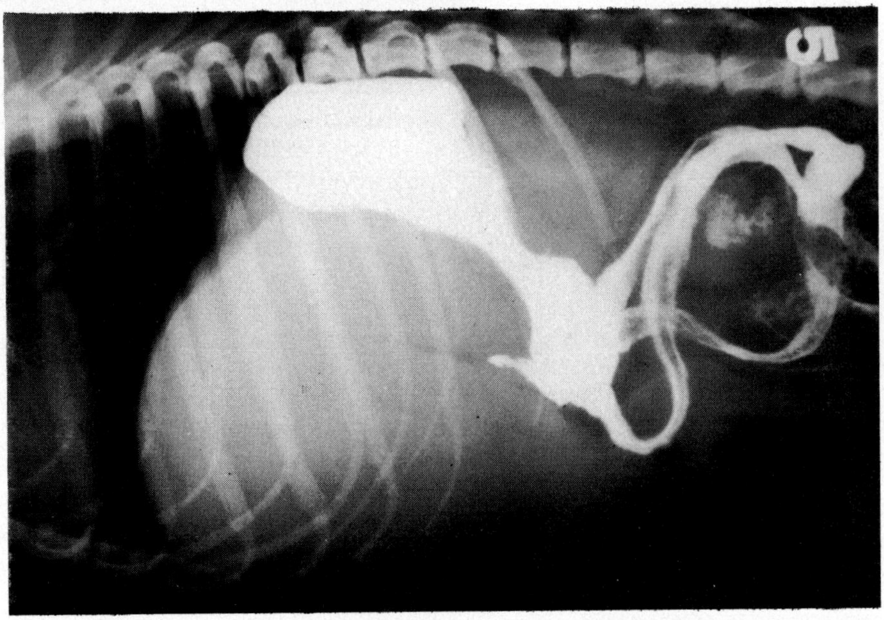

FIG. 11.30.

mass. However the use of barium is not necessarily conclusive as, in the acutely vomiting animal, it may be completely voided before it reaches and demonstrates an obstruction. When an intestinal obstruction is suspected the amount of barium administered should be reduced, so as not to overload the bowel immediately prior or subsequent to surgery.

Radiography can also be of value in showing displacement of the bowel by an intra-abdominal mass or extrusion of the intestines through a diaphragmatic rupture or into a hernial sac. The administration of barium can be helpful in these circumstances if the bowel cannot be definitely identified.

Pathological Conditions

Intestinal Foreign Body

While there is no difficulty in visualising stone and metal objects within the bowel, some foreign bodies of less radio-density (e.g., some rubber articles) can easily be missed unless a very precise radiographic technique is adopted (compression of the abdomen, the use of a grid, careful processing). Some other swallowed objects (e.g., cloth, stockings, etc.) are unlikely to be directly demonstrated in plain films. Where the presence of a foreign body is not obvious its presence may sometimes be inferred from the recognition of dilated gas-filled bowel immediately in front of the obstruction. This feature is likely to become more obvious the longer the object has been present, and the recognition of many gas-filled loops would suggest that the trouble was located a considerable distance along the bowel. The use of barium

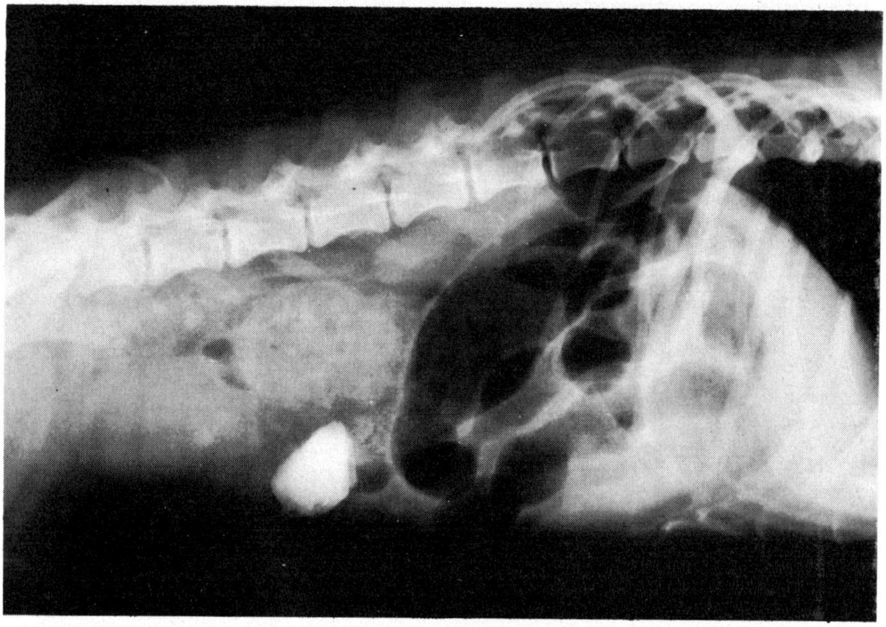

FIG. 11.31. Intestinal obstruction by a stone (note typical gas-filled loops of bowel anterior to the obstruction).

is likely to show obstruction by foreign bodies located in the duodenum but the contrast medium may be vomited before it reaches objects situated further along the intestines.

Should radiography reveal the presence of free gas within the abdominal cavity, it would suggest that perforation of the bowel had occurred as a complicating factor.

If the foreign body is of such a nature (e.g., a piece of tubing or a folded portion of rubber) that it does not cause a complete obstruction it is unlikely that the typical features of retention of gas or barium will be demonstrated, but a distortion and slowing of the column of barium could be expected.

Unless any operative interference follows shortly after radiography, it is important, particularly with the smaller objects, to appreciate that the foreign body may have moved along the alimentary tract. In these circumstances a further radiograph obtained some hours later will occasionally show that the object is likely to be passed naturally and that operation is no longer required.

Intestinal Stricture

This term is used to cover all lesions of the intestinal wall which may result in compression of the bowel lumen. The main causes of this are the presence of neoplasia, or of adhesions and fibrosis following traumatic damage to the bowel wall. It is unlikely that plain radiography will demonstrate lesions of this nature before they become advanced unless the dog has eaten indigestible material which has become impacted anterior to the stricture. While the administration of barium is likely to be

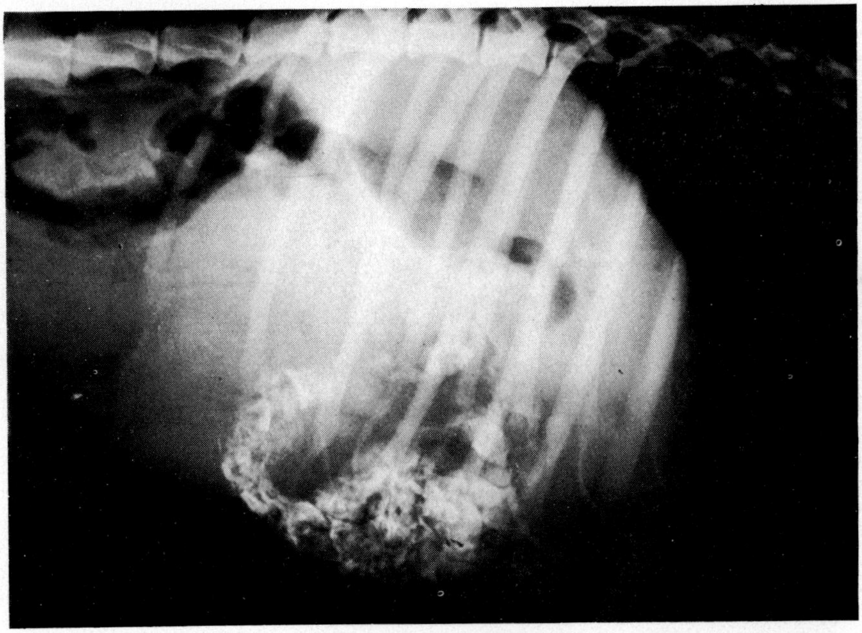

FIG. 11.32. Accumulation of bone and other indigestible material in front of a stricture of the small intestine.

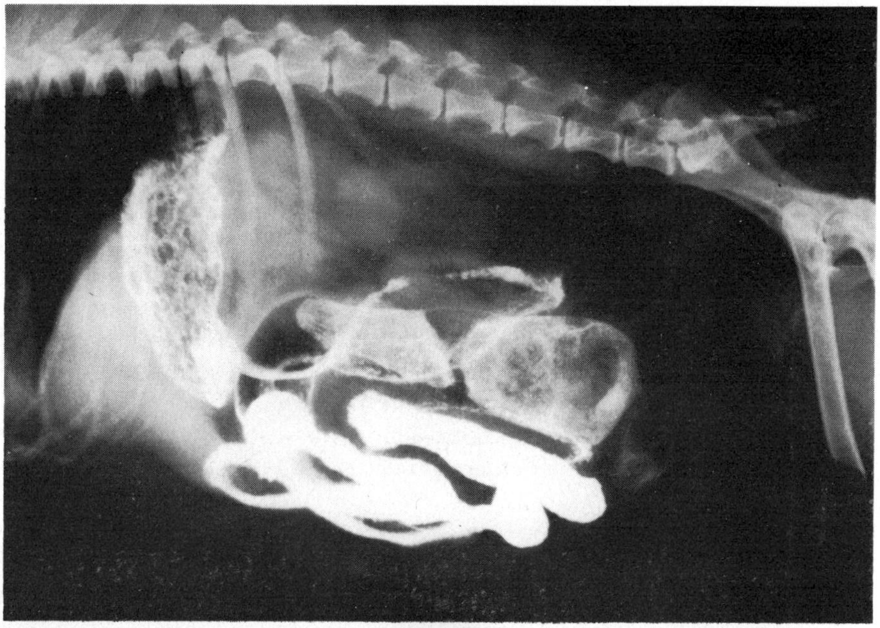

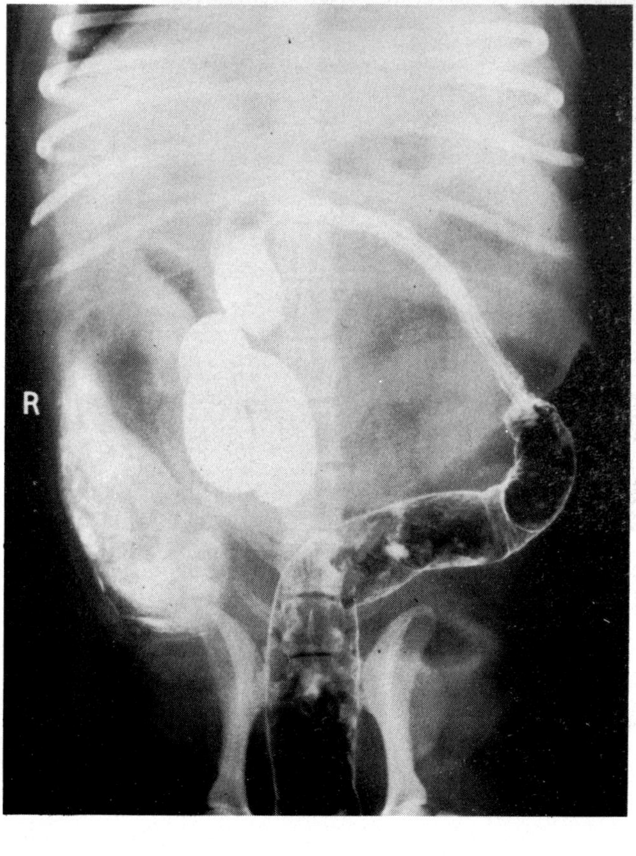

FIG. 11.33. (a) Accumulation of non-radiopaque material in front of a bowel stricture visualised by barium.

FIG. 11.34. (b) It was not clear from the previous radiograph whether the lesion was situated in the small or large bowel. A barium enema showed that it did not involve the large bowel.

of value in visualising such a lesion, it must be borne in mind that any constrictions of the column of barium seen in a single radiograph may be the result of peristaltic contraction. Only a consistent narrowing which can be recognised in a series of films is likely to be of significance.

Intussusception

Owing to lack of contrast it is difficult to demonstrate an intussusception in an abdominal radiograph and definite recognition of such a lesion will only be possible in films showing maximum detail. Under these circumstances it may be possible to appreciate the slightly increased radio-density of the sausage-shaped mass and, more typically, outlining of the layers of the intussusception by very thin layers of gas. When the lesion protrudes into the large bowel it is sometimes possible to visualise its posterior border by means of a barium enema.

When conclusive demonstration of an intussusception is not possible it is likely that at least the general evidence of intestinal obstruction, which has been discussed above, will be seen.

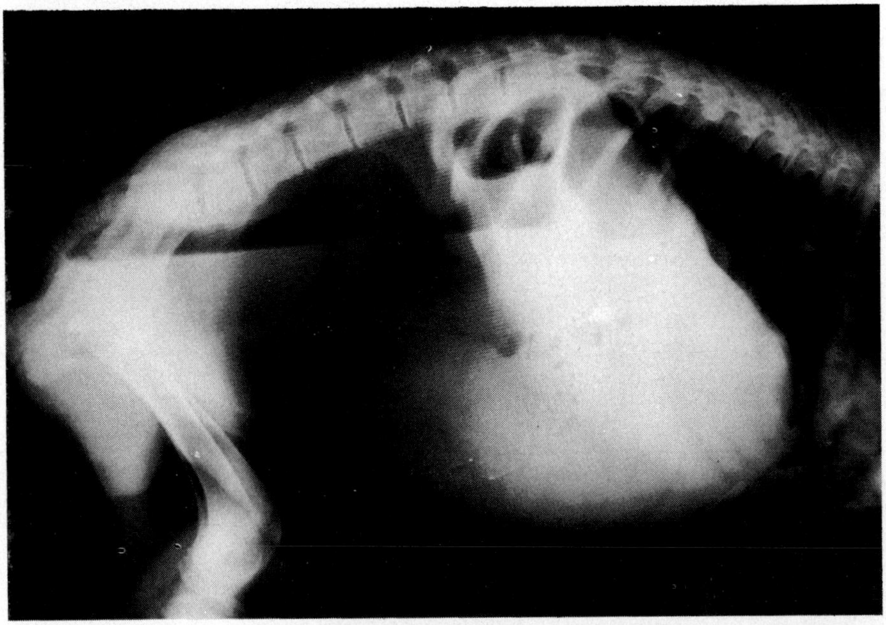

FIG. 11.35. The presence of an intussusception (barely perceptible) has resulted in obstruction of the small bowel and typical fluid levels are demonstrated. Note that the fluid is entirely within the bowel and that operation confirmed that there was no fluid within the abdominal cavity.

Enteritis

This term is used rather vaguely for any inflamed condition of the intestinal tract. The radiological features which would suggest the presence of enteritis are:

(a) An absence of food material within the bowel.

(b) An increased amount of gas dispersed throughout the intestinal tract.
(c) The particularly rapid passage of barium.

Most of these findings are of a comparative nature, and while they are likely to be seen in films of acute enteritis (which would in any case be recognised on clinical grounds), they are seldom conclusive enough to provide much assistance in evaluating cases showing milder inflammation of the bowel.

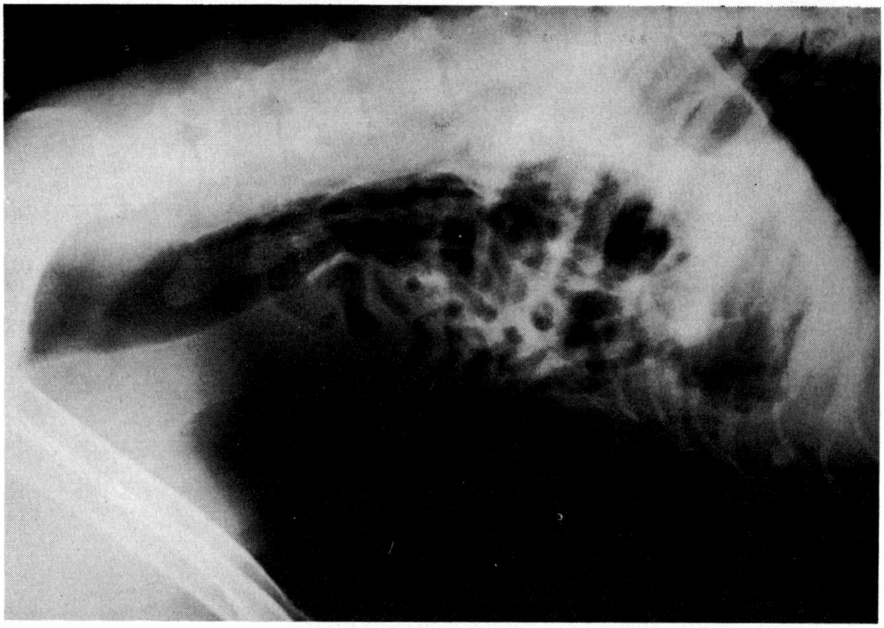

FIG. 11.36. Gas shadows throughout the intestines associated with enteritis.

THE LARGE INTESTINE

Radiography

The large bowel usually contains some faecal material which can assist in its general visualisation. For a more detailed examination of this structure, however, it is important to first wash out all faeces (radiography should not be carried out immediately after administration of an enema as the bowel may still contain additional gas and fluid). Complete emptying of the colon is particularly important if barium is to be used. This is best introduced in a dilute form (10–20 per cent.) as an enema. The introduction of such an enema will distend the bowel and produce a particularly dense outline in a radiograph. For visualisation of fine detail in the colonic and rectal wall most of the barium should be evacuated and gas introduced (usually air) until it slightly distends the tract. This will produce a double contrast effect in which the fine layer of barium dispersed over the mucous membrane of the bowel contrasts with the gas contained in its lumen.

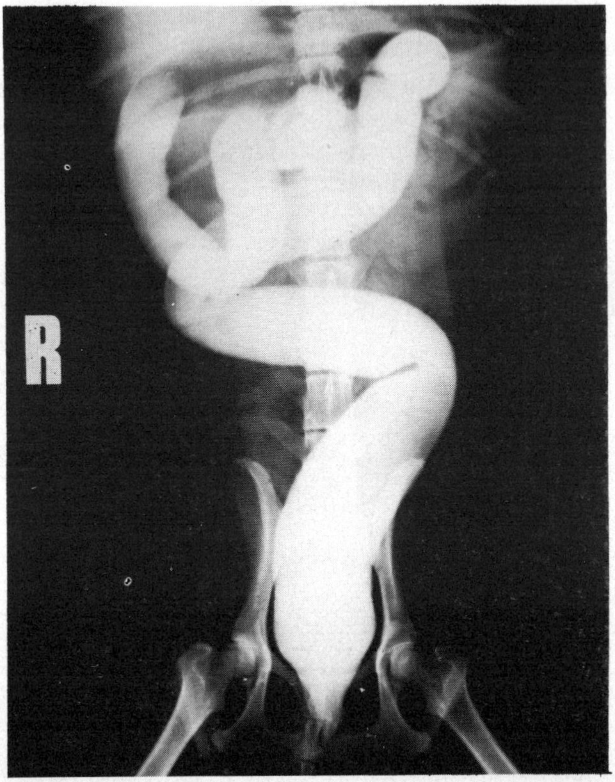

FIG. 11.37.

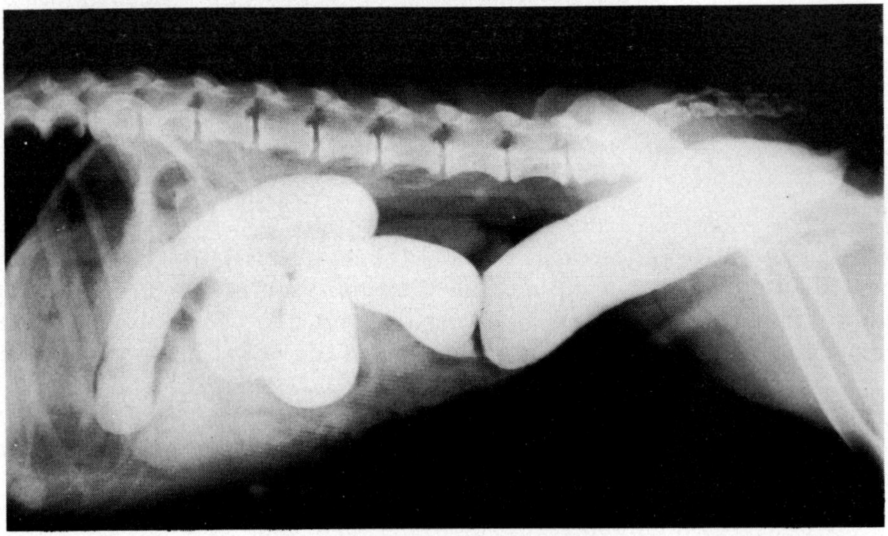

FIG. 11.38.

FIGS. 11.37 and 11.38. Ventro-dorsal and lateral projections of the abdomen to show the position of the normal colon after filling with barium.

Radiology

Usually little difficulty is experienced in identifying the large intestine in an abdominal radiograph because of its wider diameter, its faecal content and its constant position. In ventro-dorsal films this organ shows a hook-like shape to the left of the abdomen which reverses the "hook" formed by the duodenum on the other side. In lateral projections the two loops of the colon tend to overlap and occupy the upper portion of the abdomen. The caecum is also fairly constant in position—being located on the right side of the mid-point of the abdomen in ventro-dorsal radiographs, but it can seldom be identified unless it contains gas or barium.

The clinical indications for radiography of the large bowel are limited but it can be of value in the investigation of the following conditions.

Faecal Retention

While this condition is normally diagnosed on clinical grounds radiography can be of assistance in demonstrating the cause of the retention. Thus films may be

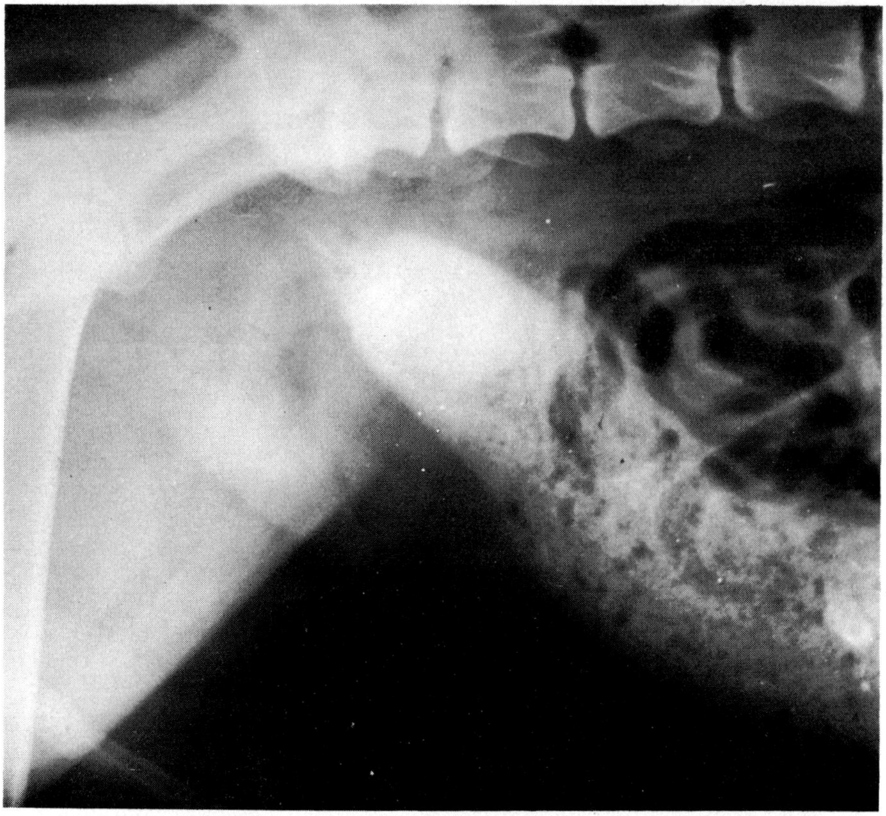

FIG. 11.39. Faecal impaction associated with compression of the terminal colon by an enlarged prostate gland.

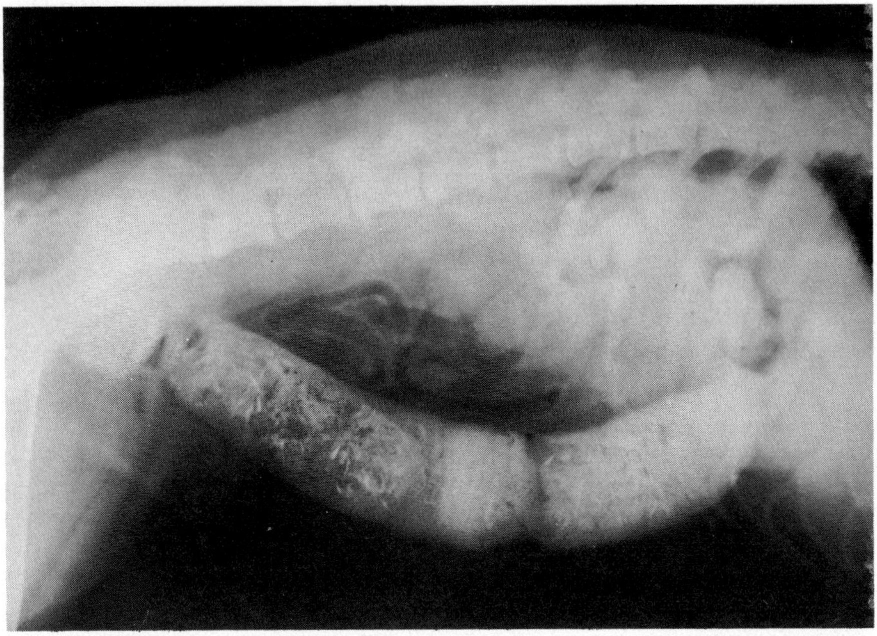

FIG. 11.40. Impaction of the colon with ingested bony material.

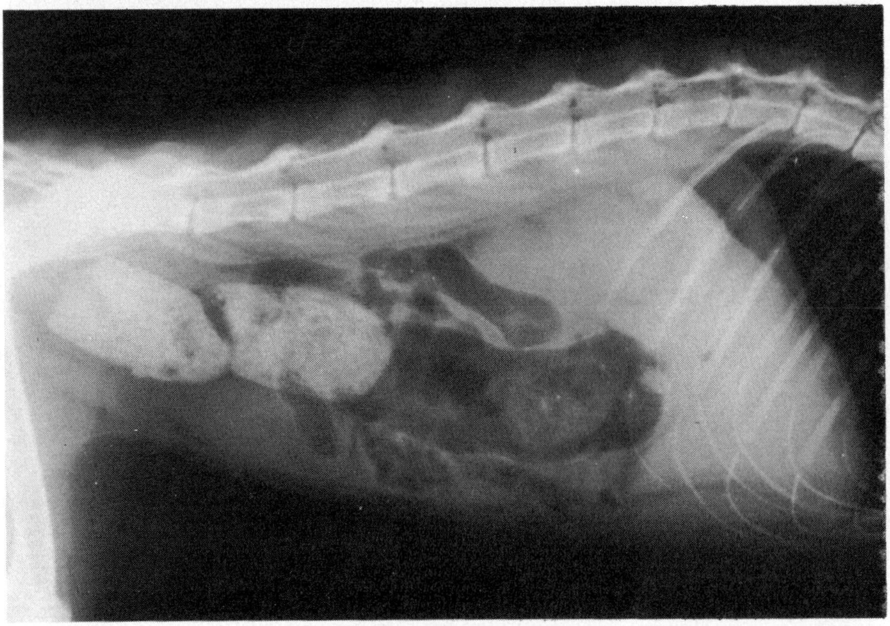

FIG. 11.41. Hairy material impacting the colon of a cat.

FIG. 11.42.

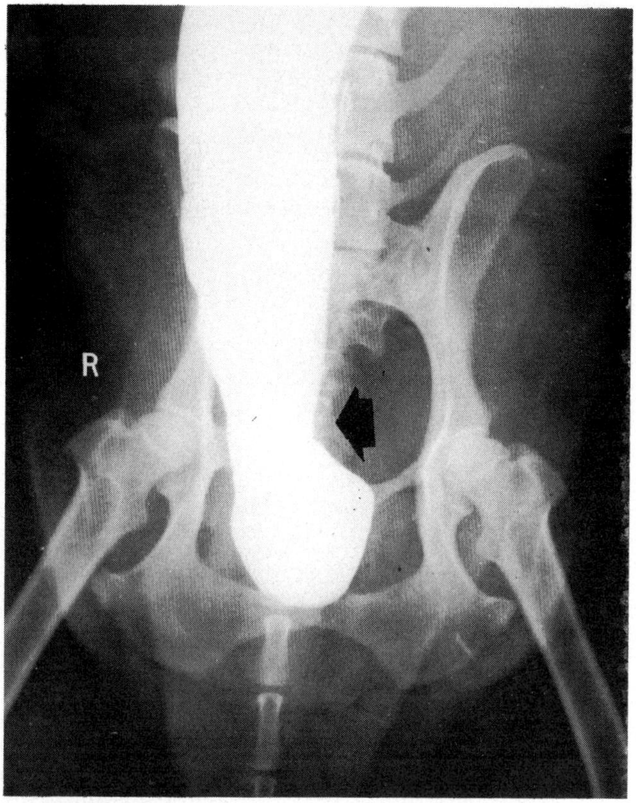

FIGS. 11.42 and 11.43. Compression and deviation of the colon by an intrapelvic neoplasm demonstrated by means of a barium enema.

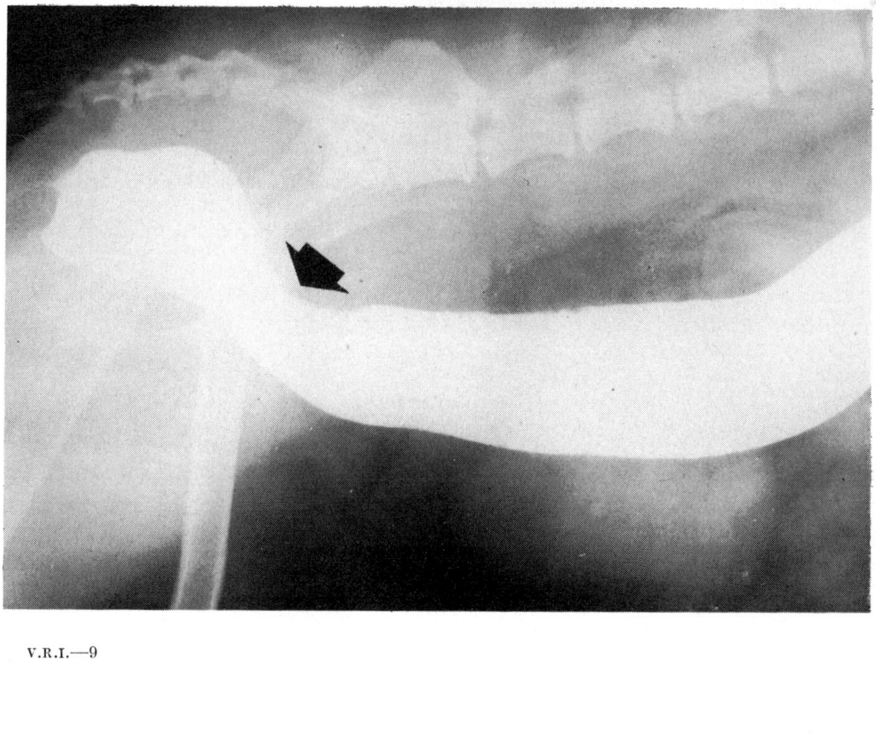

FIG. 11.43.

taken to show the nature of the faecal material (e.g., ingested bony fragments) or to demonstrate constriction of the rectum by prostatic enlargement, pelvic deformity, rectal neoplasm or other cause. When a constricting lesion is suspected it may be necessary to temporarily relieve the constipation and then to introduce barium to more accurately outline the lesion.

It is unfortunate that the terms Megacolon or Hirschsprung's Disease are sometimes applied to the very severe faecal impaction of the large bowel which may be demonstrated in a radiograph. These terms imply a paralysis or atony of the bowel wall which is not necessarily present.

Imperforate Anus

This abnormality is also likely to be diagnosed clinically, but radiography can be employed to demonstrate the thickness of the anal septum and thus the practicability

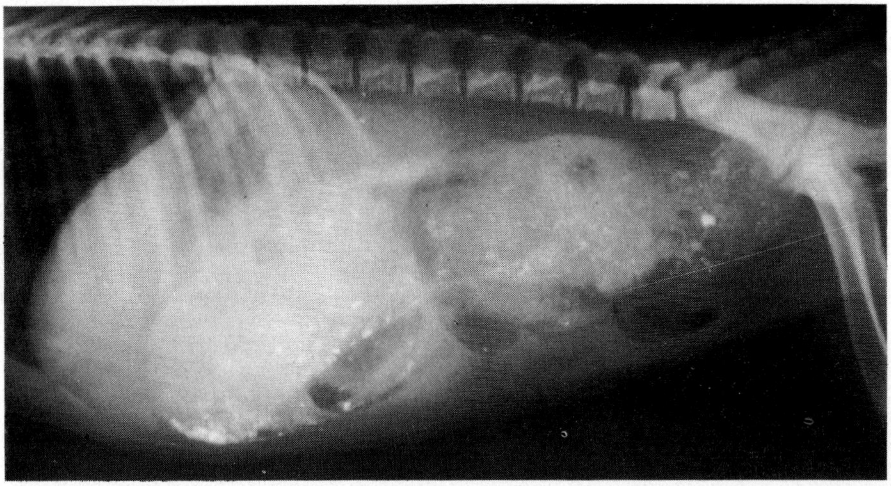

FIG. 11.44. Accumulation of faecal material in an 8 week old puppy with an imperforated anus.

of operation. If a metal probe is placed against the posterior surface of the septum, its anterior limit may be shown radiographically by rectal gas.

Intussusception

The general radiographic investigation of this condition has already been considered in relation to the small intestines. However if the intussusception protrudes into the large bowel it can often be more accurately demonstrated by means of a barium enema. On introducing the barium the significant feature would be the fact that the barium would not extend further anteriorly along the alimentary tract than the level at which the intussusception had occurred (usually at the ileo-colic junction).

On evacuating the contrast agent sufficient barium is likely to adhere to the intussuscepted portion of the lesion to visualise it.

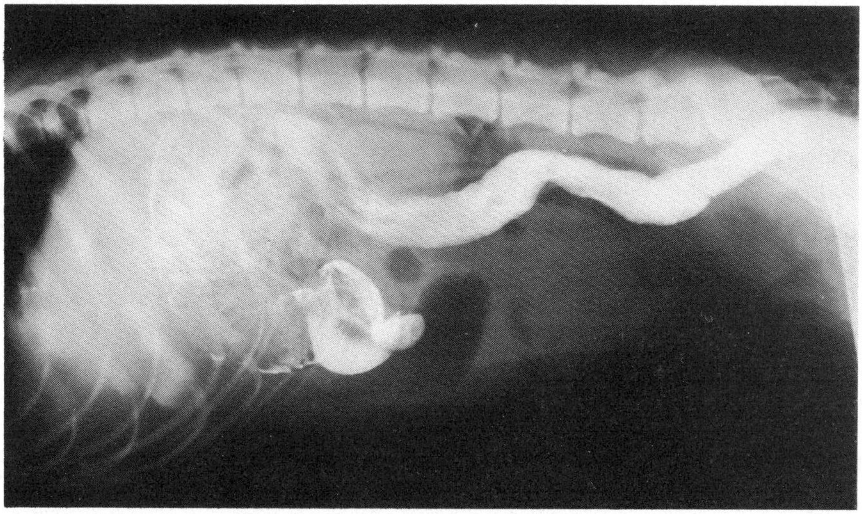

FIG. 11.45. The posterior end of an intussusception outlined by a barium enema.

REFERENCE

Cawley, A. J. and Sorrell, B. (1959), Vet. Med., **54,** 247.

CHAPTER 12

THE URINARY SYSTEM

Radiography

The difficulties listed in Chapter 10 in relation to the radiographic examination of the abdominal cavity, apply equally well to the investigation of this system and similar preparation and technique should be adopted. In particular:

(a) Food, faecal material or gas within the alimentary tract can be superimposed on the kidneys or bladder and prevent clear visualisation. In doubtful cases radiography should be repeated after suitable preparation of the patient.

(b) The use of a pressure band can assist in demonstration of the kidneys, but will often result in considerable distortion of the bladder.

Since the organs which comprise this system are separate and distinct, they will be considered individually:

KIDNEYS

Radiology

These organs are demonstrated most clearly in a lateral film, although in this plane there is likely to be considerable overlap of the two kidneys. While there can be some variation in their precise position, the right kidney is normally situated only a short distance beneath the vertebral column with its anterior end in the region of the eleventh rib. The left kidney is more variable in position and is usually located ventro-posteriorly to this.

It can be of significance to be able to judge if a particular kidney is enlarged or decreased in size. This cannot be estimated precisely and allowance must always be made for the distance of the organ from the film (e.g., the upper kidney may appear larger than the lower) and for normal variation between individuals and between breeds. However, as a very rough guide, the length of a normal canine kidney may be taken as being approximately two and a half times the length of a lumbar vertebra.

While a ventro-dorsal film should overcome the problem of superimposition of the kidneys, there is likely to be a considerable amount of overlying tissue (the lumbar muscles and the liver) and, these organs may not be visualised in this plane.

Failure to demonstrate one or both kidneys in a radiograph may be due to a number of factors and does not necessarily indicate any abnormality of the kidney. In such circumstances, one of the following contrast media techniques may be helpful:

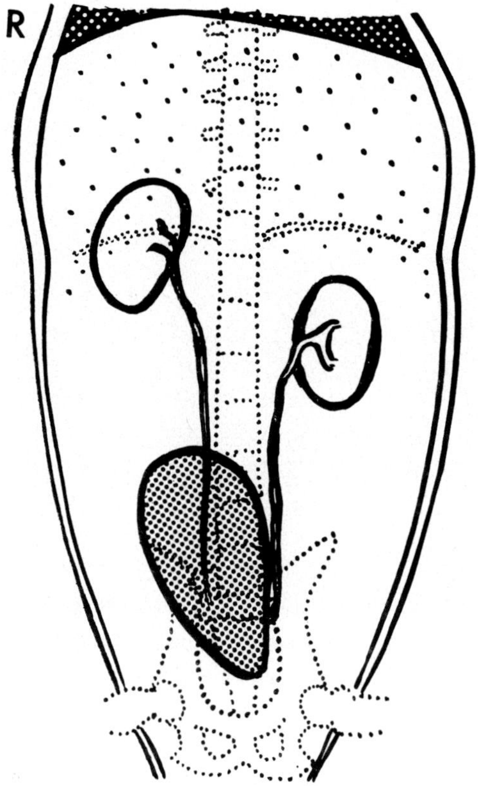

FIG. 12.1.

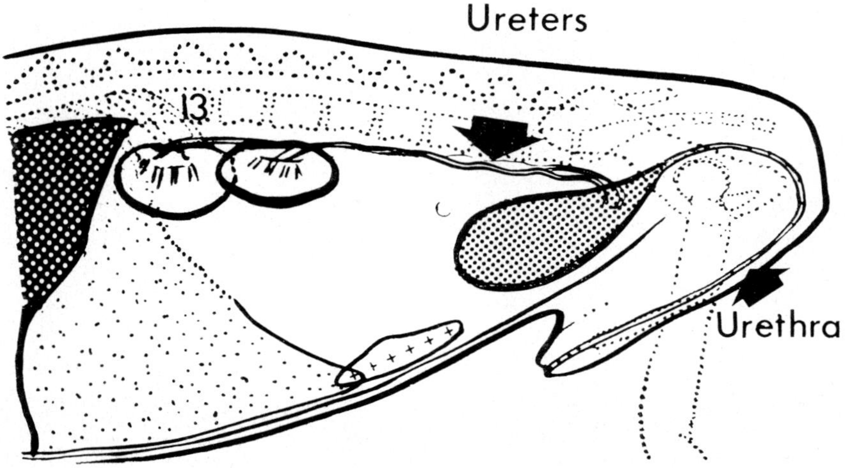

FIG. 12.2.

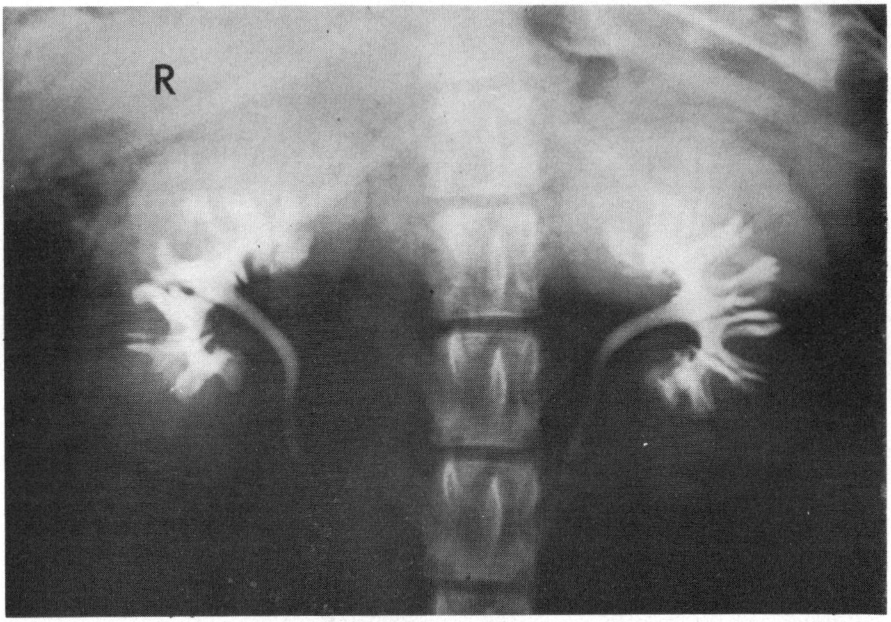

FIG. 12.3. Normal pyelogram of a dog.

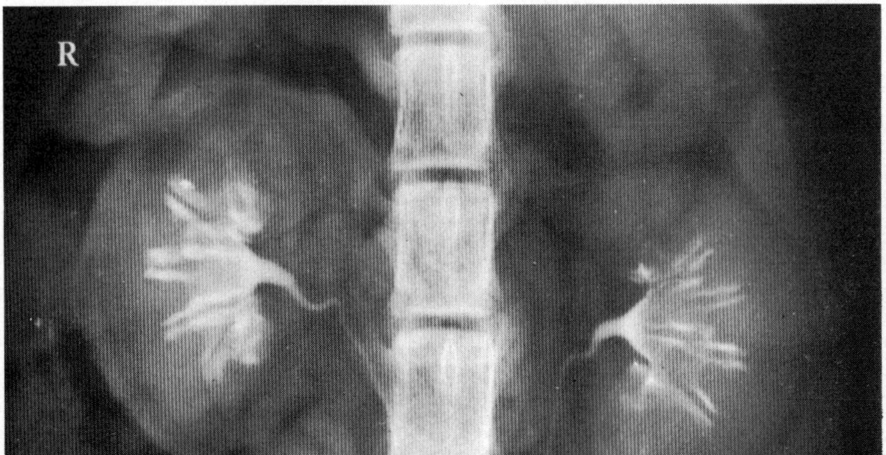

FIG. 12.4. Normal pyelogram of a cat.

(a) Pneumoperitoneum

This technique permits demonstration of the external outline of the kidneys and bladder. The procedure can be carried out on the conscious animal but the animal has to be positioned in such a way that the air rises and surrounds the organs being examined.

(b) Intravenous Pyelography

This method results in some opacification of the kidney substance and more particularly of the kidney pelvices during the excretion of suitable organic iodine preparations. The increased density produced is not always as marked as might be desired and it is advisable to use general anaesthesia: to eliminate movement, to permit the application of pressure on the ureters, and to allow for the longer exposure times required in conjunction with the use of a grid.

The use of pyelography to demonstrate kidney function is of very limited value. The contrast agent is likely to be excreted more slowly if the kidney is damaged, but such malfunction can be assessed more accurately by biochemical means, and the use of this technique in severely uraemic animals would be contra-indicated. Even in the normal animal it has been shown (Dyce, 1957) that the rate and degree of filling of the kidney pelvices can vary between the two kidneys in the same dog. However, the technique can be of value in demonstrating: whether unidentified opacities are kidney calculi, displacement or distortion of a kidney (e.g., due to neoplasia), or, complete cessation of function of one kidney.

Pathology

From the above comments concerning the radiology of the kidney, it will be apparent that only gross abnormalities of this organ can be demonstrated by radiography.

A markedly enlarged smooth outline of both kidneys could suggest acute nephritis, while a small irregular contour would be indicative of chronic interstitial nephritis, but in most instances these conditions can be demonstrated more accurately by other means.

In investigating the nature of intra-abdominal masses visualisation of the kidneys by one of the above contrast methods can confirm that these organs are, or are not, involved.

One or both of the kidneys can be a site of neoplasia (primary or secondary) and in these circumstances pyelography should demonstrate an irregular outline and a distorted pelvis.

Hydronephrosis

This condition comprises a cystic dilatation of the entire kidney usually due to obstruction of the ureter. Radiologically it should be possible to demonstrate a large mass with a smooth outline in the anterior abdomen. Being fluid filled the mass will appear of homogenous density.

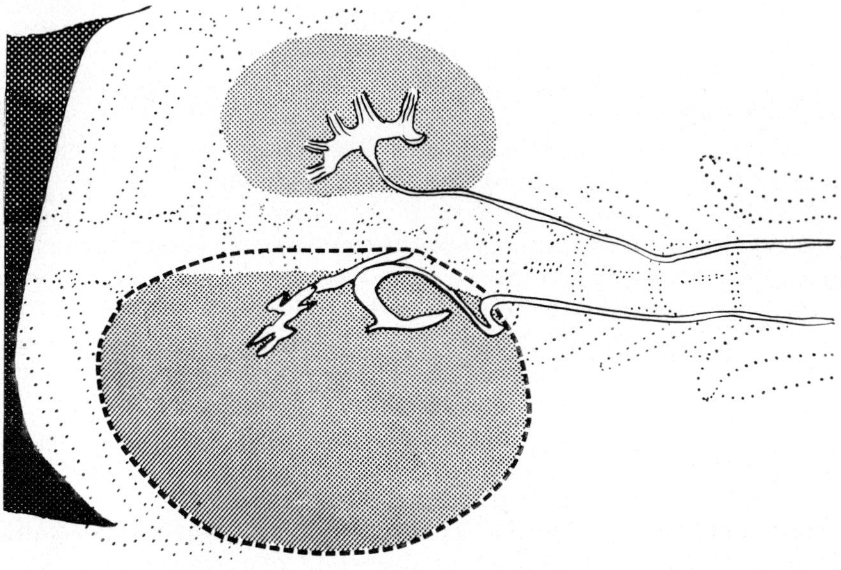

FIG. 12.6.

FIGS. 12.5 and 12.6. Neoplasia (carcinoma) of the right kidney resulting in enlargement of the kidney outline and distortion of the pelvis.

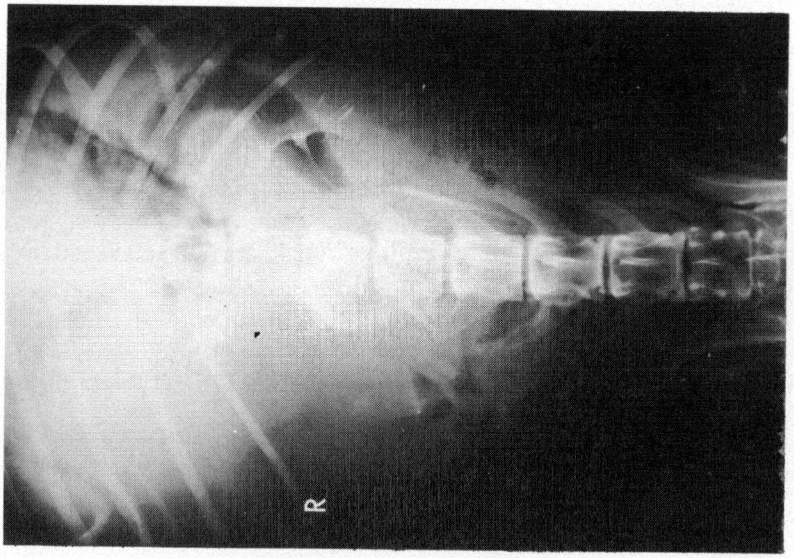

FIG. 12.5.

The radiographic investigation should be completed by employing pyelography. This would confirm the position and function of the second kidney, but the contrast agent would not opacify the cystic kidney.

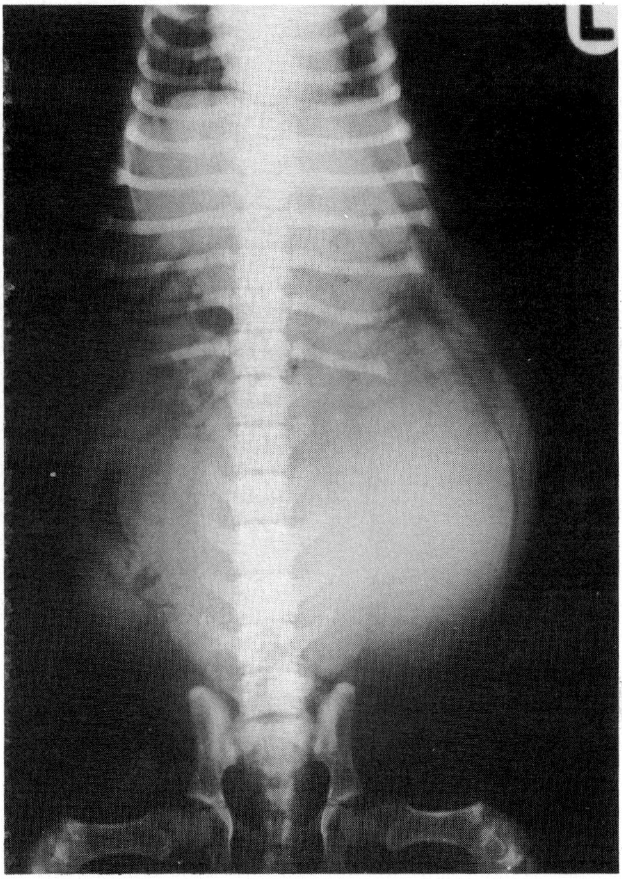

FIG. 12.7. Hydronephrosis of the left kidney in a young Dachshund due to congenital absence of the ureter.

Cystic Kidney

Carlson (1967) has reported that multicystic conditions of the kidney can be demonstrated by intravenous pyelography, as the contrast agent opacifies normal kidney tissue but not the cystic areas.

Kidney Calculi

The size and density of such calculi can vary considerably, but they will normally be recognised in radiographs as small irregular dense areas roughly central to the kidney outline. Particularly large calculi are likely to correspond in shape with the kidney pelvis but small ones may be blurred by respiratory movement and therefore missed or mistaken for material within the bowel. Intravenous pyelography could be of assistance in showing that a particular density is related to a kidney or (with large calculi) to show if the associated kidney is still functioning.

This condition has been misdiagnosed on a number of occasions in the bitch, because of superimposition of the dense shadow of a mammary gland. In such

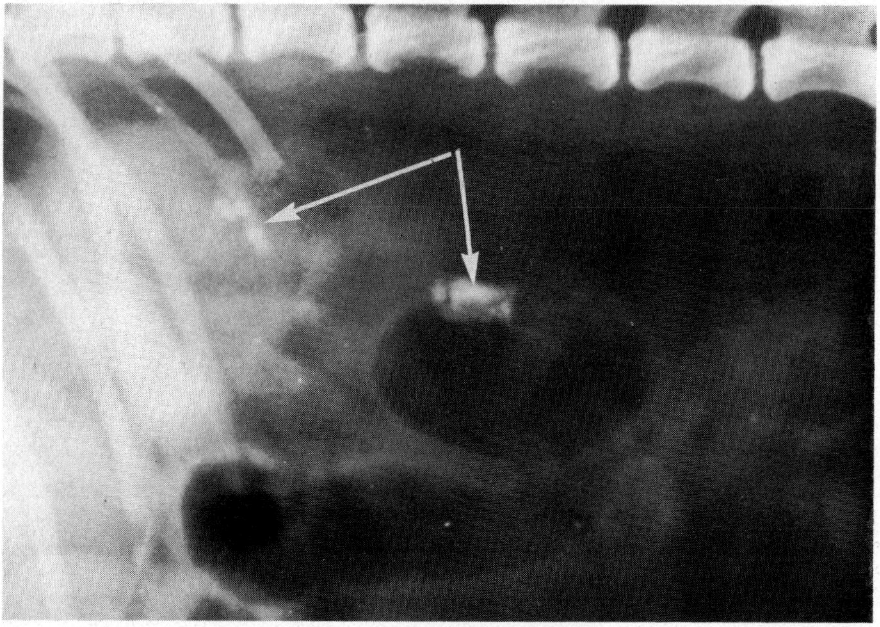

FIG. 12.8. Kidney calculi.

circumstances a careful examination of the radiograph will show a series of similar densities corresponding with the other glands, and a detailed search should be made for these, whenever the condition is suspected in a bitch.

URETERS

Radiology

The ureters cannot be identified in a normal abdominal radiograph.

Contrast media techniques may enable these structures to be recognised but cannot be relied on for this purpose. Pneumoperitoneum seldom visualises this portion of the urinary tract. The anterior ends of the ureters are usually demonstrated during intravenous pyelography and if a further radiograph is taken immediately after release of the abdominal pressure it is probable that the posterior ends will be recognised. If contrast media (air or iodine preparations) are introduced into the bladder under some pressure they sometimes overflow into the ureters and visualise the lumen of these structures.

Pathology

Pathological conditions of these structures are rare but radiography might show cystic dilatations and calculi. The demonstration of an ectopic ureteral orifice by such means has been reported by Olsson (1962).

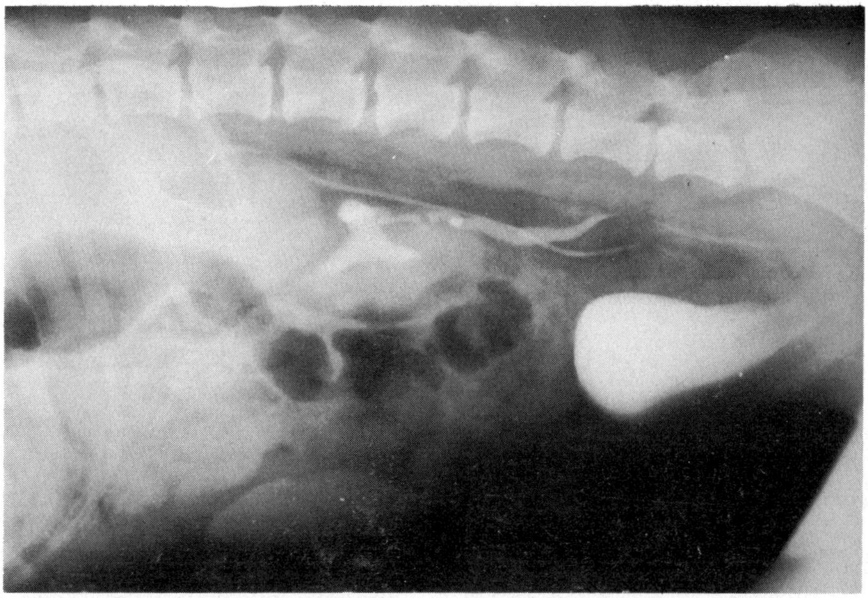

FIG. 12.9. Pyelography performed subsequent to removal of a calculus from the left kidney. The procedure indicated that the kidney was still functioning, but that there was some enlargement of the pelvis and of the ureter.

URINARY BLADDER

Radiology

The empty bladder is seldom perceptible in a radiograph but if it contains an appreciable amount of urine it is easily recognised. This structure has a smooth rounded outline becoming slightly pear shaped as it passes backward to the urethra. This rounded contour is easily flattened or distorted by pressure from adjacent masses (e.g. an impacted colon) or by the use of pressure bands during radiography and variations in the shape of the bladder are not often of significance.

When it is necessary to show the external surface more precisely, pneumoperitoneum can be employed. More frequently however, contrast media are introduced into the bladder in order to identify its position or to show internal abnormalities. These two techniques can be combined for simultaneous demonstration of the internal and external bladder surfaces.

If for any reason it is difficult to catheterise the bladder (e.g., in the cat) suitable contrast agents can be introduced into this organ by intravenous injection and subsequent excretion through the urinary system.

Pathology

Cystic Calculus

The majority of cystic calculi are radiopaque and obvious in a radiograph. But in some circumstances calculi may be less obvious:

(a) If there is only one small calculus in an empty bladder the organ is likely to be contracted and situated within the pelvic canal. In these circumstances a calculus can be missed if the film does not include the pelvic region, or if colonic faeces are superimposed on the area.

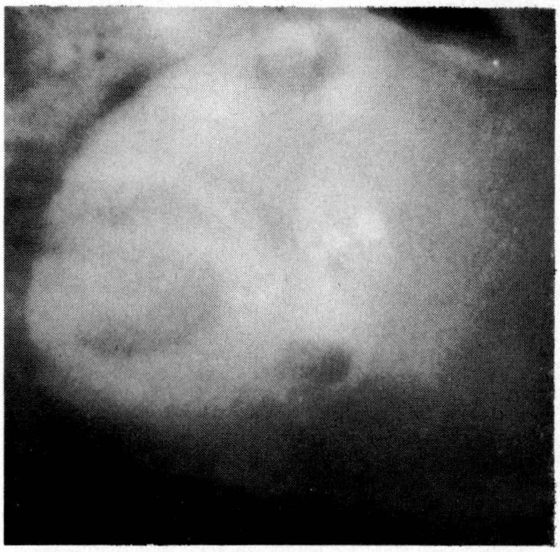

FIG. 12.10.

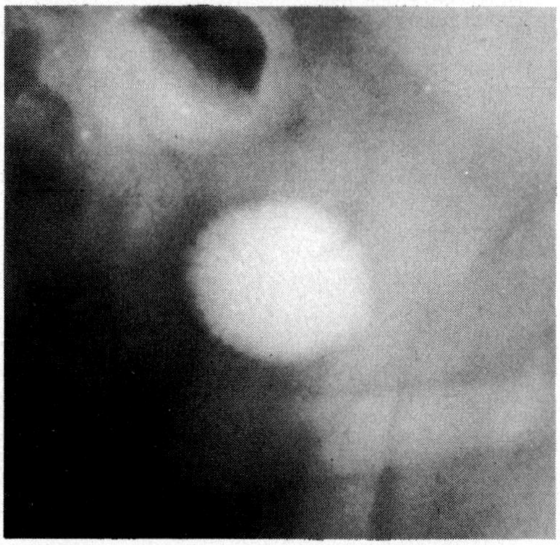

FIG. 12.11.

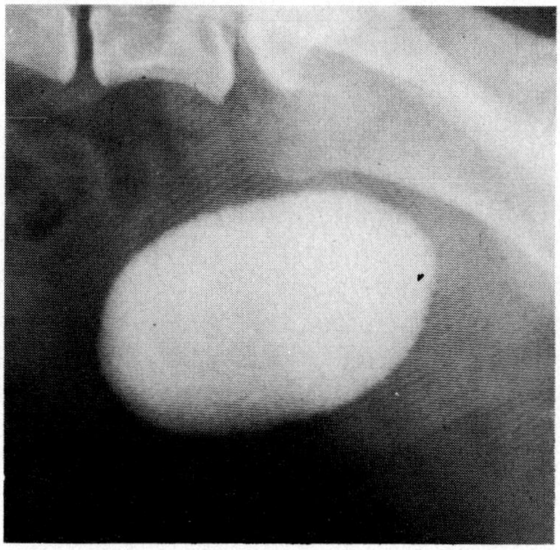

FIG. 12.12.

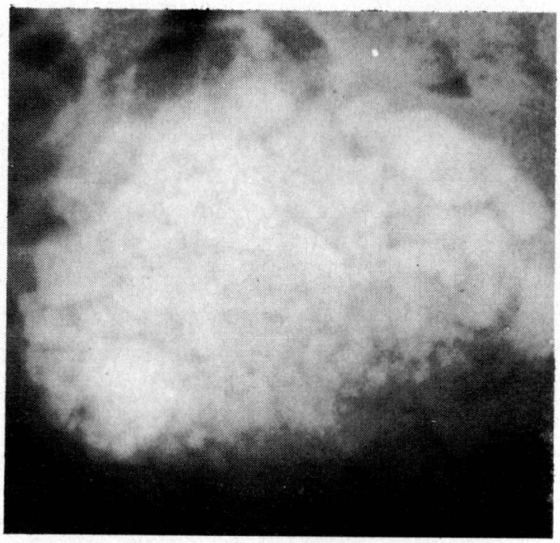

FIG. 12.13.

FIGS. 12.10 to 12.13. Various types of cystic calculi.

(b) When particularly small "gravel-like" calculi are present in a relatively full bladder they can be dispersed and show little contrast with the surrounding urine. They do, however, tend to gravitate and can usually be recognised as an accumulation in the centre of the bladder if lateral recumbent positioning is employed, or on the floor of the bladder if the animal is X-rayed in the standing position. Particularly fine "sandy" calculi will be encountered in the cat, although larger calculi also occur.

(c) It is usually considered that uric acid calculi are only slightly radiopaque and may not be demonstrated.

Pneumocystography might be necessary in any of the above circumstances to permit more accurate demonstration of the calculi (the use of dense contrast agents can mask their presence).

Neoplasia

Neoplasms (both benign and malignant) arising from the bladder wall and extending into the lumen of this organ are not uncommon. They can seldom be recognised without the use of contrast media techniques but in a few instances obvious thickening of the bladder wall or irregular dense masses within the lumen can be shown sufficiently clearly to suggest the probability of tumours being present. Superimposition of bowel or other abdominal contents on the bladder wall can give rise to a false effect or irregularity of the wall and the possibility of this artefact must be born in mind when examining radiographs for lesions in this region.

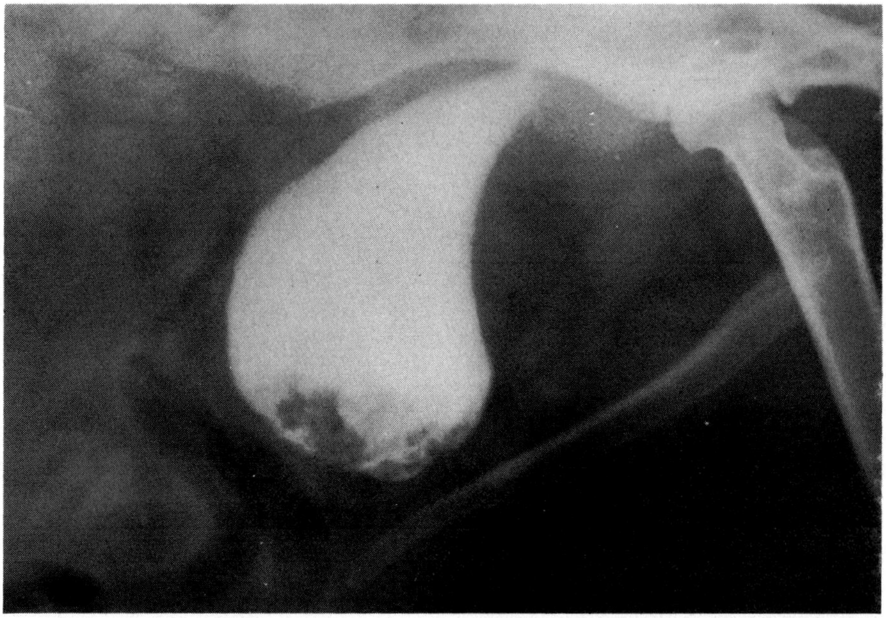

FIG. 12.14. Neoplasia of the anterior wall of the bladder (note indentation of the posterior ventral wall by an enlarged prostate gland).

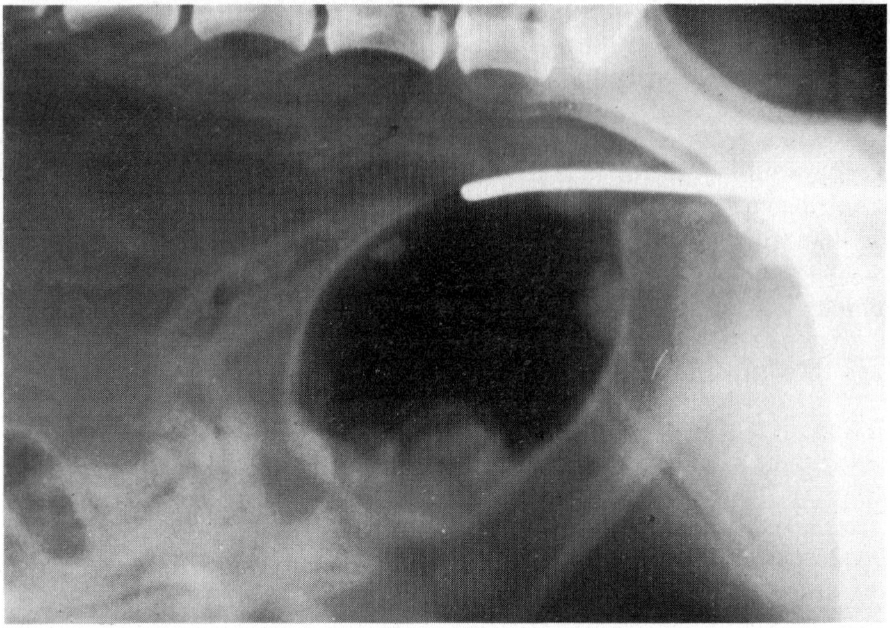

FIG. 12.15. Multiple tumors protruding into the lumen of the bladder.

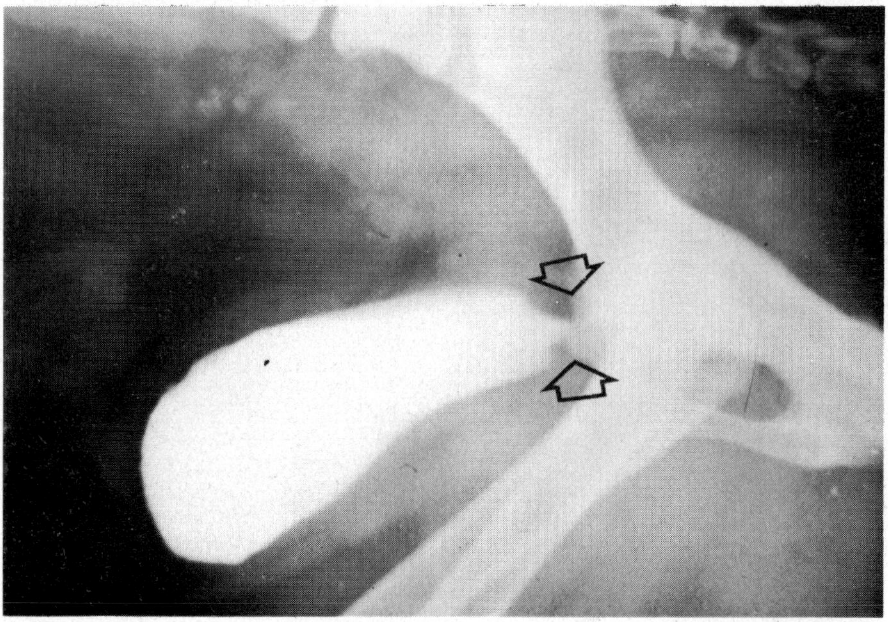

FIG. 12.16. Neoplasia of the neck of the bladder outlined by contrast agent.

Blood clots within the bladder can be mistaken for neoplastic masses and, if haematuria is present, it is particularly important that the bladder should be thoroughly washed out and completely emptied before introducing contrast agents. For the purpose of this examination these agents may be either air or iodine preparations. They should outline the inner wall of the bladder and may permit differentiation between pedunculated papillomata and irregular, more diffuse, malignancies.

While lateral and ventro-dorsal projections will reveal most neoplasms it may be necessary to obtain oblique views to show the full extent of the lesion, particularly if surgery is contemplated.

Ruptured Bladder

Radiography would be of assistance in investigating suspected leakage of urine into the abdominal cavity following traumatic injury or surgery. Such leakage cannot be demonstrated in a plain film, but visualisation of a normal fluid-filled bladder would indicate that it was not occurring.

Catheterisation and the introduction of contrast material directly into the bladder would be the best method of showing any such lesion of the bladder wall. Obviously any such investigation should be undertaken cautiously, to prevent tearing of an already weakened bladder, and to avoid the introduction of irritant or contaminated material into the abdominal cavity.

Filtered air or low dilutions of the aqueous organic iodine preparations would be suitable contrast agents. A small quantity (e.g., 5 ml.) of the agent should be introduced and the catheter left in position during radiography. This should enable the position of the catheter and the contrast material to be identified, but in doubtful cases small additional quantities might need to be injected until retention or leakage from the bladder could be definitely confirmed.

URETHRA

Radiology

The urethra cannot normally be visualised radiographically in a plain film but the os penis will indicate the position of the terminal portion in the male dog. When other portions need to be demonstrated this can be achieved by inserting a radio-paque probe or by radiography during the injection of a contrast agent through a catheter, either with the catheter in situ, or as it is withdrawn.

Pathology

The main reason for radiographing the urethra is the demonstration of urethral calculi. Since individual calculi are only slightly radiopaque it is important that positioning should be so arranged that the X-ray beam will have to traverse the minimum of extraneous tissue. In general, little difficulty should be experienced in demonstrating calculi situated at the lower end of the urethra, but those occurring in the region of the ischeal arch will be less clearly visualised and this area must be

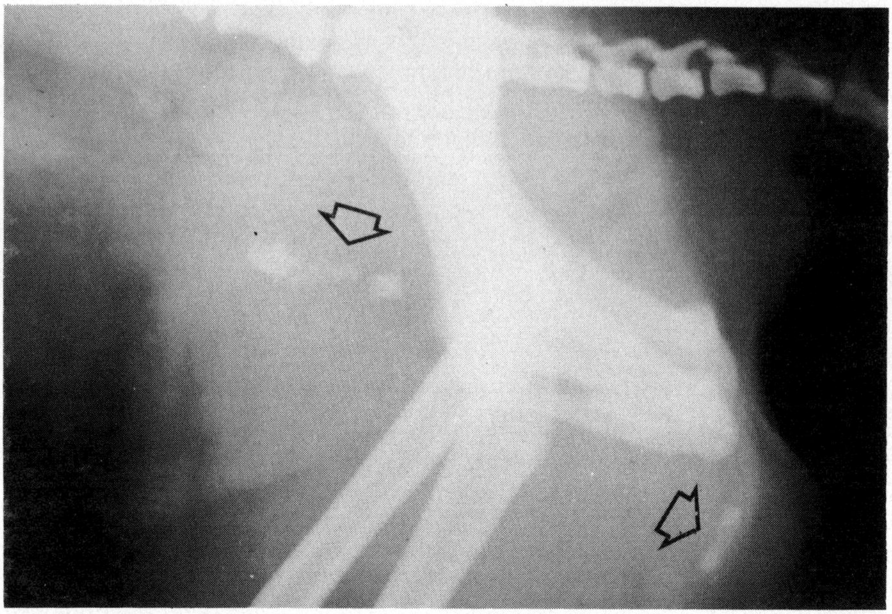

FIG. 12.17. Urethral calculi situated within an enlarged prostate gland and at the ischeal arch.

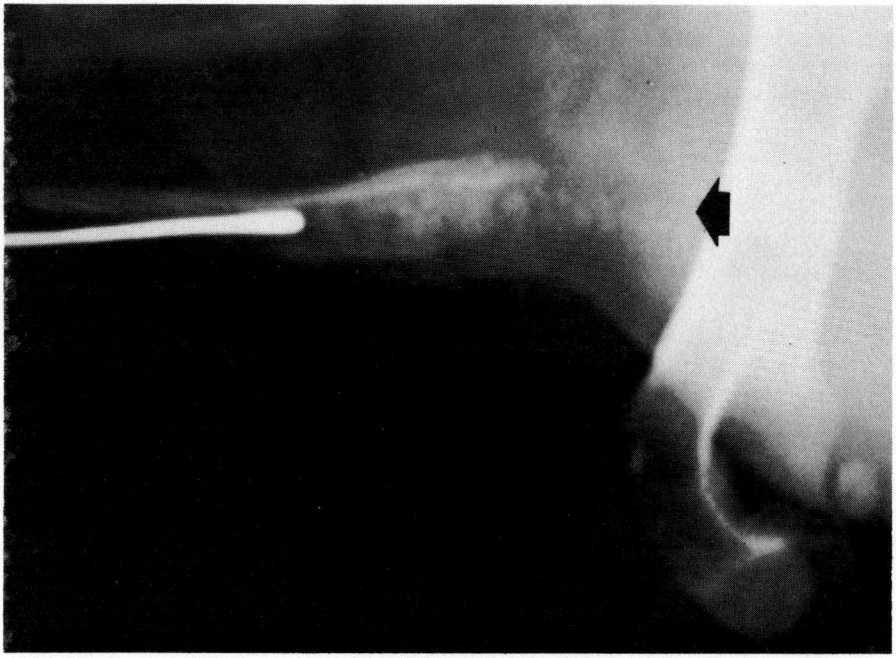

FIG. 12.18. Multiple urethral calculi lodged at the posterior end of the os penis.

very carefully examined. Where indefinite shadows are seen, it may be necessary to show the position of the urethra by one of the methods suggested above, before it can be decided whether such opacities are within the urethra or not.

It should also be noted that if the urethra is positioned over the dog's stifle joint the fabellae at the back of the femur can be mistaken for calculi.

OS PENIS

Because this bone is very thin, it is commonly over-penetrated and can be barely perceptible in a film. The area is usually only examined when looking for calculi but it should not be forgotten that this bone can be a site of fractures.

PROSTATE GLAND

It is doubtful if the prostate gland can be demonstrated radiologically unless it is enlarged, and in the majority of instances considerable enlargement with forward displacement has to occur before it will be recognised.

In some circumstances, however, enlargement of the intra-pelvic prostate gland will cause sufficient compression of the rectum for this to be recognised in a radiograph (aided if necessary by giving a barium enema).

The larger gland which has passed forward into the abdomen is shown on a lateral abdominal radiograph as a relatively dense mass (just anterior and ventral to the pelvic brim) in the position normally occupied by the urinary bladder, which is displaced

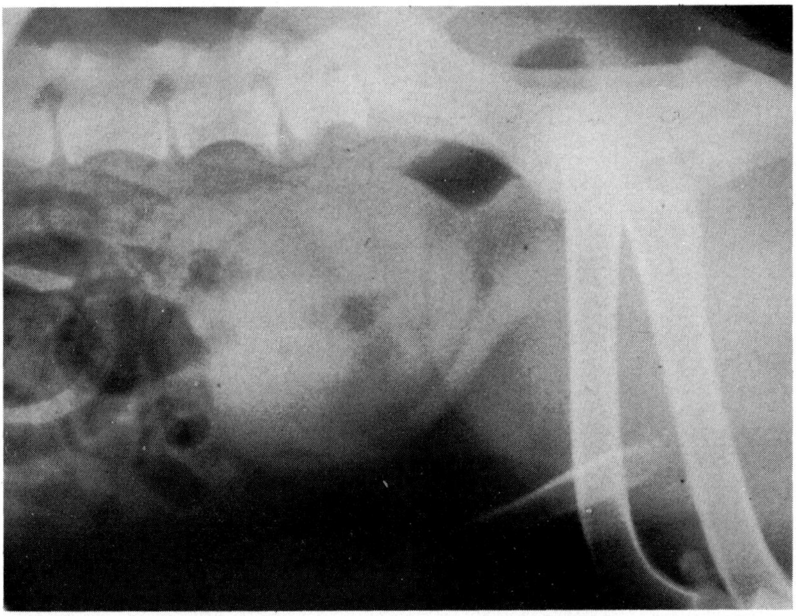

FIG. 12.19. (a) Radiography revealed a circular mass which might be either a full bladder or an enlarged prostate gland.

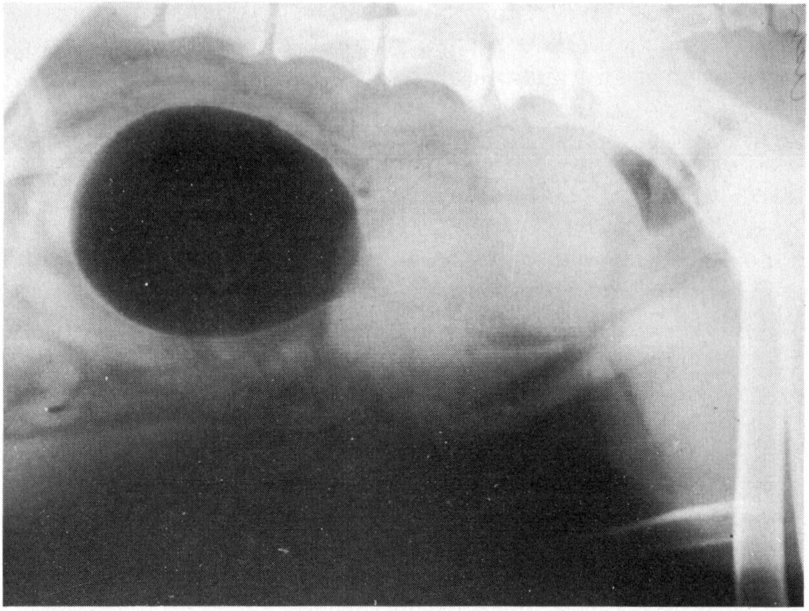

FIG. 12.20. (b) The same area after the introduction of air has outlined the bladder and shown that the mass was the prostate gland.

FIG. 12.21. Displacement of the rectum by an intrapelvic prostate gland.

forward. Where difficulty is experienced in distinguishing these two structures it may be necessary to definitely identify the bladder by the introduction of contrast agent.

It is unlikely that radiography of the prostate gland will permit a more definite diagnosis than the fact that the gland is enlarged and displaced.

The development of radio-opaque prostatic calculi has been reported (Carlson, 1967) but appears to be rare.

REFERENCES

Carlson, W. D. (1967), Veterinary Radiology. Second Edition. London: Bailliere, Tindall and Cassell.
Dyce, K. M. (1957), X-ray Focus, p. 2, Ilford, Essex: Ilford, Limited.
Olsson, S.- E. (1962), J. small Anim. Pract., **3**, 75.

CHAPTER 13

THE GENITAL SYSTEM

This chapter is concerned exclusively with the female genital system and in particular with the uterus, as those portions of the male genital system which may need to be examined radiologically (prostate gland, urethra and os penis) have been considered in Chapter 12.

Radiography

The general advice given in Chapter 10 concerning the radiography of the abdominal cavity applies equally to the examination of the genital system.

Preparation of the patient by emptying the alimentary tract is probably not necessary when gross lesions are present, but could be of significance when films are to be examined for slight enlargement of the uterus or for the first evidence of pregnancy.

The use of all aids to increased definition is also of importance since the components of this system are not easily distinguished from adjacent structures. In all but the smallest animals it will be necessary to employ a grid and it is usually advisable to use a compression band (obviously any pressure should be applied cautiously when marked distension of the uterus is suspected).

When endeavouring to demonstrate the normal or only slightly enlarged uterus, it can be of assistance to be able to apply local pressure to the appropriate portion of the abdomen. A useful way of doing this is to use an ordinary wooden kitchen spoon. The blade of the spoon is used to compress the posterior portion of the abdomen while the animal is being radiographed in lateral recumbency. This local pressure helps to push the bladder and any other abdominal contents to one side, leaving only the uterus in the particular area. It is helpful if a radiopaque marker is attached to the spoon to indicate the area on the film where the uterus is likely to be visualised.

Contrast media techniques have not been shown to be of much practical value in the demonstration of clinical conditions of this system, but in particular circumstances their use might be considered. Pneumoperitoneum could possibly be of assistance in visualising the outline of the uterus and ovaries. The more specific techniques involving the introduction of contrast agents through the uterine cervix have been described by various authors (Cobb, 1959; Cobb and Archibald, 1959; Dyce, 1961). At present, however, these methods appear to have little clinical application. The common uterine condition, pyometra, can usually be diagnosed by a combination of clinical examination, plain radiography and laboratory investigation; and the use of hysterography when this condition is present could involve an unnecessary risk.

Contrast media techniques might be of value in visualising non-inflammatory lesions of the uterus (e.g., neoplasia) but these are not commonly encountered.

Radiology

It is seldom that any part of the normal female genital tract can be visualised in a radiograph (unless pregnancy is present), although under ideal conditions the posterior portion of the uterus might be just perceptible.

THE UTERUS

The main clinical reason for radiographing this organ is to visualise uterine enlargement. While marked dilatation of this organ (associated with closed pyometra or the later stages of pregnancy) is fairly easily recognised in a radiograph, the early stages of uterine thickening are less obvious and are difficult to distinguish from bowel shadows. Features which help to differentiate between these structures are:

(a) In lateral abdominal projections the uterus occupies a fairly constant position and other abdominal structures can often be moved to one side by the application of pressure to the area. This will sometimes enable the uterus to be identified at the pelvic inlet where it is situated ventral to the colon and dorsal to the neck of the bladder and extends forward and downward following the curve of the posterior abdominal wall.

(b) Gas shadows will not be seen within the uterus (except when gas-producing organisms are present).

Clinical Conditions

Normal Pregnancy

Radiography is frequently employed to confirm normal pregnancy in animals. While the stringent precautions adopted in human radiography are of less importance in animals, the marked susceptibility of foetal tissues to the harmful effects of irradiation should be borne in mind, and unnecessary repetition of such examinations should be avoided.

In some circumstances it may be possible to recognise the early evidence of uterine enlargement associated with pregnancy. Visualisation of such changes is, however, very variable and depends not only on high radiographic standards but also on uncontrollable factors, particularly the size and condition of the animal. In any case, unless a series of foetal swellings can be recognised, no specific diagnosis beyond "uterine enlargement" can be made, and radiologically the appearance of the uterus at about the fifth week of pregnancy may be indistinguishable from that associated with closed pyometra.

Usually it is only when the foetal bones can be distinguished that pregnancy can be definitely confirmed. Definite recognition of such ossification will not be possible before the forty-second day of foetal development and often not until a few days later. The most characteristic feature is a curved "dotted line" of the vertebral column terminating in a larger denser area representing the skull. The main limb bones and ribs can also be appreciated at the same time or shortly afterwards.

When multiple pregnancy is present calcification and visualisation of the skeletal system does not necessarily take place simultaneously in all the foeti. There can be a delay of several days before all the foeti can be definitely identified.

The value of radiography in diagnosing pregnancy in the bitch may be summarised as follows:

(a) During the fourth, fifth and sixth weeks it may be possible to demonstrate an increase in size of the uterus, but it is unlikely that pregnancy can be distinguished from other causes of uterine enlargement.
(b) During the seventh week ossification of the foetal bones first becomes apparent but early recognition of this will depend on good radiographic technique.
(c) During the eighth and ninth weeks foeti will be easily visualised and no difficulty should be experienced in determining the presence or absence of pregnancy.

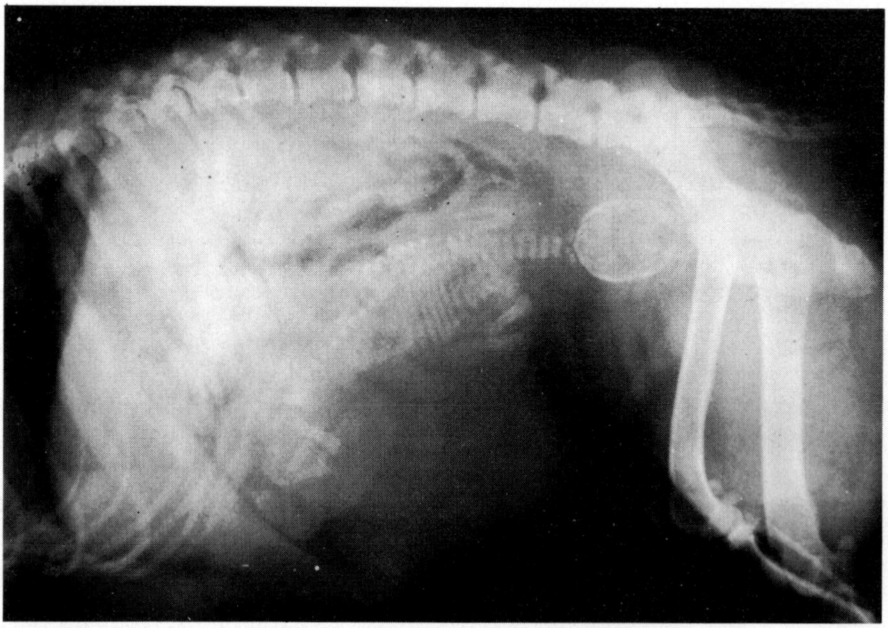

FIG. 13.1. Normal full term foetus.

Since pregnancy can usually be confirmed by palpation in the cat it is seldom necessary to use radiography for this purpose. Foetal bones can be demonstrated at approximately the same stages of pregnancy in this species as in the dog.

Abnormal Pregnancy

In cases of dystocia radiography can be of assistance in showing the presentation of the first foetus and the number of other foeti within the uterus.

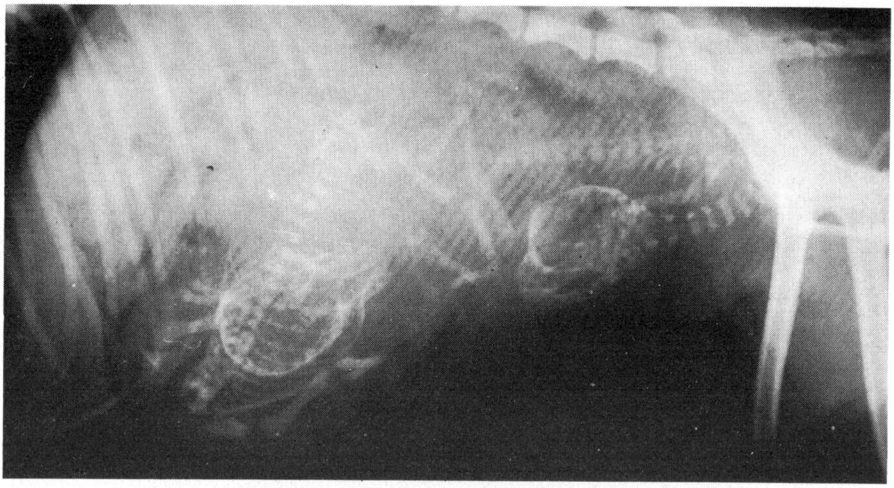

FIG. 13.2. Dystocia—displacement of the head of the presented foetus.

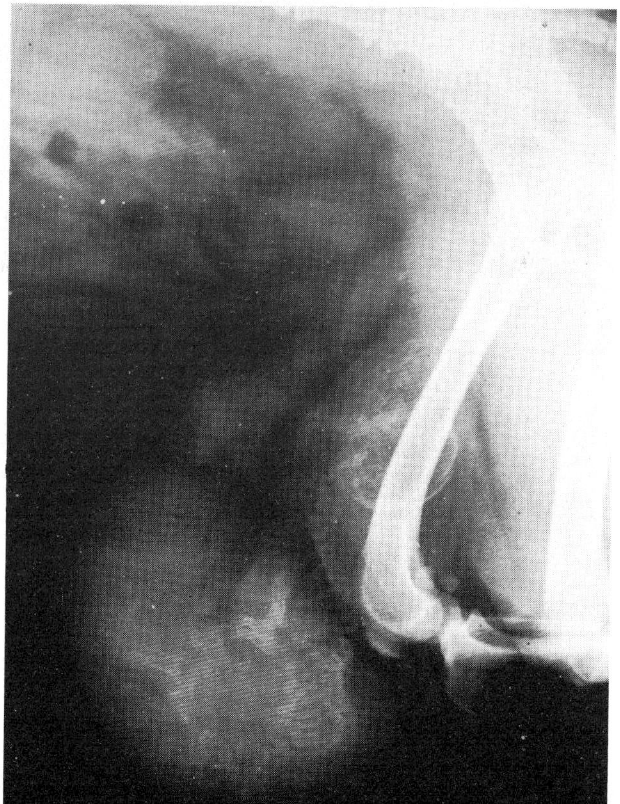

FIG. 13.3. Retention of a foetus within an inguinal hernia.

Radiography may in some circumstances provide evidence that a foetus is dead, but the characteristic features are slow to develop and it is never possible to prove the converse (i.e., that a foetus is still alive) from films alone.

If a retained foetus becomes infected it is likely that gas shadows will be recognised within the uterus.

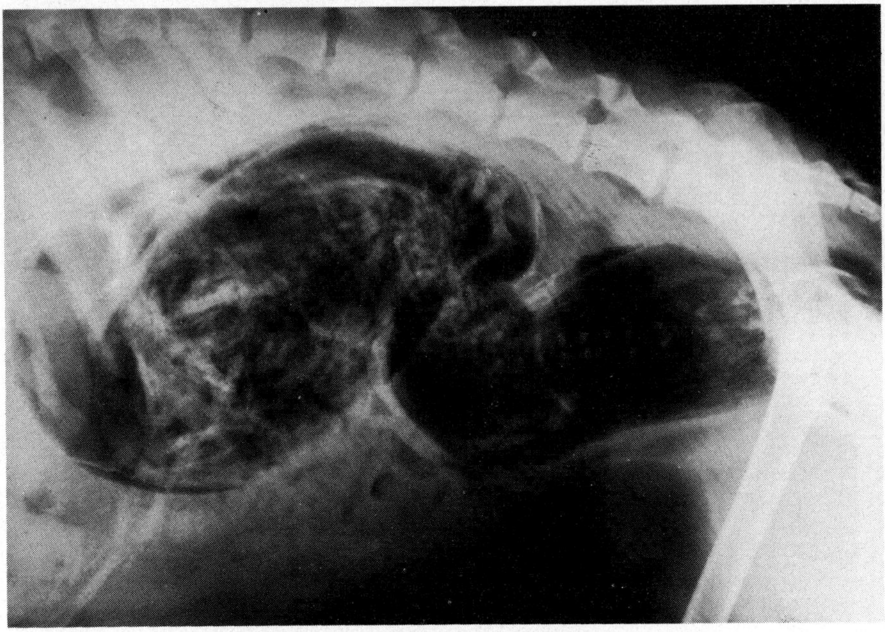

FIG. 13.4. Gross infection of a retained foetus.

In those instances in which the foetus remains sterile no marked changes will be noted for some time. As the fluids are absorbed and the foetus becomes mummified the bones will appear more distinct and somewhat "bunched up" in a radiograph. Very occasionally, overlapping of the cranial bones, which is a characteristic feature of foetal death and collapse, can be demonstrated.

Ectopic Pregnancy

The presence of an ectopic foetus or foeti within the abdomen may be suspected on clinical grounds or may be an incidental finding when radiography is performed for other reasons. The skeleton is usually well ossified and clearly perceptible in a film. A slow process of disorganisation occurs, however, and with the passage of time bony detail may be lost and the foetus appear as a roundish mass of irregularly calcified tissue. The main radiological features which help to differentiate ectopic from intrauterine foeti are:

(a) The foetal outline is round and tightly curled, in contrast to the more moderate curve seen in normal pregnancy.

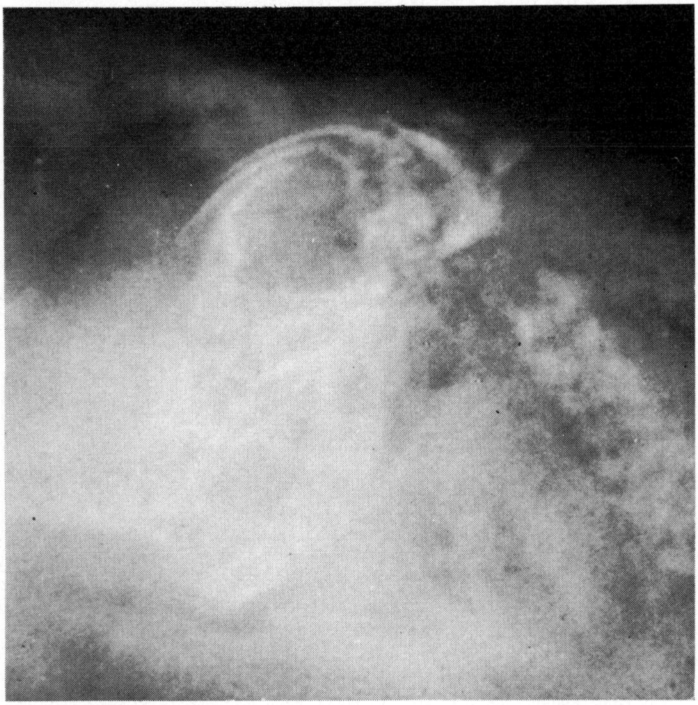

FIG. 13.5.

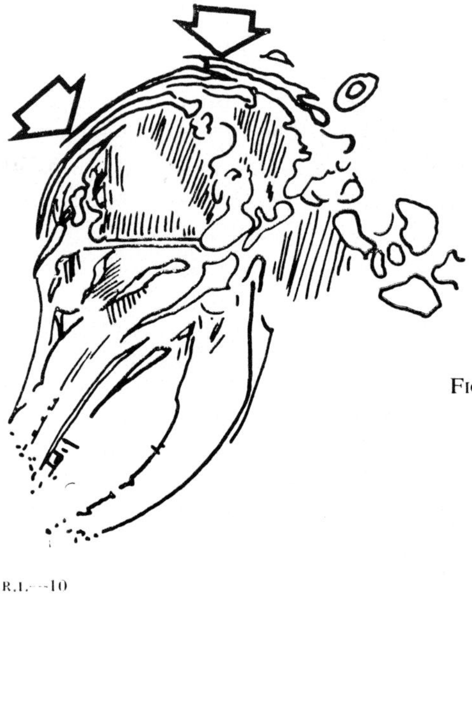

FIG. 13.6.

FIGS. 13.5 and 13.6. Overlapping of the cranial bones associated with intrauterine death of a foetus.

(b) Since there is no fluid present to mask detail, the foetal bones are more obvious and contrast clearly with surrounding tissues.
(c) The foetal units are usually bunched together in the mid-portion of the ventral abdomen and their position may not be related to that of the uterus.
(d) There should be no change in the appearance and development of a foetus if radiography is repeated after 7 to 14 days.

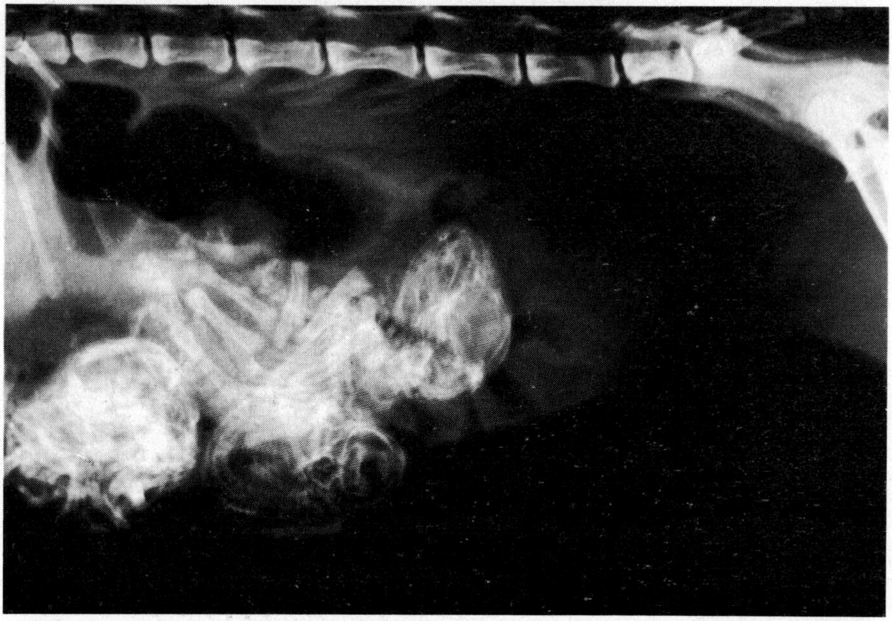

FIG. 13.7. Ectopic pregnancy in a cat—foetal units free in the abdominal cavity.

Metritis and Pyometra

The slight thickening and enlargement of the uterus which occurs in association with milder forms of metritis and open pyometra can be difficult to demonstrate in a film on account of the lack of contrast between the uterus and adjacent loops of bowel. The characteristic position in lateral projections (passing forwards and downwards from the pelvis) and the absence of gas or faecal matter within its lumen may, in some films, enable the uterus to be identified and the enlargement to be appreciated.

It is in the investigation of the closed case of pyometra that the use of radiography is of the greatest value, and in these circumstances the radiological findings are usually more typical. The uterus is seen as a dilated, homogenous, and often saccular structure originating from the pelvic area. The size and extent of the uterus can vary considerably but when particularly large it will be seen to be doubled over and to be displacing the rest of the abdominal contents.

As mentioned above, the middle period of pregnancy (30–40 days) may be indistinguishable from pyometra on radiological evidence alone.

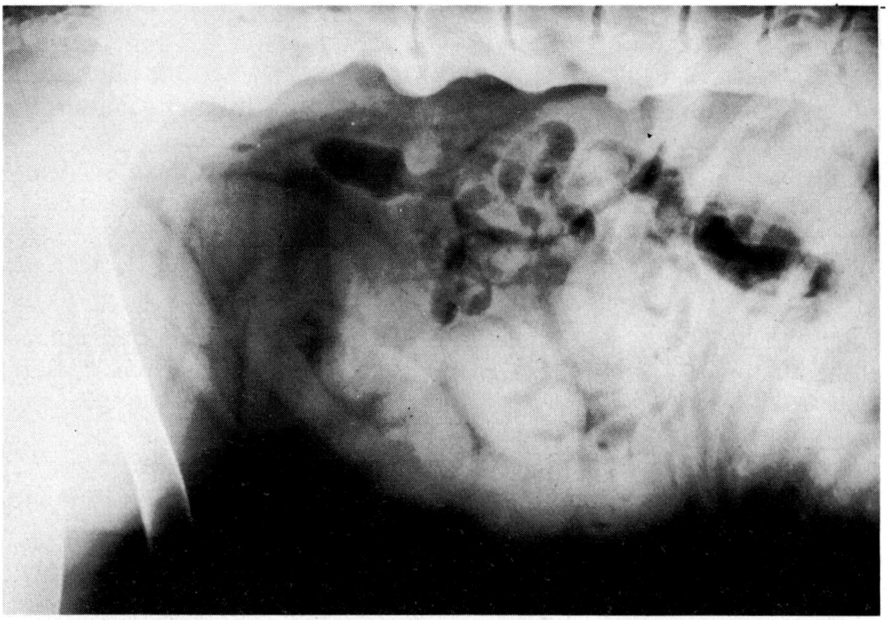

FIG. 13.8. Uterine enlargement in a closed case of pyometra.

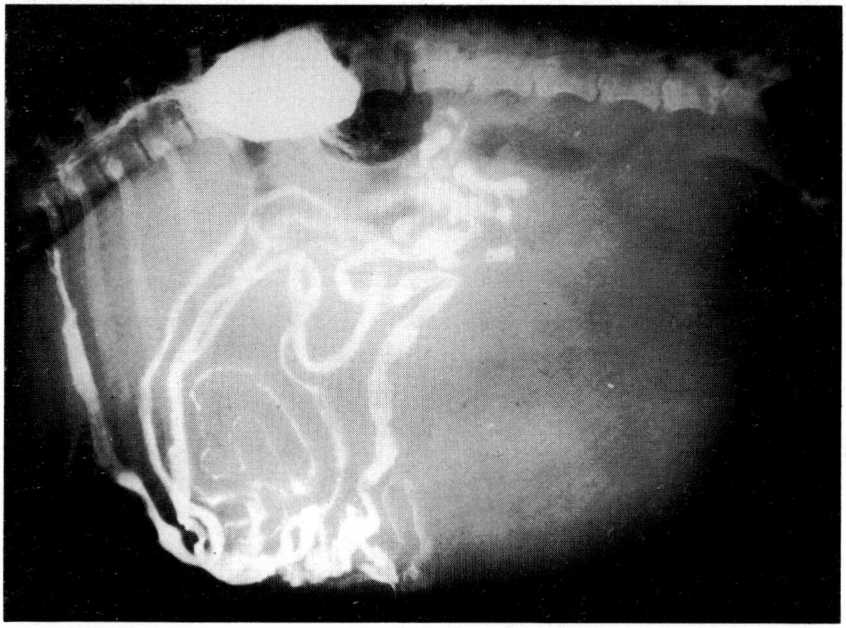

FIG. 13.9. Displacement of the alimentary tract by an unusually large ovarian cyst.

THE OVARY

The normal ovary cannot be identified in a radiograph. If this organ becomes sufficiently enlarged (usually as the result of neoplastic changes) it can be recognised in lateral abdominal films as a dense mass, possibly resulting in some displacement of the alimentary tract.

It is unlikely that this structure can be definitely recognised as an ovary but it should always be considered when attempting to identify unexplained localised structures seen in abdominal radiographs of the bitch.

THE SHEEP

Radiography has been used to a limited extent to confirm pregnancy and to identify the number of foeti in the ewe. From published papers (Benzie, 1951; Ford, Clark and Gallup, 1963) it would appear that there can be considerable variation in the stage at which pregnancy is confirmed.

In this species radiological detail is obscured by the presence of the rumen and by a thick (and often dirty) fleece and there are practical difficulties in obtaining good

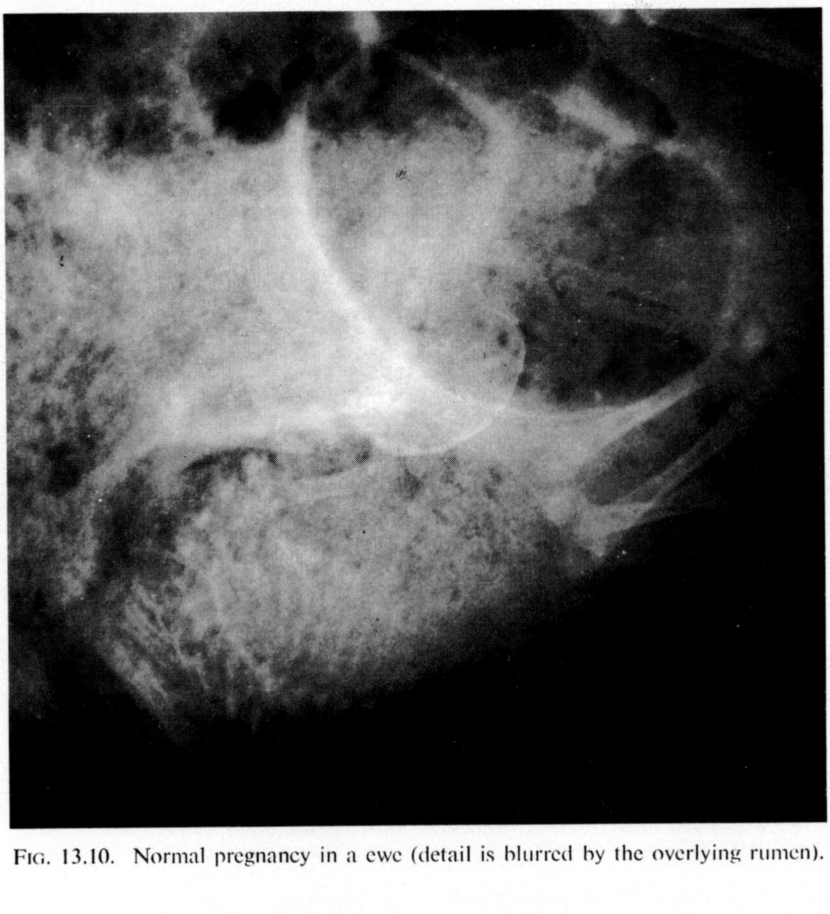

FIG. 13.10. Normal pregnancy in a ewe (detail is blurred by the overlying rumen).

radiographs in the larger breeds of sheep. There is also some evidence that foetal bone becomes radiopaque at an earlier stage in the smaller than in the larger breeds.

In addition, it has been shown that, when twins or triplets are present, there may be a delay of some 10 days after recognition of the first foetus before the others can be identified.

In the paper mentioned above Ford, Clark and Gallup conclude "that the number of lambs *in utero* can be determined by X-ray examination in Clun ewes with an accuracy of 90 per cent. or more provided the animals are examined later than the ninetieth day of gestation, and provided that the radiologist has had some experience in examining this type of X-ray negative. With smaller breeds in which foetal bones seem to become radio-opaque earlier in pregnancy there is a probability of accuracy approaching 100 per cent." From their own limited experience of this species the authors would subscribe to these conclusions and feel that the reference to Clun ewes should probably include the other larger breeds.

REFERENCES

Benzie, D. (1951), Br. vet. J., **107,** 3.
Cobb, L. M. (1959), Vet. Rec., **71,** 66.
Cobb, L. M. and Archibald, J. (1959), J. Am. vet. med. Ass., **134,** 393.
Dyce, K. M. (1961), X-ray Focus, pp. 2, 3, 19, Ilford, Essex: Ilford, Limited.
Ford, E. J. H., Clark, J. W. and Gallup, A. L. (1963), Vet. Rec., **75,** 958.

CHAPTER 14

THE CENTRAL NERVOUS SYSTEM

Since nervous tissue is of low radiopacity, and the central nervous system is always surrounded and very largely obscured by the denser bone, this system cannot be directly visualised in a radiograph. Lesions can only be demonstrated indirectly by (a) noting abnormalities of the adjacent skeletal system, or (b) outlining a portion of nervous tissue by the use of contrast media. Each of these methods can be employed for the radiological investigation of the two principal portions of the central nervous system.

THE BRAIN

The Cranial Cavity

The general shape and outline of the cranial cavity can be appreciated in a skull radiograph and the radiologist should be aware of the marked variation in shape which occurs in different breeds of dog.

In human radiology the demonstration of the detailed structure of the cranium (particularly of the pituitary fossa) is of considerable clinical importance and is achieved by very precise positioning of the tube and the patient, and by the use of tomography. Similar techniques do not appear to have been employed to any extent in animals.

At present, the only lesions of this region that are likely to be demonstrated in animals by radiography are fractures of the skull and gross cases of hydrocephalus.

Cranial Fractures

Fractures involving the cranial bones can be difficult to recognise because there is seldom much displacement and the area involved is likely to be obscured by superimposition of other portions of the skull. Provided that the radiograph shows good definition, it is likely that the fracture site will be shown as a line of radiotranslucency extending across the skull (this must be differentiated from unossified suture lines in the young dog). "Sky-line" projections can be of assistance in demonstrating depression and displacement of portions of bone.

Hydrocephalus

Radiography is likely to be of limited value in diagnosing cases of hydrocephalus and will be conclusive only in the more severely affected animals. The evidence of this condition which might be seen in a radiograph would comprise:

(a) Enlargement and distortion of the cranial cavity. Unfortunately the breeds of dogs considered to be most prone to congenital hydrocephalus (e.g., Chihuahuas) have a cranium which is naturally prominent. Recognition of this feature, particularly in the young puppy, will therefore be difficult unless normal litter mates are available for comparison.
(b) Thinning of the bones comprising the cranium. Again it will be particularly difficult to appreciate this in the young, unless normal animals are available for comparison.
(c) The presence of fluid within the cranial cavity. Since such fluid is of equivalent radiopacity to brain tissue, its presence cannot be appreciated unless contrast media techniques are employed.
(d) Delay in closing of the cranial suture lines or of the fontanelles (unossified areas at the junction of several suture lines). Unfortunately there is considerable variation, even in the normal animal, of the dates at which such closure occurs.

Contrast Media Techniques

There are two main methods by which contrast media are employed to visualise the whole or part of the brain. In one (cerebroangiography), the vascular pattern is temporarily opacified, in the other contrast agents are introduced directly around the brain (encephalography) or into the ventricules (ventriculography). To date, while all of these techniques have been employed in normal experimental animals, very little use has been made of such methods in clinical cases.

Cerebroangiography

The details of this procedure have been described by James and Hoerlein (1960) and by Spooner (1961). Essentially it involves a surgical dissection of the neck to permit the introduction of one of the usual angiographic agents into the internal carotid circulation and the rapid exposure of a series of films to record the vascular pattern produced. In suitable circumstances brain neoplasia may be demonstrated by the fact that the affected area has an increased blood supply or because contrast agent remains in the particular area after it has cleared from the rest of the brain.

This method could have definite clinical applications in the dog, but it requires a careful surgical and radiological technique and considerable experience is necessary to interpret the radiographs.

Encephalography and Ventriculography

Contrast agents which are intended for introduction around the meninges of the brain must be completely non-irritant or they will cause severe reactions and often the death of the patient. For this reason the agents usually employed for these purposes are air, or the oily preparations of iodine. These substances are introduced around the brain or, more particularly, into the ventricles, to demonstrate distortion due to congenital or neoplastic conditions. Two techniques for undertaking these procedures in the dog have been investigated by Cobb (1960) and by Hoerlein and Petty (1961). One method involves the subarachnoid injection of the contrast agent

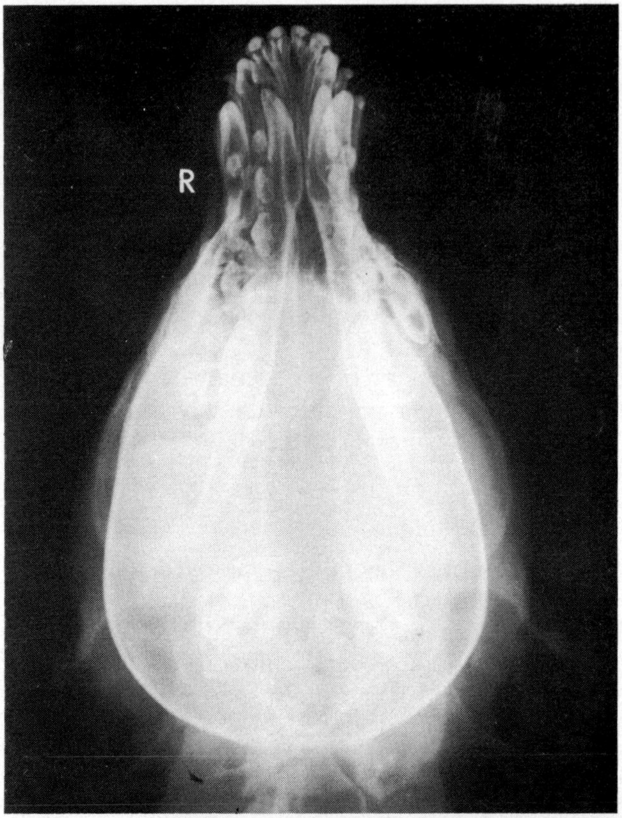

FIG. 14.1.

FIGS. 14.1. and 14.2. Hydrocephalus in a five month old Poodle. Note the enlargement of the cranial cavity and that the fontanelle has not closed.

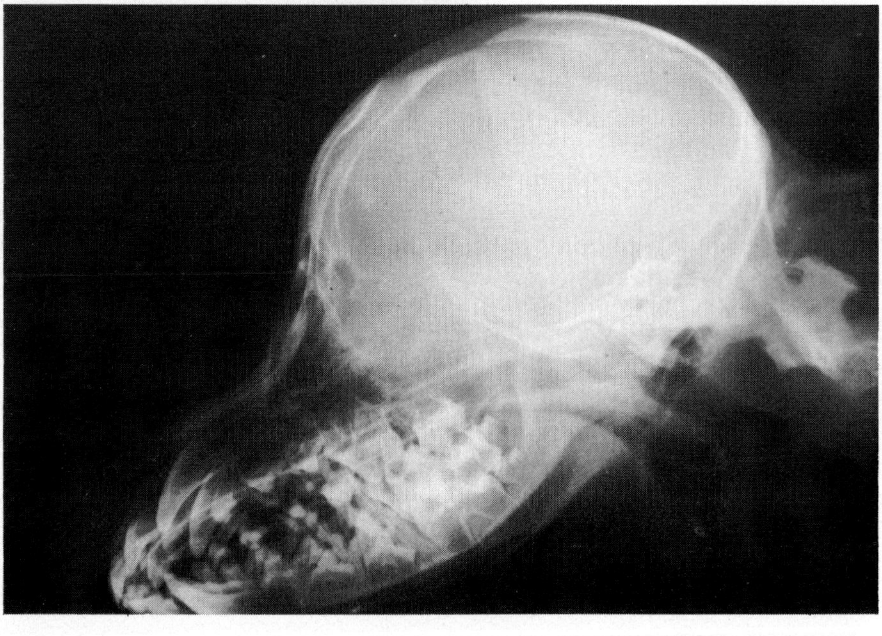

FIG. 14.2.

(usually air) by lumbar or cisternal puncture and its introduction into the cranium and ventricles by positioning and manipulation of the patient. The other method necessitates the direct introduction of a needle into one of the ventricles after drilling a hole through the appropriate portion of the skull. It is reported that the second method is the only reliable way of visualising the ventricles and that air is not a very satisfactory contrast agent for this purpose.

While interesting films showing the value of the intraventricular injection of air in demonstrating hydrocephalus have been published (Carlson, 1967), it would appear that considerable more experience of the use of these techniques is required, both in the normal animal and in the clinical case, before they can be adequately evaluated.

THE SPINAL CORD

The Vertebral Column

The principal abnormalities of the vertebral column which may result in lesions of the spinal cord are either deformities of the bone, or intervertebral disc lesions. The former have been discussed and illustrated in Chapter 5, but must be referred to again here.

Deformities of the Vertebral Column

The majority of the significant traumatic injuries to the vertebral column result in fracture of a vertebral body and the displacement is usually obvious in a radiograph, provided that two projections of the area are obtained. Dislocation of a vertebra may also be demonstrated by evident displacement. In some instances, however, the displacement is minimal and the presence of the injury is shown by complete collapse and narrowing of an intervertebral space or by separation of the articular facets.

Compression and angulation of a vertebra is usually the result of bone disease. This occurs most frequently in association with juvenile osteoporosis but could be a sequel of neoplasia or osteomyelitis. At the same time it must be remembered that in Bulldogs and similar breeds, radiography may reveal compression of the bodies of thoracic vertebrae which is not associated with any clinical symptoms. Thus it must not be assumed that demonstration of lesions of this nature is necessarily the explanation of nervous symptoms shown by the animal.

Another abnormality of the vertebral column which is frequently seen in a radiograph, but which is of doubtful clinical significance, is ankylosing spondylosis. It is sometimes considered that the active development of this condition is associated with mild pain and discomfort, but it is only when radiography shows that the new bone formation extends so far latero-dorsally as to compress the emerging nerves that symptoms of paralysis can be ascribed to this lesion.

Soft Tissue Lesions

Neoplasia

In addition to the bony lesions mentioned above, neoplasia arising from the spinal cord or its associated tissues could occur and result in nervous symptoms.

Such a lesion would not be demonstrable in a plain radiograph, but the occurrence of a lipoma within the thoracic neural canal and its demonstration by the use of contrast media, has been recorded by Funkquist (1961).

Ossifying Pachymeningitis

This chronic inflammatory condition (termed osseus pachymeningitis by Carlson 1967) is probably the only lesion of the spinal cord which can be directly visualised in radiographs. It is associated with the development of bony layers or plaques in the meninges. Because these layers are extremely thin they are not easily demonstrated within the vertebral column. They are only likely to be recognised in lateral films of the spine within the intervertebral foramina, as extremely thin lines of bony tissue at the upper and lower margins of the spinal cord.

Intervertebral Disc Lesions

The investigation of suspected intervertebral disc protrusions is probably the commonest reason for radiographing the spine of the dog but only a percentage of such lesions can be effectively demonstrated in a plain film.

The normal intervertebral disc is, when compared with the adjacent bony structures, completely radiotranslucent. Provided that precise radiography is undertaken, the size and position of such an intervertebral disc is represented by the space between the vertebral bodies. In a number of instances the nucleus pulposus or centre of the disc becomes calcified and demonstrable in a radiograph. Such calcification may occur in a single disc or in a series of discs in the same vertebral column. These changes are not in themselves associated with any symptoms, but the presence of a number of such calcifications usually indicates that the particular dog has a predisposition to intervertebral disc protrusion.

When radiographing a dog for evidence of an intervertebral disc protrusion lateral views of a small area of the spine are essential. Films taken in other projections are

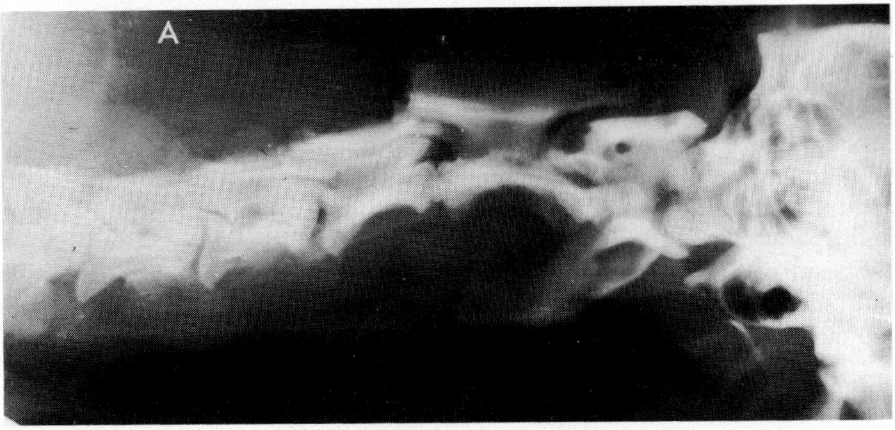

FIG. 14.3. (A) It is not possible to examine the intervertebral spaces in this radiograph of the neck of a conscious dog (muscular spasm associated with pain has resulted in marked narrowing of the spaces).

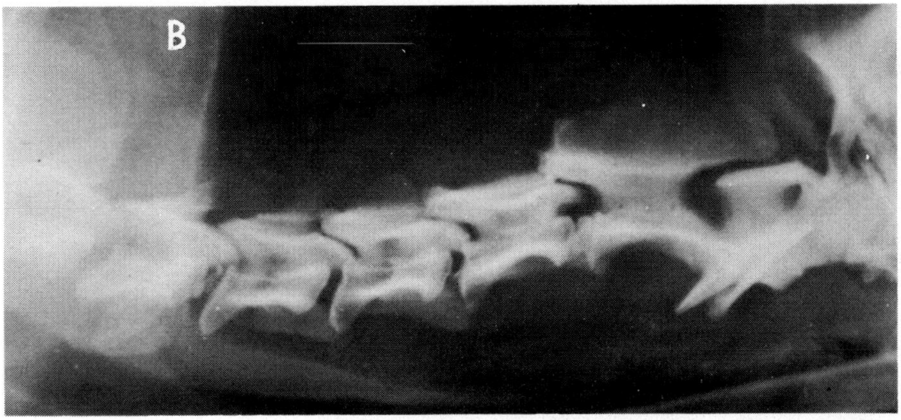

FIG. 14.4. (B) The same dog radiographed after anaesthetisation.

of less value but may occasionally provide additional information. There are really only two radiographic features which, in a plain film, provide evidence of such a protrusion having occurred.

(a) Narrowing of the intervertebral space. In the conscious animal, pain or extreme nervousness can result in muscular contraction and marked compression of these spaces. In these circumstances the size of the discs cannot be accurately assessed unless analgesics, sedation or general anaesthesia are employed.

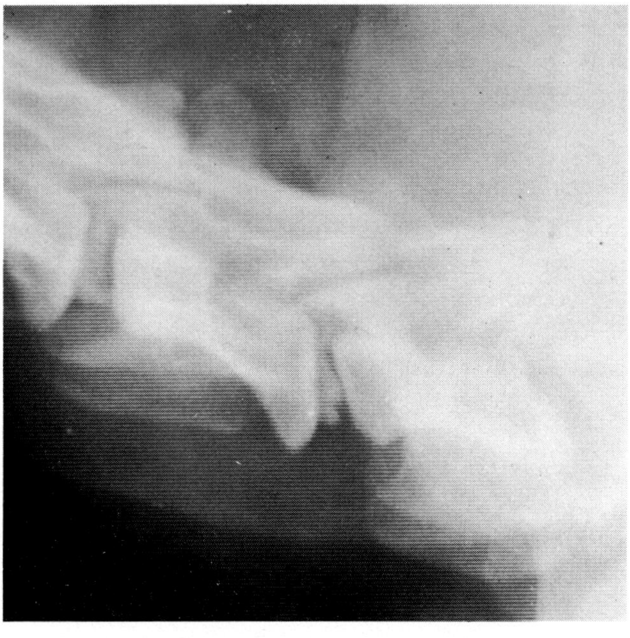

FIG. 14.5. Narrowing of the upper portion of the 4th cervical intervertebral space as a result of an intervertebral disc protrusion.

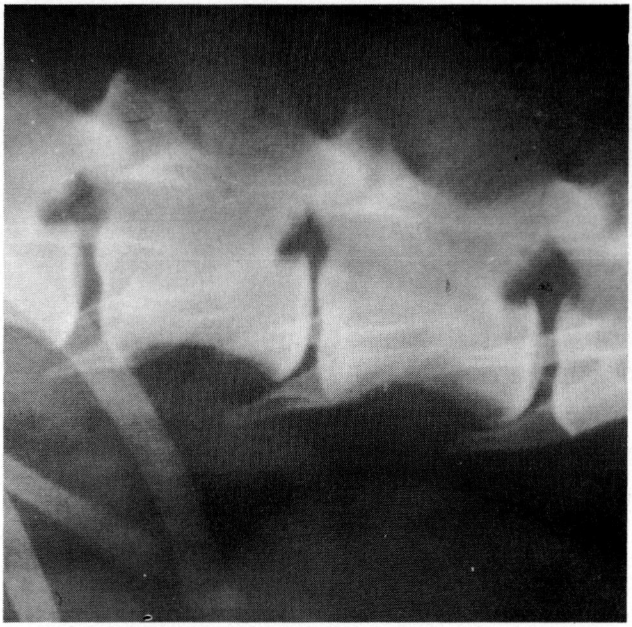

FIG. 14.6. Protrusion of the 2nd lumbar intervertebral disc shown by obvious narrowing of the space.

Similarly, if the X-ray beam which traverses the intervertebral space is an oblique one (i.e., if the space is situated at the edge of the film, or if the spine is not parallel with the film), this will again produce a false effect of narrowing. Therefore, narrowing of an intervertebral space should be considered of radiological significance only if it can be clearly recognised that the spaces on either side are fully visualised and of normal width. In doubtful cases radiography should be repeated to check if the narrowing of the particular disc is a consistent feature of other films. In a few instances this feature may comprise narrowing of the upper end of the intervertebral space and result in angulation rather than uniform narrowing of the space.

(b) Calcification of the displaced disc material. When this feature is present it may be recognised as a small irregular calcified mass situated in the intervertebral foramina just dorsal to the intervertebral disc. In the cervical region such protrusions may be more difficult to appreciate because the transverse processes of these vertebrae lie across and obscure the intervertebral foramina.

In some instances this feature may be less obvious and comprise dorsal displacement of the calcified centre of the disc which impinges on, or slightly protrudes into, the floor of the neural canal.

While demonstration of one or both of these features may be considered diagnostic of an intervertebral disc protrusion, in many cases neither are present and if it is important to show the lesion precisely the use of myelography has to be considered.

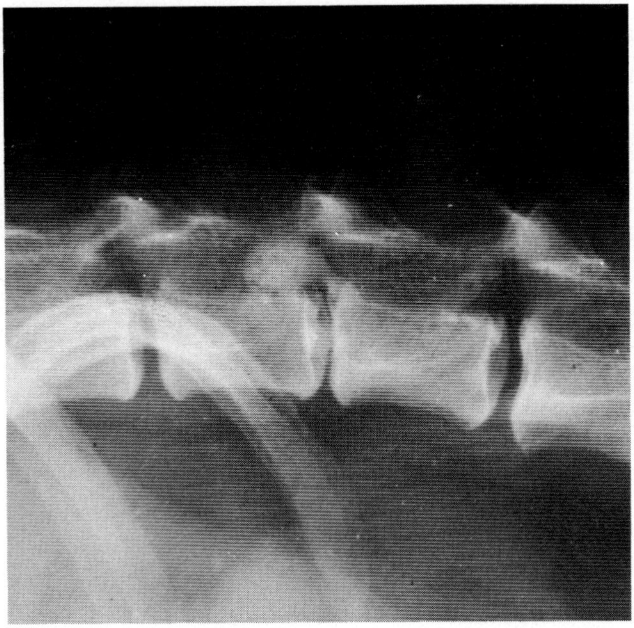

FIG. 14.7. Protruded material of the 1st lumbar intervertebral disc visible over the neural canal.

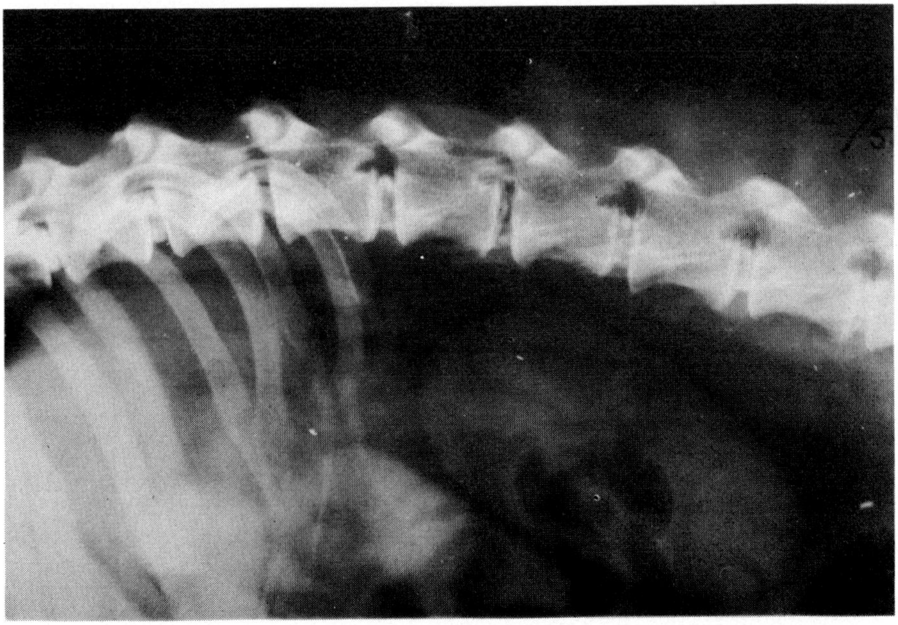

FIG. 14.8. Calcification of a large number of intervertebral discs with evidence of protrusion of the 2nd lumbar disc.

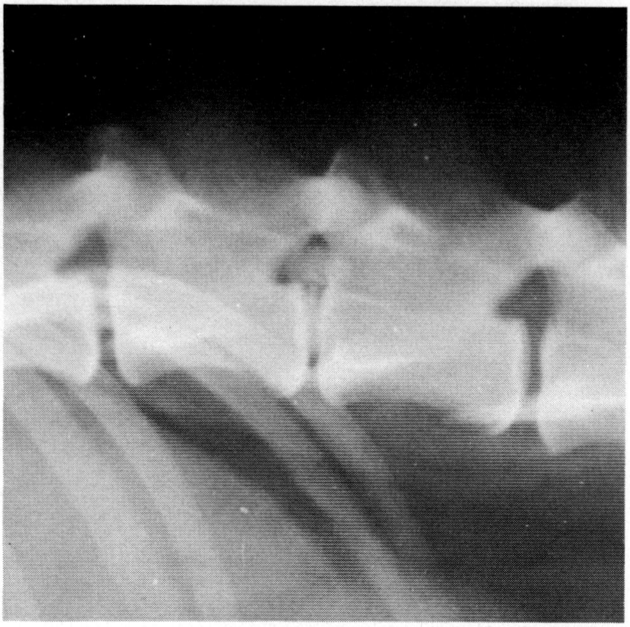

FIG. 14.9. Protruded intervertebral disc material visualised at the 1st lumbar intervertebral foramen.

Usually intervertebral disc protrusions are only recognised in the dog. They do occur in the cat, but as they are not commonly associated with clinical symptoms they are seldom investigated by radiography.

Contrast Media Techniques

The use of myelography to outline the spinal cord could be of considerable value in the demonstration of intervertebral disc protrusions not perceptible in a plain radiograph and for the investigation of compression of the cord by neoplasms or other lesions. This procedure has been used quite extensively in the dog. It can be undertaken by either of two methods, neither of which is a simple technique and each has certain disadvantages.

Both procedures involve the introduction of a contrast agent into the subarachnoid space (epidural injection does not accurately outline the spinal cord) and may be summarised as follows:

(a) The introduction of an oily agent through the cisterna magna. The use of this method in the dog was first reported by Brook (1936) and has since been employed by a number of other workers. The contrast agent is introduced by cisternal puncture and then the animal is placed on a steep slope so that the material gravitates along the subarachnoid space until radiography shows that it is indented or completely held up by a lesion pressing on the cord. The use of an oily contrast agent obviates the dangerous reactions caused by the irritant properties of most other agents. It has very real disadvantages however, in that the viscous nature of the material results in a slow passage along the canal, a tendency to false arrests and a not very precise outlining of compressions of the cord. Furthermore the material remains within the spinal canal for a long period after its introduction.

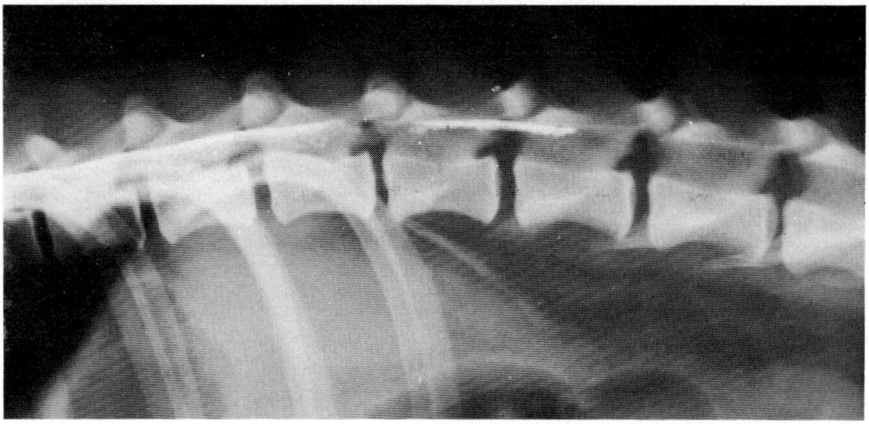

FIG. 14.10. A protrusion of the 1st lumbar intervertebral disc demonstrated (but not clearly outlined) by a break in the column of oily contrast agent.

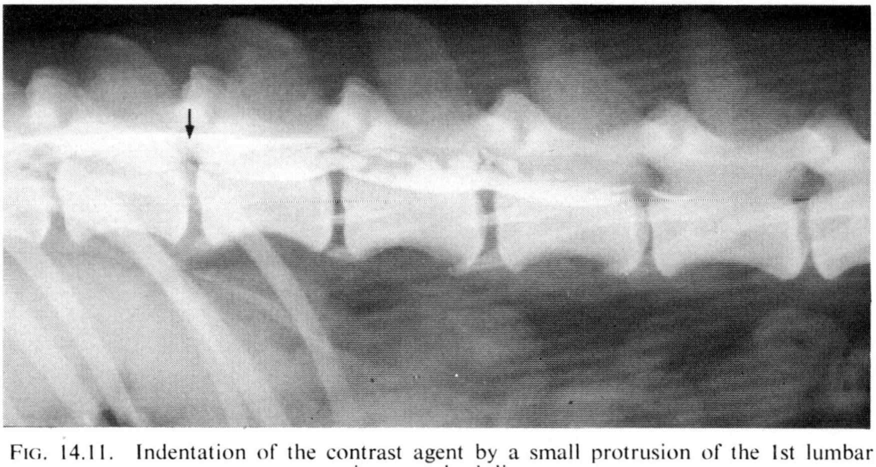

FIG. 14.11. Indentation of the contrast agent by a small protrusion of the 1st lumbar intervertebral disc.

(b) The introduction of a water-soluble agent by lumbar puncture. This method, which was introduced by Funkquist (1962), is an attempt to overcome some of the disadvantages of the methods described above. The use of a water-soluble contrast agent, Kontrast U (Leo) results in immediate and accurate outlining of the compression and in rapid elimination of the material. However, the irritant nature of this contrast agent can cause serious side-effects on injection. This can be prevented by combining the medium with a local anaesthetic before its introduction and by employing a relaxant as part of the general anaesthesia necessary to carry out the examination.

The injection is made into the ventral subarachnoid space after passing a fine needle directly downwards through the spinal cord between the fourth and fifth or fifth and sixth lumbar vertebrae. This transfixion can cause damage to nervous tissue, but the risk is claimed to be slight. Contrast material introduced by this route does not outline the cervical region unless cisternal puncture and drainage of cerebrospinal fluid is also carried out.

REFERENCES

Brook, G. B. (1936), Experimental and Clinical Studies of the Spine of the Dog, Baltimore, Wm. Wood & Co.
Carlson, W. D. (1967), Veterinary Radiology. Second Edition. London: Bailliere, Tindall and Cassell.
Cobb, L. M. (1960), Can. vet. J., **1**, 444.
Funkquist, B. (1961), J. Am. vet. med. Ass., **138**, 302.
Funkquist, B. (1962), J. small Anim. Pract., **3**, 53 and 67.
Hoerlein, B. F. and Petty, M. F. (1961), Am. J. vet. Res., **22**, 1041.
James, C. W. and Hoerlein, B. F. (1960), Vet. Med., **55**, 12, 45.
Spooner, R. L. (1961), J. small Anim. Pract., **2**, 243.

CHAPTER 15

THE MUSCULAR SYSTEM AND ASSOCIATED TISSUES

The value and practicability of the use of radiography in the investigation of this system is obviously limited, but there are, nevertheless, a few clinical circumstances in which it can be of assistance.

Radiography

The exposure factors chosen for radiographing a particular portion of an animal are usually selected in relation to the bony rather than the muscular tissues. If the maximum value is to be obtained from the investigation of soft tissues, it is important to reduce these exposure factors considerably (usually the mAS is halved). This can assist in the appreciation of subtle differences in radiodensity and permit visualisation of such features as muscle lines, fat, gas, etc., while still showing denser structures (e.g., foreign bodies, calcification of tissues).

Radiology

When examining radiographs for evidence of traumatic and inflammatory injuries there is a natural tendency to concentrate on the more obvious lesions of the skeletal

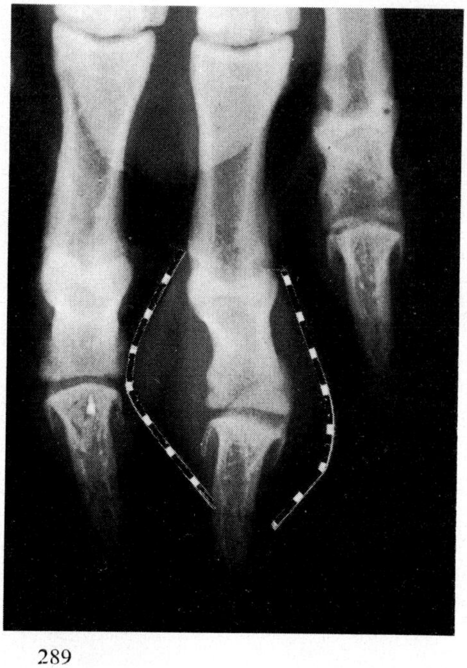

FIG. 15.1. Soft tissue swelling (and absence of bony injury) demonstrated in a "knocked-up" toe of a Greyhound.

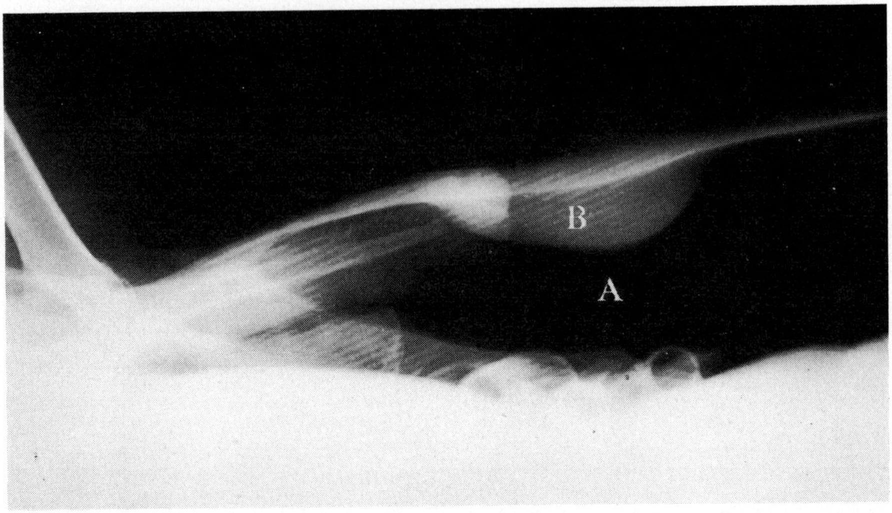

FIG. 15.2. A lateral projection of a Boxer dog positioned on its back in order that pneumoperitoneum might be used to delineate a neoplastic mass arising on the inner surface of the rectus muscle.

A—pneumoperitoneum
B—neoplastic mass.

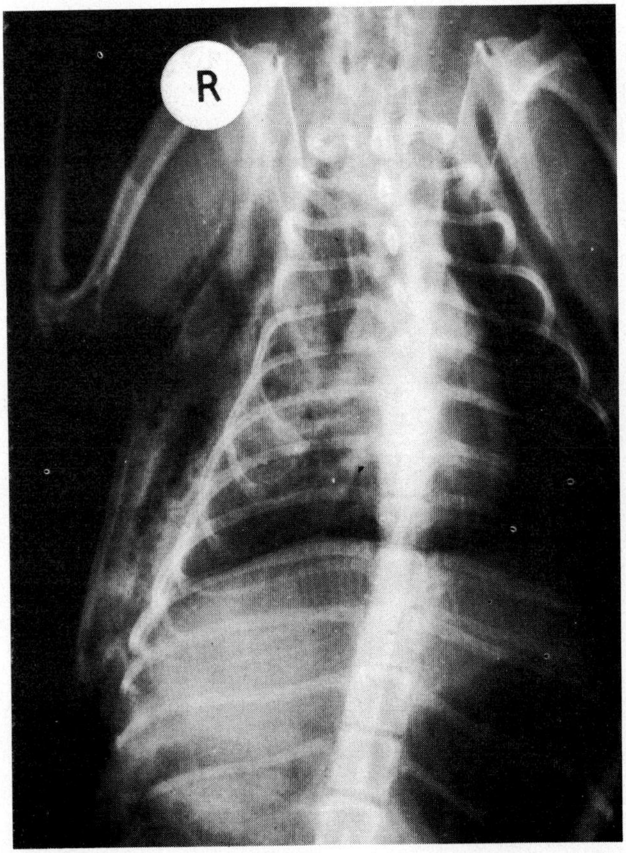

Fig. 15.3. Emphysema of the subcutaneous tissues in association with a chest injury.

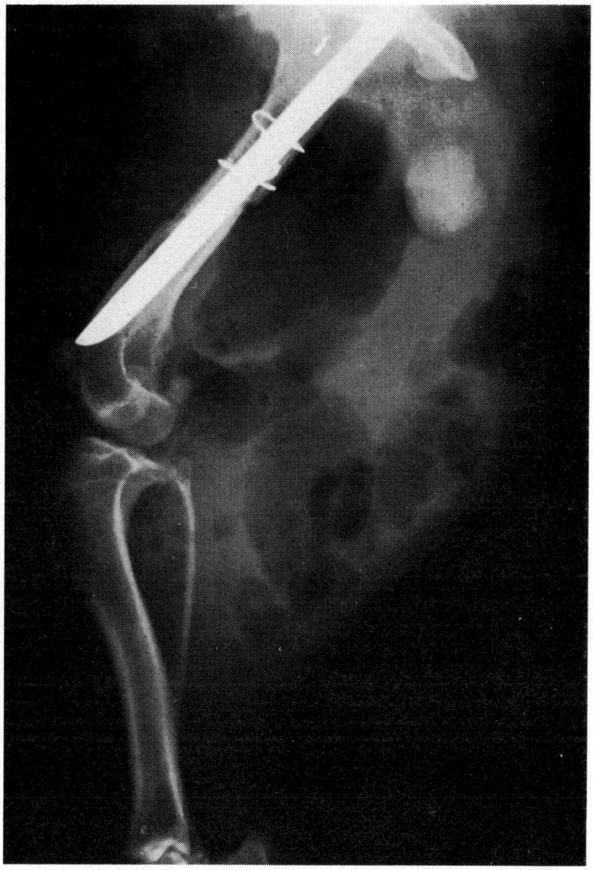

FIG. 15.4. Gas shadows due to contamination of a surgical wound by gas-producing organisms.

system and to overlook the additional information which may be obtained from an examination of the associated soft tissues. Visualisation of the enlargement and distortion of the soft tissues shows the extent of the involvement of these tissues in the injury and may indicate the site of other injuries not actually involving bone.

When investigating swellings involving the deeper layers of the abdominal muscles the introduction of pneumoperitoneum before radiography, may permit the amount by which the swelling protrudes into the abdominal cavity to be demonstrated.

The recognition of dark gas shadows within soft tissues adjacent to the chest can be associated with thoracic injuries or, in other situations, with the presence of gas-forming organisms.

Foreign Bodies

The value of radiography in demonstrating foreign bodies within soft tissues will depend on the radiopacity of the object. Metallic substances and pieces of grit will be easily visualised, although the shadow of thin wire may be blurred by movement or easily lost behind dense bone. Grass seeds will not be perceptible and thorns, portions of wood, and fragments of glass are unlikely to be recognised unless they are particularly dense or located in very thin tissues.

Provided that the object can be distinctly visualised, radiography can be of considerable assistance in judging its nature, size and precise location. The fact that the exact position of the foreign body is not known usually results in it being positioned obliquely and thus produces a distorted or foreshortened image on the radiograph. Provided that a second film has been taken at right angles to the first, such distortion can normally be recognised and allowance made for it in identifying the object. In cases of doubt these preliminary films will make it possible to repeat radiography with the object placed parallel to the cassette and thus produce an accurate reproduction.

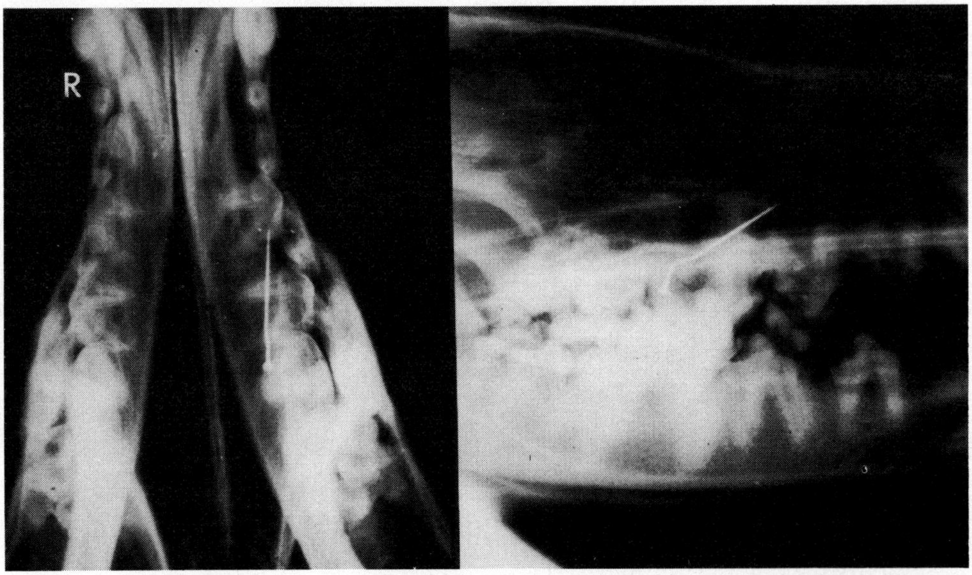

FIG. 15.5. Two radiographic projections are required for localisation of this foreign body.

Exact identification of the position of the object with a view to its location by surgery can be a more difficult matter. There are several radiographic techniques by which the depth of a foreign body beneath the surface of a body can be calculated. In one of these the level of the patient's skin is first identified by means of a radiopaque marker. The area is radiographed using exposure factors reduced by about fifty per cent. This exposure is then repeated after moving the X-ray tube in a plane parallel with the film but without disturbing the patient or the film. By measuring the distances the images of the foreign body and the skin marker have moved with the second exposure, it is possible by means of a geometrical formula, to calculate the exact distance the foreign body is situated beneath the skin surface.

Reference to more detailed explanations of these techniques are given at the end of this chapter, but in general such involved methods are seldom of much practical use, particularly if the patient, or even the skin marker, are moved before surgery is attempted.

In the majority of instances all that is necessary to permit adequate localisation for surgery is to take sufficient radiographs of the area to permit a reasonably accurate localisation of the position of the object in relation to an adjacent bone to be established. If the object is not situated sufficiently close to a bone it may be necessary to use skin markers (needles inserted in the skin or other small radiopaque objects stuck to the skin) as a fixed point to which the foreign body may be related. If the latter method is used, it must be remembered that if the skin is loose, such a marker can move considerably on handling the region.

Calcification within Soft Tissues

Calcification of soft tissues may be demonstrated radiologically when investigating abnormal swellings or thickenings, or may be an incidental finding when radiographing for other purposes. Such changes may be encountered under the following circumstances.

(a) **Calcinosis Circumscripta** This is a definite clinical entity, although of unknown etiology, in which there is a local accumulation of amorphous calcified material. It involves the skin or superficial tissues and has been reported as occurring in the pads of the feet, over body prominences, and in the mouth and tongue. Radiography may be employed to show the extent and nature of the lesion. The condition is usually easily recognisable on account of its clearly demarcated outline, its uniform but considerable density, and its somewhat lobular pattern.

(b) **Calcification of Haematomata** The tendency for unabsorbed haematomata to become calcified with time can be the explanation for unexpected areas of calcification noted in a radiograph. Such changes are more likely to be encountered in the deeper parts of the body (e.g., within the abdominal cavity) because the more superficial haematomata will be recognised clinically and dealt with at the time of their occurrence. Radiologically this condition should be suspected when an otherwise unexplained calcification is encountered in an area where it would have been possible for a haematoma to have developed.

(c) **Calcification of Tendons** While not commonly encountered, small areas of calcification may occasionally be demonstrated along the course of tendons and probably represent senile and chronic inflammatory changes. They should be distinguished from the osteophytic outgrowths which may extend outwards from bone at the site of tendinous insertions in some chronic inflammatory conditions.

(d) **The Mammary Gland** This heading is added here merely as a reminder that the presence of milk within the mammary glands can give rise to areas of density in abdominal radiographs. The formation of bony tissues which occurs in association with some mammary tumours can also be demonstrated radiologically.

(e) **Calcification of Lymphatic Glands** Calcification of the intra-abdominal lymphatic glands was mentioned in Chapter 10. Similar changes can occur in the more superficial lymphatic glands and nodes.

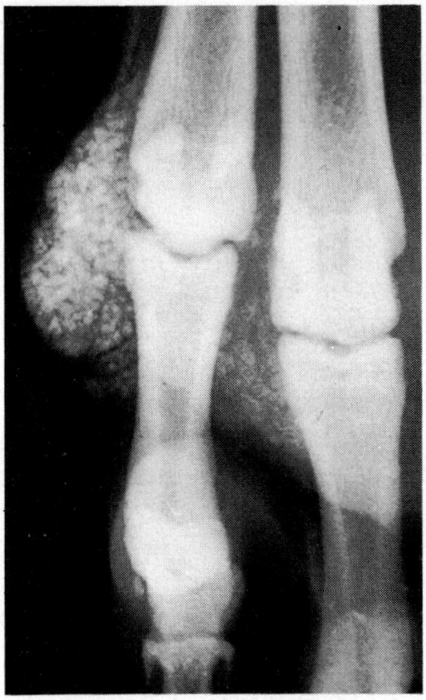

FIG. 15.6.

FIGS. 15.6 and 15.7. Lesions of calcinosis circumscripta.

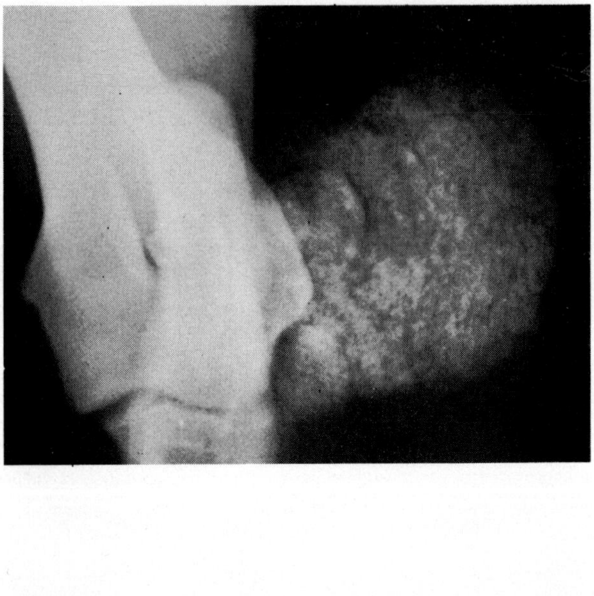

FIG. 15.7.

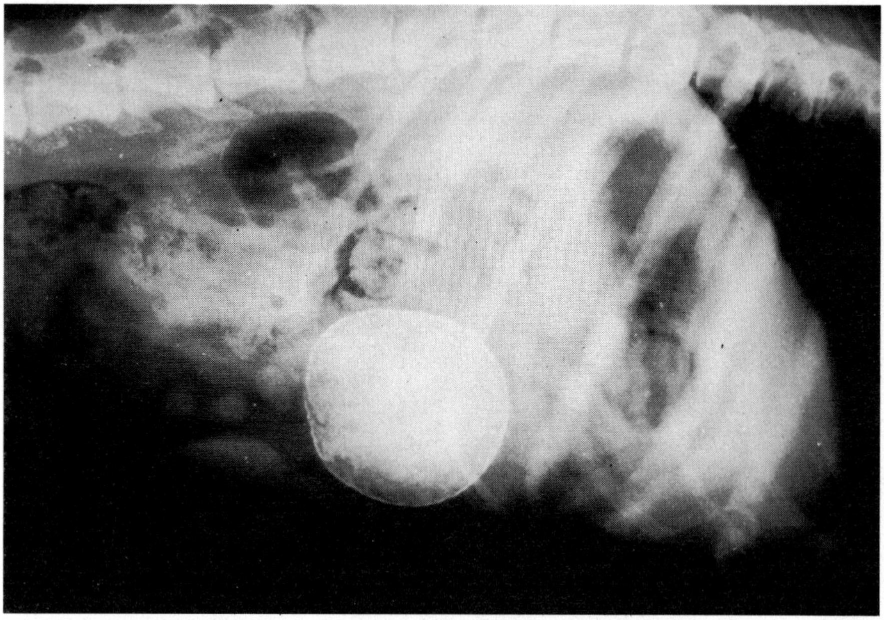

FIG. 15.8. A calcified haematoma in the abdominal mesentry.

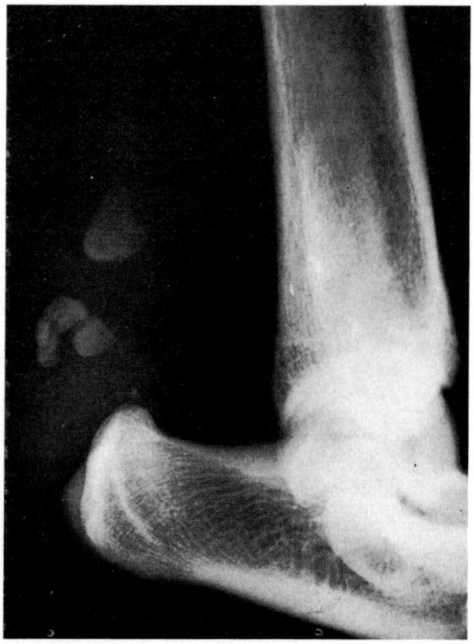

FIG. 15.9. The development of localised calcified lesions within the gastrocnemius tendon.

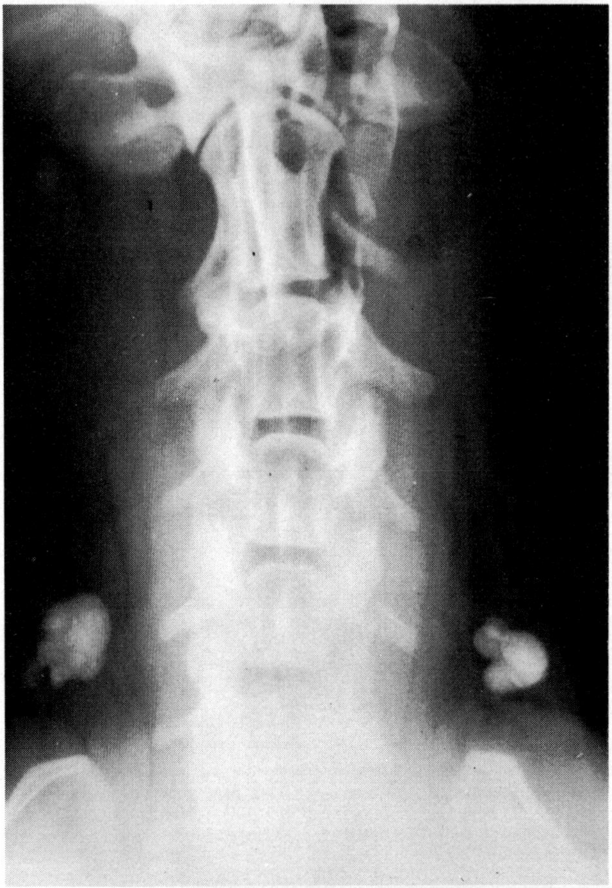

FIG. 15.10.

FIG. 15.10 and 15.11. Calcification of the lymphatic glands in the neck.

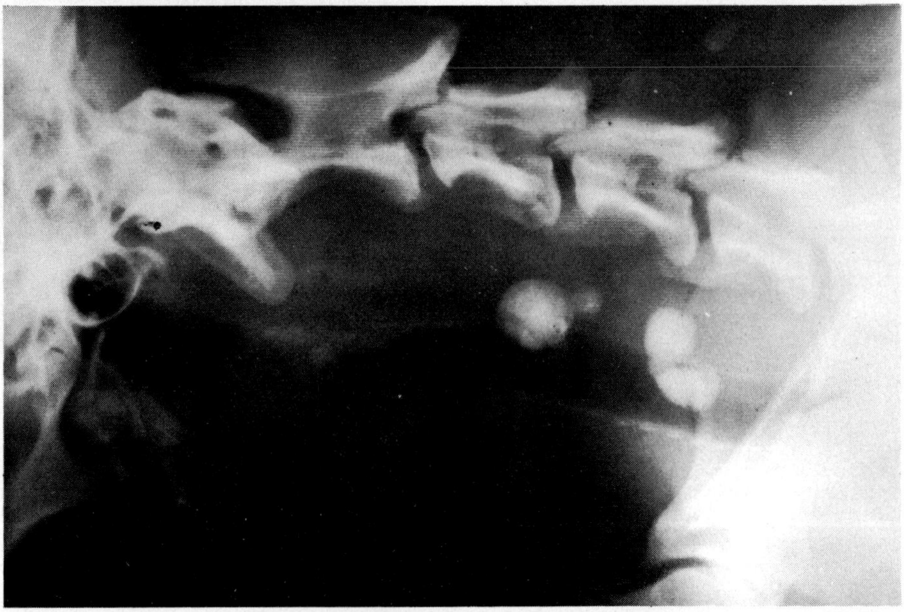

FIG. 15.11.

The Investigation of Sinus Tracts

While radiography can be of assistance in demonstrating the extent of such tracts, the procedure is not always practicable and its value is somewhat limited. Usually it is necessary to use contrast media but a preliminary plain radiograph should always be taken, as this may show the cause of the sinus (e.g., a foreign body or infection of adjacent bone) or the presence of gas shadows. The contrast agents commonly used

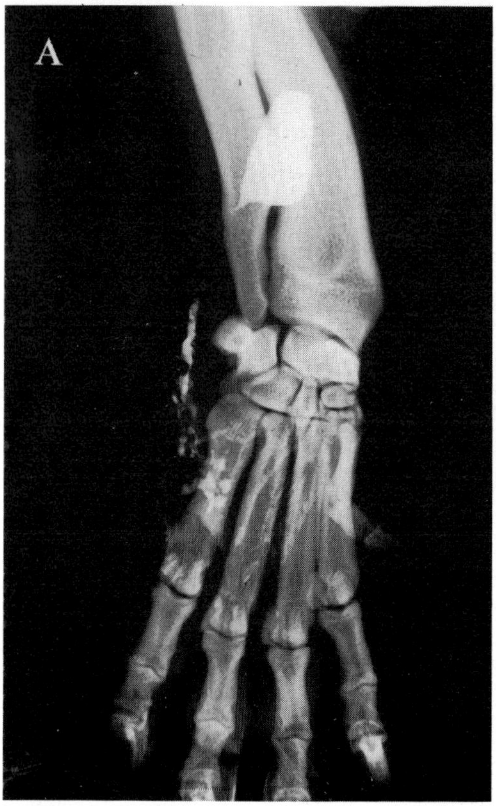

FIG. 15.12.

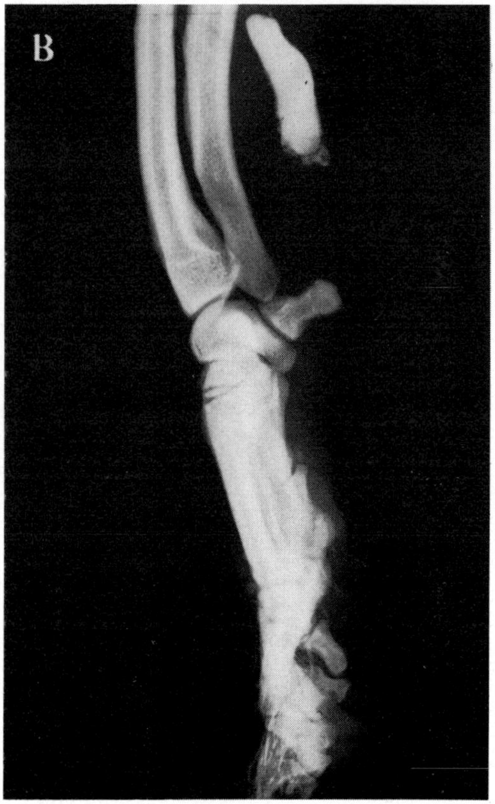

FIG. 15.13.

FIGS. 15.12 and 15.13. Visualisation of a sinus cavity by filling it with contrast agent.

to outline sinus cavities are the oily preparations, since these are not irritant and they are not easily absorbed and removed from the site. However, because they are of a viscous nature they do not flow easily and they may fail to outline the cavity precisely. Therefore an attempt should always be made to remove discharge and debris from the sinus, and the contrast material should be introduced as far as possible into the cavity, using a syringe with a long narrow nozzle. Finally any contrast agent spilt on to the skin should be carefully removed before radiographing the area.

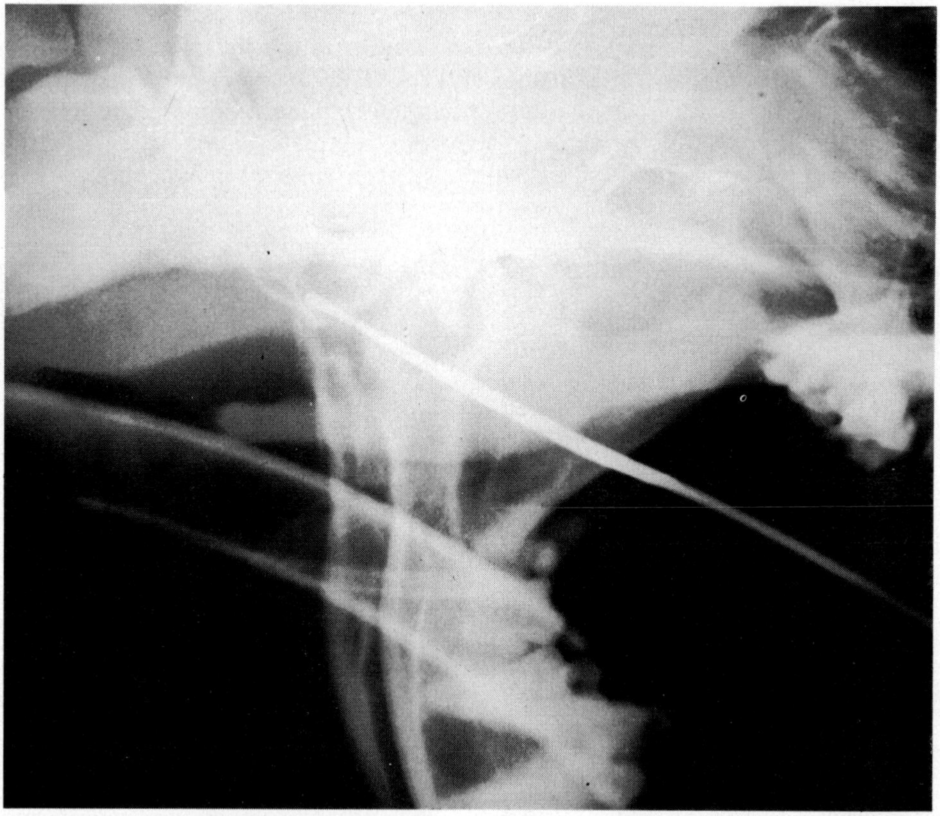

FIG. 15.14. Communication of a sinus with the tympanic bulla demonstrated by radiography after insertion of a metallic probe.

Since the contrast material may not fully outline the cavity, the extent of the tract can sometimes be demonstrated more simply by introducing a metallic probe and then radiographing the part.

REFERENCES

References to methods of localisation of foreign bodies:

Jaundrell-Thompson, F. and Ashworth, W. J. (1965), X-Ray Physics and Equipment. Oxford: Blackwell Scientific Publications, p. 30.

Kemp, L. A. W. (1964), Mathematics for Radiographers. Oxford: Blackwell Scientific Publications, p. 63.

Young, M. E. J. (1967), Radiological Physics. London: Lewis & Co., p. 319.

INDEX